Introduction to
Health Services

WILEY SERIES IN HEALTH SERVICES
Stephen J. Williams, Sc.D., *Series Editor*

Health Care Economics
  Paul J. Feldstein

Issues in Health Services
  Stephen J. Williams

Introduction to Health Services
  Stephen J. Williams and Paul R. Torrens

**National Priorities for Health:
  Past, Present, and Projected**
  Robert F. Rushmer

Introduction to Health Services

Edited by

STEPHEN J. WILLIAMS

Associate Professor and Associate Director
Graduate Program in Health Services
    Administration and Planning
Department of Health Services
School of Public Health
    and Community Medicine
University of Washington

PAUL R. TORRENS

Professor and Chairman
Division of Health Services
    and Hospital Administration
School of Public Health
University of California at Los Angeles

A WILEY MEDICAL PUBLICATION
JOHN WILEY & SONS
New York • Chichester • Brisbane • Toronto

Library of Congress Cataloging in Publication Data

Main entry under title:

Introduction to health services.

    (Wiley series in health services)
    Includes index.
    1. Medical care—United States. 2. Health services administration—United States. I. Williams, Stephen Joseph, 1948–   II. Torrens, Paul R.
III. Series, [DNLM: 1. Health services—United States. W84 AA1 W65i]
RA395.A3I57   362.1'0973   79-22401
ISBN 0-471-04612-4

Printed in the United States of America

10 9 8 7 6 5

For D. and N. Williams and
C., J., C., J.C., and N. Torrens

Contributors

Patricia A. Armstrong, M.P.H.
Formerly, Research Associate
Department of Health Services
School of Public Health
 and Community Medicine
University of Washington
Seattle, Washington

Thomas W. Bice, Ph.D.
Professor
Department of Health Services
School of Public Health
 and Community Medicine
University of Washington
Seattle, Washington

Robert H. Brook, M.D., Sc.D.
Associate Professor of Medicine
 and Public Health
University of California at Los Angeles
Senior Health Services Researcher
The RAND Corporation
Santa Monica, California

William L. Dowling, Ph.D.
Professor and Director
Graduate Program in Health Services
 Administration and Planning
School of Public Health
 and Community Medicine
University of Washington
Seattle, Washington

Robert L. Kane, M.D.
Associate Professor of Medicine
Associate Director
U.C.L.A. Health Services Research
 Center
University of California at Los Angeles
Senior Health Services Researcher
The RAND Corporation
Santa Monica, California

Rosalie A. Kane, D.S.W.
Lecturer, School of Social Work
University of California at Los Angeles
Consultant
The RAND Corporation
Santa Monica, California

Charles E. Lewis, M.D., Sc.D.
Professor of Medicine and Public
 Health
Director
U.C.L.A. Health Services Research
 Center
University of California at Los Angeles
Los Angeles, California

James P. LoGerfo, M.D.
Associate Professor
Department of Health Services
School of Public Health
 and Community Medicine
Associate Professor of Medicine
School of Medicine
University of Washington
Seattle, Washington

Lawrence A. May, M.D.
Assistant Professor of Medicine
University of California at Los Angeles
Director, Health Services Research
  Center
Wadsworth V.A. Hospital Center
Los Angeles, California

Mary Richardson, M.H.A.
Instructor, Department of Health
  Services
Administrator, Clinical Training Unit
Child Development and Mental
  Retardation Center
University of Washington
Seattle, Washington

William C. Richardson, Ph.D.
Professor of Health Services
Associate Dean
School of Public Health
  and Community Medicine
University of Washington
Seattle, Washington

Robert F. Rushmer, M.D.
Professor
Center for Bioengineering
University of Washington
Seattle, Washington

Stephen M. Shortell, Ph.D.
Professor
Department of Health Services
Director, Center for Health Services
  Research
School of Public Health
  and Community Medicine
University of Washington
Seattle, Washington

Paul R. Torrens, M.D., M.P.H.
Professor and Chairman
Division of Health Services
  and Hospital Administration
School of Public Health
University of California at Los Angeles
Los Angeles, California

Stephen J. Williams, Sc.D.
Associate Professor
Associate Director
Graduate Program in Health Services
  Administration and Planning
Department of Health Services
School of Public Health
  and Community Medicine
University of Washington
Seattle, Washington

Foreword

In recent years, health care services in the United States have been characterized by immense growth and expansion—growth in the range of services offered, in the costs of those services, and in the number of personnel providing them. This rapid expansion has forced health care policymakers in all parts of the country to ask some critical questions.

How much effort and money should our country spend on health care? What proportion of those resources should be spent on treatment and what proportion on health promotion or prevention? What types of technologies should be developed and what systems of evaluation should be applied to those technologies before they are introduced widely into the system? What methods of planning and priority setting should be established to ensure the most productive use of our resources?

As these questions become increasingly complex and difficult to resolve, it becomes ever more important for health care professionals to understand the environment in which these questions arise. The major trends in health services, the factors that influence the receipt of services, the capacity of the system to respond to people's needs, and the impact of the services on the health of the people—all these must be understood by everyone working in the system.

This book attempts to provide a better basis for that understanding by bringing together a wide-ranging set of ideas and opinions on health care in this country. The result of a collaborative effort of the faculty of the School of Public Health at the University of California, Los Angeles, and the School of Public Health and Community Medicine at the University of Washington, the text reflects the insight and experience of many of the nation's leading teachers and researchers in the field of health services. It is our sincere hope that, as a result of this book, we can all develop a better understanding of the problems facing us and move strongly towards their fair and swift solution.

Lester Breslow, M.D., M.P.H.
Dean, School of Public Health
University of California at Los Angeles

Robert W. Day, M.D., Ph.D.
Dean, School of Public Health
    and Community Medicine
University of Washington

Preface

Since the end of World War II, health services in the United States have undergone rapid and dramatic changes. New and more powerful technologies have been developed, generations of more specialized personnel have been educated, and more elaborate and expensive facilities have been constructed. At the same time, a complex network of new programs has been developed to handle the financing, planning, monitoring, and regulating of all aspects of health care.

By any measure, this country's health services system is huge and complex. It is also frequently confusing and discouraging to those who must work within its many programs. Indeed, it is sometimes so difficult to understand and so frustrating to change that the people within the system not only stop trying to understand why it is the way it is but also stop trying to improve it. They simply withdraw and concentrate their energies on their particular part of the system, trusting that someone else will make the right judgments for the system as a whole.

Unfortunately, this isolationism is a luxury we can no longer afford. It is essential, now more than ever before, that all those within the system understand its workings and concentrate their efforts towards making it work better.

This book is divided into five parts, the first of which is an introduction to the health services system of this country. It discusses the major trends that have characterized health care in the United States. This introduction is designed to set the stage for the detailed discussions of the various aspects of the system that follow.

Part Two discusses the factors associated with the utilization of health services. The bases for the needs and demands for health services are examined in two chapters. The first of these, Chapter 2, outlines the biological bases of disease, including both physiological and psychological trends. The second chapter in this part, Chapter 3, describes the primary patterns of health service utilization and presents frameworks to help us understand better why these patterns have developed.

The providers of health services are discussed in Part Three of this book. Chapter 4 covers ambulatory and community services, while Chapter 5 discusses inpatient services and the role of the hospital in the health services system. Chapter 6 examines some of the sweeping issues of long-term care, with a particular focus on the nursing home. Finally, Chapter 7 focuses on services to meet mental health needs.

The organizations and programs that provide health care require a variety of resources to carry out their mission, and these resources are the subject of Part Four. The technological resources for health are discussed in Chapter 8, while the subject of health personnel is taken up in Chapter 9. The finances and financial systems for health care are discussed in Chapter 10, and are considered both as a resource and as a mechanism for regulating the behavior of individuals and organizations within the health care system. As such, this chapter serves as a link to Part Five, which is devoted to assessment and regulation of the health services system.

Chapter 11 in Part Five discusses the setting of priorities for health services and the use of regulatory and planning mechanisms to achieve social goals. The assessment of the effectiveness of health care services, and particularly the evaluation of the quality of care, is discussed in Chapter 12.

Thus, this book addresses the reasons for providing health services, the organizations and programs that provide care, the resources needed to provide the services, and the systems of assessment and modification needed to alter the direction of the system in the years to come.

Throughout the various chapters, certain common concerns will repeatedly appear. Assuring easy access to health services for all who need them, maintaining a level of care that is of acceptable quality, understanding and controlling the factors causing the rapid rise in the cost of care, and establishing a more rational method of priority setting and planning—all these form a common thread that runs throughout all the chapters in the book.

This book has the dual purpose of both describing the health services system of this country and critically assessing various aspects and component parts of that system. The reader should develop an appreciation for the complexities and subtleties of health services, and understand that there are many biological, behavioral, and organizational factors affecting the use of health care resources.

Much of the existing empirical research in health services has been incorporated into this book, yet much more remains to be done before all the components of the system and all their interrelationships are completely understood. It is hoped that the reader will be challenged not only to better understand the present structure of health services in this country but also to develop an analytical framework for understanding new developments as they occur in the future. In that way, as new issues or new forces appear on the scene, they can be easily integrated into a framework that has already been worked out.

It is our feeling that everyone involved in providing health services has a duty to read about and reflect on the nature and structure of our health services system. At the same time, it is important for each of us to consider and understand our values and our biases, since they will affect our thoughts about health care. As the reader progresses through this book, it is important to keep these values and biases in mind and to look for their effects on his or her opinions and conclusions about health care.

It is also important to keep in mind the values of our society, particularly as they are expressed through politics and the political system. Although there is no separate chapter in this book on the politics of health care, the influence of politics is suggested throughout the text. The reader should be continuously aware that politics is a major force shaping the present and future health services system of this country.

Finally, the health services system is immense, and no single textbook could cover all of its aspects. As a result, many of the organizations, trends, and influences that are involved in health care in the United States are mentioned only briefly and some are omitted entirely. The objective has been to focus attention on those institutions of most significance or on those from which the most can be learned, while at the same time recognizing that a number of others have had to be omitted because of the realities of limited space.

For the reader who seeks a more extensive elaboration of this *Introduction to Health Services,* the Wiley Series in Health Services also includes a companion volume, *Issues in Health Services,* edited by Stephen J. Williams. All the chapters in this present volume, except one, were written especially for this book. The *Issues* volume, however, is a collection of articles from the health services literature, designed to complement and parallel the parts and chapters of this volume. Both of these books, *Introduction,* and the companion *Issues,* are intended for use by advanced undergraduate and graduate students in any of the health fields, including health services administration, medicine, nursing, and the allied health professions. They are also intended to be comprehensive primers on health services for clinicians, administrators, planners, policy analysts, and policymakers who seek a better understanding of the health services system and their roles in it.

This book has benefited substantially from assistance provided by Barbara Anderson, Colleen Gawle, Annette Lefcourt, Billee Lewis, Bernice Goldberg Maslan, Diane McKenzie, Cheryl Michels, Jan Peterson, and Marilyn Taber. Artwork in the book was drawn by Dale Leuthold of the University of Washington. Cathy Somer of John Wiley & Sons has been a most pleasant and responsive editor. Scott Klein assisted greatly in the production of this book.

Finally, in addition to the participation of our colleagues as contributors to this book, many associates and students over the years have stimulated our thinking about health services and encouraged the book's development. To all of them, we owe a significant debt of gratitude, which we hope is partially met by their satisfaction with our efforts.

Stephen J. Williams

Paul R. Torrens

Contents

PART ONE: OVERVIEW OF THE HEALTH SERVICES SYSTEM   1

CHAPTER 1: Historical Evolution and Overview of Health Services in the United
States   3
Paul R. Torrens

Section I. Historical Evolution of Health Services in America   3

Section II. Overview of Health Services in the United States   15

Health Services: A Summary of Perspectives   29

PART TWO: CAUSES AND CHARACTERISTICS OF HEALTH SERVICES
UTILIZATION IN THE UNITED STATES   33

CHAPTER 2: The Physiologic and Psychologic Bases of Health, Disease, and Care
Seeking   35
Lawrence A. May

Defining Illness and Disease   35

Disease Processes   37

The Physiological Bases of Changing Disease Patterns   41

Social and Cultural Influences on Disease and Behavior   43

CHAPTER 3: Factors Associated with the Utilization of Health Services   48
Stephen M. Shortell

Analytical Categories and Conceptual Distinctions   49

Analytical Models and Key Findings   62

Broader Frameworks for the Study of Health Services Utilization   79

Special Issues in Health Services Utilization   81

An Assessment of Utilization   85

PART THREE: PROVIDERS OF HEALTH SERVICES   91

CHAPTER 4: Ambulatory and Community Health Services   93
          Stephen J. Williams

Private Office-Based Practice: Solo Practice   96

Private Office-Based Practice: Group Practice   99

Institutionally Based Ambulatory Services   111

Governmental Programs: Health Centers   113

Non-Institutional and Public Health Services   115

Organization of Ambulatory Care Systems   118

CHAPTER 5: The Hospital   125
          William L. Dowling and
          Patricia A. Armstrong

Historical Development of Hospitals   126

Characteristics of the Hospital System   133

Internal Organization of Community Hospitals   143

Trends and Issues in the Hospital Industry   150

CHAPTER 6: The Nursing Home: Neither Home Nor Hospital   169
          Robert L. Kane and
          Rosalie Kane

Historical Development   170

Descriptive Data on Nursing Homes   172

Paying for Nursing Home Care   177

Medical Care in Nursing Homes   182

Quality of Nursing Home Care   183

Quality of Life   187

Medical Versus Social Models   189

Conclusions   193

CHAPTER 7: Mental Health Services: Growth and Development of a System
197
    Mary Richardson

Definitions of Mental Illness   197

Extent of Mental Disorders   200

Development of the Mental Health System in the United States   203

Mental Health Personnel   209

The Organization of Services   214

Issues and Trends in Mental Health   218

PART FOUR: RESOURCES FOR HEALTH SERVICES   225

CHAPTER 8: Technological Resources for Health   227
    Robert F. Rushmer

Historical Heritage of Health Technologies   228

Development of Diagnostic Technologies   234

Monitoring Methods   245

Emergency Medical Services   245

Therapeutic Technologies   246

Technology Assessment: The Broad View   251

Future Forecasts   253

CHAPTER 9: Health Care Personnel   256
    Paul R. Torrens and
    Charles E. Lewis

Trends in Health Care Personnel in the Twentieth Century   257

Special Issues for Health Personnel   272

Optimizing Health Care Personnel Resources   279

CHAPTER 10: Financing Health Services   287
    William C. Richardson

Health Care Expenditures   287

Financial Arrangements and Economic Relationships   292

Health Insurance Coverage in the United States   303

Public Policy Issues   316

PART FIVE: ASSESSING AND REGULATING SYSTEM PERFORMANCE
          323

CHAPTER 11: Health Services Planning and Regulation 325
             Thomas W. Bice

             Planning and Regulation 325

             Origins and Development of Health Services Planning 328

             Origins and Development of Health Services Regulation 340

             An Assessment of Planning and Regulation 347

CHAPTER 12: Evaluation of Health Services and Quality of Care 355
             James P. LoGerfo and
             Robert H. Brook

             Generic Issues of Program Evaluation of Health Services 356

             Quality Assessment in Health Care 365

             Measurement Issues 366

             Quality Assessment Methods 369

             Patient Satisfaction and the Quality of Care 377

             Access to Care 377

             Illustrative Studies of the Quality of Care 378

             Quality Assurance in Medical Care 381

             Performance-Based Assurance Approaches 383

             Malpractice as a Quality Assurance Mechanism 386

             An Assessment of Quality of Care 387

INDEX 391

Part One
Overview of
the Health
Services System

CHAPTER 1

Historical Evolution and Overview of Health Services in the United States

Paul R. Torrens

This chapter introduces the development, background, concepts, and issues of health care in the United States. The first section of the chapter presents the historical evolution and development of health services in this country; the second section describes the current organization of services. Combined, these sections set the stage for the detailed analyses of the latter chapters in the book.

SECTION I.
HISTORICAL EVOLUTION OF HEALTH SERVICES IN AMERICA

In *The Tempest,* a Shakespearean character is portrayed as saying, "What's past is prologue," suggesting that the events of the past merely set the stage for the future. In a more pertinent sense, George Santayana has written, "Those who cannot remember the past are condemned to repeat it." This is particularly true of the American health care system, since many of the issues and forces which have shaped and formed it in the past continue to influence us today. If we are to better understand the future, it seems appropriate to look at the past first.

This chapter is adapted from material previously presented in *The American Health Care System: Issues and Problems,* Paul R. Torrens, St. Louis, The C. V. Mosby Company, 1978.

The modern American health care system has had three important periods of development and now seems to be entering into a fourth. The first period began in the mid-nineteenth century (1850) when the first large hospitals, such as Bellevue Hospital in New York City and Massachusetts General Hospital in Boston, began to flourish. The development of hospitals symbolized the *institutionalization of health care* for the first time in this country. Prior to this time, health care in the United States was a loose collection of individual services functioning independently and without much relation to each other or to anything else. By today's standards, the first hospitals were not very remarkable, but they did provide the first visible focus around which health care services could be organized.

The second important historical period began around the turn of the century (1900) with the *introduction of the scientific method into medicine* in this country. Prior to this time, medicine was not an exact science, but was instead a rather informal collection of unproved generalities and good intentions. After 1900, stimulated by the opening of the new medical school at the Johns Hopkins University in Baltimore, medicine acquired a solid scientific base that eventually transformed it from a conscientious but poorly-equipped art into a detailed and closely-defined science.

With the coming of World War II, the United States underwent a major social, political, and technological upheaval whose effect was so marked that it ended the second and signaled the beginning of the third period of health care development. The scientific advances continued unabated, but now they were paralleled by a *growing interest in the social and organizational structure of health care*. During this time, attention was first directed toward the financing of health care, with the resultant formation of health insurance plans such as Blue Cross and Blue Shield. This was also the time of increasing concentration of power in the federal government, as witnessed by the Hill-Burton Act (Hospital Survey and Construction Act), by the huge research budgets of the National Institutes of Health, and, more recently, by the passage of Medicare. Finally, during this period the principle of "health care as a right, not a privilege" was widely discussed and generally accepted.

In only the last few years, it has appeared that this country is moving into a new, fourth phase in its development, an era of *limited resources, restriction of growth, and regulation of effort*. Before this period, it had been presumed that the health care system would always be encouraged to grow and expand, both in size and complexity, and that there would always be sufficient resources to support that expansion. Now it seems that the limits of our resources are being approached and that the health care system is forced to consider options or alternatives to unrestricted growth and expansion. This might even be called the era of the cost-benefit analyst, the health planner, and the government regulator.

PREDOMINANT HEALTH PROBLEMS OF THE AMERICAN PEOPLE

Since the dawn of recorded history, human beings have repeatedly suffered the sudden and devastating appearance of epidemics of infectious disease. Plague, cholera, typhoid, smallpox, influenza, yellow fever, and a host of other diseases raged almost at will creating havoc wherever they struck.

During the period 1850 to 1900 in this country, these epidemics of acute infectious diseases were still the most critical health problem for the majority of Americans. Of particular importance were those diseases related to impure food, contaminated water supply, inadequate sewage disposal, and the generally poor condition of urban housing. During this time, for example, a widespread cholera epidemic occurred throughout the country, resulting in an official death toll of 5,071 in New York City alone and an unofficial toll of several times higher. During this same period, yellow fever killed 9,000 in New Orleans in 1853, 2,500 in 1854 and 1855, and another 5,000 in 1858. Abraham Lincoln regularly sent his family away from the White House during the summer months to escape the "fevers," probably malaria, which swept through Washington.

By 1900, the epidemics of acute infectious disease had been brought under control due to improving environmental conditions. In the latter years of the nineteenth century, cities had begun to develop systems for water purification, for sanitary disposal of sewage, for safeguarding the quality of milk and food, and for monitoring the quality of urban housing. Health departments had begun to grow in numbers and in strength, and had begun to apply the methods of case-finding and quarantine with satisfying results. Indeed, by 1900, as Table 1–1 shows, those epidemic scourges which had held mankind in their power for centuries were now eliminated as major causes of death in the United States.

Since 1900 the predominant health problems which attracted the attention of the health services system were those acute events, either infectious or traumatic, that affected individuals one by one. The pendulum had swung away from epidemics of acute infections that affected large numbers of people and now had begun to swing towards conditions of an individual nature that require individualized treatment. As Table 1–1 shows, pneumonia and tuberculosis were the primary causes of death in 1900, with heart disease, nephritis, and accidents close behind.

Relieved from the burden of the epidemic illnesses, the newly-developed medical sciences turned their attention to better surgical techniques, the discovery of new sera for the treatment of pneumonia, and the development of new tests for more accurate and rapid diagnoses. Hospitals began to grow rapidly, medical schools flourished, and there was a general air of excitement that suggested the world was on the brink of significant advances in the treatment of individual illnesses.

Significant advances *were* being made. In Baltimore and Boston, the students of William Halsted, the pioneer surgeon at Johns Hopkins Hospital, began to operate on cases that had previously been beyond the abilities of surgeons. Advances in obstetrics now made it safer for women to have babies, and for the first time women did not approach childbirth with the fear of dying in delivery. Research work by two physicians, Banting and Best, in the laboratories of the University of Toronto led to the discovery of insulin in 1922, and for the first time diabetes could be effectively treated. Other research by Whipple, Minot, and Murphy into the causes of pernicious anemia led to successful medical treatment for that condition, and further spurred the rush to find new treatments for other age-old conditions.

There were new discoveries on all fronts, each of which contributed some new advance in medical treatment. In 1928, however, in a cluttered laboratory at St.

TABLE 1–1. Death Rates for Leading Causes of Death, 1900 and 1972, United States

1900		1972	
Cause of Death	Death Rate per 100,000 Population per Year	Cause of Death	Death Rate per 100,000 Population per Year
All Causes	1,719	All Causes	942
Pneumonia and influenza	202.2	Diseases of the heart	361.3
Tuberculosis	194.4	Malignancies	166.6
Diarrhea, enteritis, and ulceration of intestine	142.7	Cerebrovascular disease	100.9
Diseases of the heart	137.4	Accidents	54.6
Senility, ill defined or unknown	117.5	Influenza and pneumonia	29.4
		Suicide and homicide	20.8
		Diabetes mellitus	18.8
Intracranial lesions of vascular origin	106.9	Certain diseases of early infancy	16.4
Nephritis	88.6	Arteriosclerosis	15.8
All accidents	72.3	Cirrhosis of the liver	15.7
Cancer and other malignant tumors	64.0	Bronchitis, emphysema and	
Diphtheria	40.3	asthma	13.8

Source: *Vital Statistics of the United States*, U.S. National Center for Health Statistics, Washington, D.C., August 1973.

Mary's Hospital in London, a Scottish researcher, Alexander Fleming, produced the first of several discoveries that were to lead to the treatment of patients with penicillin for the first time in 1941. This discovery absolutely revolutionized medical care and totally changed the patterns of disease that threatened mankind. Within a few years after the treatment of the first patients with penicillin, antibiotics became readily available and acute illnesses which had previously meant serious illness and possible death, now meant nothing more than the discomfort of an injection and a few days of disability. Many older people experienced the incredible effects of the antibiotic era. When they had contracted pneumonia as children, their families admitted them to hospitals and despaired for their lives; now, as older adults they were told they had "a little pneumonia," given an injection of penicillin, and treated at home.

With the arrival of the antibiotic era in the 1940s and the subsequent conquest of acute infectious disease, the American people's predominant health problems became chronic illnesses. Since acute infections were no longer snuffing out the lives of children, people were living longer and beginning to show the presence of long-term chronic diseases, such as heart disease, cancer, and stroke. As shown in Table 1–1, these three conditions alone now account for two-thirds of all deaths. A similar review of the causes of disability would show arthritis, blindness, arteriosclerosis, and other chronic diseases as the predominant causes of morbidity and limitation of function.

For the future, chronic illnesses will probably continue to be the predominant health problem for the American people. Increasingly important will be chronic illnesses related to personal life styles and the environment. Evidence is rapidly accumulating to suggest that many of the more important chronic illnesses are either self-inflicted (albeit without that intent), or are the result of hazards introduced inadvertently into the environment.

The predominance of chronic illness as the major threat to health in the future raises a number of relevant issues for health professionals. First, as May points out in Chapter 2, the entire method of defining a chronic illness and determining its prevalence must be reexamined to obtain a more accurate picture of the situation. At the present time, a chronic disease is identified or documented based on the first appearance of symptoms or on positive laboratory tests. In most cases, however, it is known that the disease process started long before the appearance of those symptoms. In a practical sense, this forces one to ask the question: when should a chronic disease be considered to be present? The implications of the answer to this question for the planning and financing of health services could be enormous.

Chronic illnesses also have two important characteristics that directly affect both prevention and treatment. First, as was just pointed out, they often begin early in life, long before overt symptoms appear; the exact starting date for a chronic disease is never known. For example, a study of apparently healthy young soldiers, who were suddenly killed in combat in the Korean War, showed that almost one-fourth had already started to develop early microscopic evidence of coronary artery disease before age 20. Second, once a chronic illness is present, it remains with the patient forever; it is not the *disease* that is "cured" by medical treatment, but rather its more prominent *symptoms* or external manifestations are "treated."

Unfortunately, while the pattern of predominant illnesses has changed from epidemics of acute infections in the 1850s, to individual acute conditions in the 1900s, and finally to chronic illnesses in the 1950s, thinking about prevention and treatment has been slow to catch up. Acute infections very conveniently have a clear-cut beginning, middle, and end; as a result, they are amenable to one-shot solutions. If there is an epidemic caused by contamination of the water supply, the construction of a sewage treatment facility will eliminate it completely. If there is a threat of poliomyelitis infection, the ingestion of polio vaccine once or twice will permanently protect a population.

With chronic illnesses, however, prevention and treatment cannot be a one-shot affair, even though this is still how our health care system approaches them. Arteriosclerotic heart disease, for example, begins early in life and is probably affected by diet, cigarette smoking, stress, obesity, and several other factors that are directly related to personal habits and life-style. Prevention of these conditions cannot be accomplished by giving a person a single lecture on the evils of high-cholesterol food or the dangers of heavy cigarette consumption. Rather, prevention must be long-term, continuous, and aimed at bringing about major changes in an individual's knowledge of disease, personal values, and behavior patterns. Unfortunately, that understanding has been slow in coming and most of our preventive efforts are focused on one-time activities or are aimed at very limited aspects of life sytle.

Optimal treatment for long-term, continuous illness requires a system of health care that is, in itself, long-term and continuous. Unfortunately, the organization of our health services is still modeled on the disease patterns that were predominant in the 1900–1945 period and concentrates on individual episodes of illness as if they were separate and distinct entities. As a result, the health care system is primarily short-term and discontinuous in nature, and it treats chronic illness as if it were merely a series of separate acute episodes. This trend is further reinforced by the current method of financing of health services, with its great emphasis on paying for individual services rendered rather than on the long-term, continuous nature of the underlying disease process.

It is entirely possible (and indeed, probable) that the predominant disease patterns will be changing again in the future, bringing forth an entirely different set of conditions which may require an entirely different array of services and interventions. It will be important for future generations of health professionals to watch for changes in predominant disease patterns to ensure a health care system that is genuinely pertinent and responsive to the problems of the day.

TECHNOLOGY AVAILABLE TO THE AMERICAN PEOPLE FOR HEALTH CARE

During the three developmental periods of the American health care system, what technology was available to handle the diseases which affected the American people? What tools were available to health workers to conquer these conditions?

In the period from 1850 to 1900, only a very rudimentary technology was available for the treatment of disease. The scientific base of medicine was still very narrow, and the number of effective medical treatments was very limited. Indeed, a great deal of energy and effort was expended in the appearance of treatment, but whether a patient recovered from an illness or not usually depended more upon the patient and the disease rather than the treatment.

Physicians during this period of time were poorly-trained. They usually obtained their skills by serving apprenticeships with physicians already in practice and then going on for short courses at very simple medical colleges. What physicians had to offer was usually contained in their black bags which they took with them wherever they went. They spent a good deal of time in patients' homes and almost no time at all in hospitals. In general, their entire practice was little different from the practice of their predecessors for centuries before them.

Nurses during the period 1850 to 1900 were not much better trained. Generally they were members of religious groups who volunteered to work in the few hospitals that existed, or they were poor, desperate, discarded women who frequented these institutions anyway and were pressed into service. Their work was non-scientific in the extreme and consisted simply of assisting patients in their usual bodily functions in whatever way possible. Not until the first training program for nurses was organized at Bellevue Hospital in the 1860s was there any formal preparation for this important role anywhere in the country.

As for the hospitals themselves, they were merely places of shelter and repose for the sick poor who could not be cared for at home. Anyone who could stay at home usually did so, since hospitals had little to offer that would not be obtained at home if one had the money. Indeed, the hospitals of those days were often a direct threat to the lives of patients, since they were dirty, crowded, and disease-ridden. Infectious diseases frequently spread rapidly among hospitalized patients, and during the typhus epidemics of 1852 in New York City, for example, the highest mortality rates for the disease were among patients and staff of the hospitals themselves.

After 1900, conditions began to change, spurred on by the new discoveries that were emerging from the research laboratories in this country and in Europe. In 1912, for example, a Polish chemist, Casimir Funk, published a paper, *The Etiology of Deficiency Diseases,* in which he described "vitamines" and opened a whole new field of disease conditions to treatment. In 1908, James MacKenzie, in London, published his famous book *Diseases of the Heart,* and patients all over the world were the beneficiaries. In countless medical schools and hospitals throughout this country and Europe, major scientific advances were achieved, each of which contributed to easier and safer diagnosis and treatment of acutely ill patients.

The medical schools led the way in many of these advances as a result of some basic reforms which took place in the early 1900s. Prior to this time, a large number of small, poorly-staffed, free-standing medical colleges existed throughout the country, fourteen in Chicago alone in 1910, and ten each in Missouri and Tennessee. In 1910, Abraham Flexner undertook a study of medical education for the Rockefeller Foundation and in his report, *Medical Education in the United States and Canada,* recommended that medical education in this country undergo radical reform. In particular, he strongly urged that the training of physicians be made a university function and that it be based on a firm scientific foundation. On the basis of his recommendations and the support of the Rockefeller Foundation, many of the small, unaffiliated schools began to close and many of the remaining ones became part of universities with the important result that physicians began to be trained as scientists as well as practitioners.

Gradually, physicians began to have more effective tools with which to work and the range of their capabilities expanded rapidly. They still continued to spend the majority of their time in their offices or in patients' homes, but they now also began to look toward the hospital for the care of their more severly ill patients. A small, but gradually increasing number of physicians began to specialize in one particular area of medicine or another, however; by 1940, more than 80% were still in "general practice."

For their part, hospitals in the 1900s began to play an increasingly important role in health care. As more technology developed, it tended to be concentrated in hospitals, with the result that patients and physicians began going to hospitals for the technology to be found there. St. Luke's Hospital in New York City, for example, was 50 years old in 1906 when it opened its first private patient pavilion. Before that time, there was no reason for private patients to go to a hospital, because they could usually get the same type of care in their homes. Now, however, hospitals began to possess services and skills that were not available anywhere else.

Although the period of 1900 to 1940 was one of rapid growth in scientific technology, it was nothing compared to what happened with the advent of World War II. With the start of the war, this country mounted a massive effort to organize the best talents available for the care of the wounded and for the solution of the health care problems generated by the war. For the first time, relatively large efforts in research were begun under the direction of the federal government, and the results were impressive. The development of antibiotics accelerated rapidly, new surgical techniques for the treatment of trauma and burns were discovered, and new approaches to the transportation of the sick and wounded were developed. The range and breadth of problems that were subjected to organized investigation were remarkable, opening the way for an even more greatly expanded research effort after the war was over. In 1950, the size of the research commitment begun during World War II had risen to $73,000,000 per year, $35,000,000 of which was distributed through the National Institutes of Health (NIH). By 1974, this had risen to an annual research budget of $2,500,000,000 with $1,600,000,000 coming from a now greatly expanded NIH.

After World War II, hospitals were no longer the same. Previously, they had been places for the care of patients, with great emphasis being placed on the "caring" function. Now they became extensions of the research laboratories, places where medical science was practiced, and where "curing" was the order of the day. New procedures, new equipment, and new techniques all flourished to such a degree that the hospitals were now captured by their technology. The technology itself was the motivating force for hospitals and most major decisions were based on that technology.

The operation of these newly complex institutions called for waves of new workers, each more specialized and more highly skilled than the last. Before the war there had been approximately 20 major categories of health workers; by the 1970s there were hundreds. With the increasing specialization of services and skills, there was also an increasing interdependence of health workers on each other and an increasing reliance on the health care system to integrate the work of so many separate groups.

Physicians were severely affected by these trends. With the explosive growth of scientific knowledge after the Second World War, it was impossible for one physician to know everything, and so the trend toward specialization in a particular sub-area of medicine had a strong impetus. Before the war, approximately 80% of physicians were general practitioners and 20% specialists. In the years after the war these percentages were reversed. In their training and practice, physicians focused more and more on the scientific aspects of diagnosis and treatment, and as a result spent more time in hospitals and less time in the patients' homes. The hospital became the emotional center of the physician's life, since it was here that the most important, most challenging, and most interesting aspects of training or treatment occurred.

These trends affected nursing and the other health professionals to only a slightly lesser degree. The training of nurses and other health professionals became increasingly more scientific, more specialized, and more lengthy during the years after World War II. The desire to be recognized as competent in a particular area led to the proliferation of professional groups, and to formal accreditation on the basis of scientific training and ability. It also led to university-based training programs in all of the health professions.

Today the technology available to the American health care system has advanced to an incredible degree. Intrauterine diagnosis of fetal malformations, nuclear-powered cardiac pacemakers that operate for years, and sonarlike sensing devices that let blind people "see" what is in front of them are all accepted as merely the expected developments of a technological age. The merging of technologies from other fields with those of the health field, such as in the development of the computerized axial tomographic scanners, has further added to the immense range of technology available to the health care system. As Robert Rushmer points out in Chapter 8, however, this immense explosion of technology in recent years has not been without its problems. Indeed, the technology itself has *caused* a rather serious set of problems with which future generations of health care professionals must come to grip.

One of the most obvious problems raised by the new technology is its cost and the effect that it has on the entire financial structure of the health services system. The costs for providing this vast new technology increases each year, as do the costs for staffing that technology with the increasingly specialized and highly trained personnel that are needed. These increased costs are passed along to the public, to health insurance plans, and to the government, all of whom now ask, "Can we continue to spend our money in this way? Are we getting enough back for our money? Is there a better way in which we can use our resources for the people under our care?"

Possibly a more important problem of the technology is its impact on the form and configuration of the health care system and on the values and patterns of practice of the professionals in that system. In many ways, the American health services system has been captured by its technology and has been subtly and seductively shaped by its demands. Decisions regarding the design of programs and institutions, the training of personnel, and the distribution of services have been governed by technological considerations that loom larger every year.

A still more profound effect of technology is its ability to insinuate itself into the values of not just the system, but also of the people who work in the system. The student entering a health profession rapidly learns that academic success, and later, professional success, comes from mastery of the scientific technology. Increasingly, the student views excellence as being reached through technical achievements and gives decreasing importance to the more personal, nontechnical aspects of disease. By the time the student becomes a fully accepted member of the profession, a value system has been established which views illness as a series of technical problems to be solved by the application of specific technical solutions. This is then reinforced in practice by the expectations of the public and by the requirements of the regulators, both of whom have come to view "quality" in terms of technical excellence. The result, very frequently, is a professional performance which is excellent in technical terms and rather poor in human terms.

A quite different problem of technology arises not from its excessiveness, but rather from its inefficient distribution to society. If there is indeed more technology available than can be provided equitably to all people due to limits on funding, then large portions of society do not benefit as much as they should from technological knowledge. Marked differences exist, for example, in mortality and morbidity measures for white and non-white segments of society, possibly indicating an unequal access to modern health care technology. The answer, obviously, is to improve the health services system to ensure adequate distribution of available resources.

In summary, virtually no technology was available to treat disease prior to the 1900s. Technology began to appear and grow rapidly after the turn of the century. World War II fostered an incredible surge of research endeavors, with the result that the health care system began to be overwhelmed by the range and diversity of available technology. By the 1970s, the American health care system had been captured by its technology and the challenge was now to regain mastery over the giant that had been created.

SOCIAL ORGANIZATION FOR THE USE OF TECHNOLOGY

How has our society organized to use the technology available to it? What has been the predominant view about the role of society in health care? During the period 1850 to 1900, no organized program was available for the use of whatever technology might have existed. Public services were rudimentary, and were concentrated upon a very narrow range of problems. There were hospitals in a few areas, but they were generally started by religious or charitable groups for the care of those who were obviously and publicly impoverished. The predominant ethic of the time was that people should care for themselves and be self-sufficient, and if they become dependent, should take advantage of and be grateful for the various charities that were established for these specific purposes.

This philosophy of rugged individualism and relative lack of large-scale social organization for health care predominated in this country until the 1930s when the Great Depression struck with full force. At that time, economic forces beyond the comprehension of most Americans struck down many people, destroying their lives and leaving them destitute. The old ethic of an individual's being totally and personally responsible for all aspects of life was badly shaken by the events of the Depression.

With the arrival of Franklin Roosevelt in the White House, the New Deal was launched and a wide array of social programs appeared, all aimed at repairing the damage of the Depression. The importance of the New Deal in terms of American social thought cannot be underestimated since, for the first time, American society entered actively into large-scale national programs to assist those who could not assist themselves.

In health care, the governmental activity was still minimal, limited to a few specific areas of grant-in-aid programs to states to improve certain public health services such as infectious disease control and maternal and child health. Although the services were limited and aimed primarily at the poor, this small start did signify an assumption of responsibility by the national government for health care, at least for those who could not care for themselves.

The next major change in social organization and social thinking came with the arrival of World War II. As part of the mobilization effort, millions of men and women entered military service and in return received a wide array of health services simply by virtue of that service. The significance was twofold: first, the services themselves were provided without charge by salaried physicians working for the government; second, they were provided as a "right" of those in the service and were clearly not a charity for people who could no longer take care of themselves as previous governmental efforts had been.

Not only did World War II accustom the country to large-scale health care programs provided by the society to its members, but it also encouraged the growth of the health insurance industry. During the war, a "freeze" was imposed on wages and salaries so that very little collective bargaining for increases in salary could occur. However, considerable activity did occur in the development of pensions, disability programs, and health insurance plans, with the result that the health insurance industry began to flourish. The development of the health insurance industry provided the American public with a new form of social organization, the "third party" or fiscal intermediary. Before the development of health insurance, the public had no form of social organization to protect it from the sudden onslaught of medical bills. With the arrival of this new phenomenon, health insurance, the American public began to gain experience in the cooperative effort of pooling many individual contributions for a common group objective—protection from financial disaster.

The period immediately after World War II witnessed the slow, tentative growth of the "Blue" plans, Blue Cross and Blue Shield, non-profit community-based health care plans which insured against hospital and medical costs. With the success and growth of Blue Cross and Blue Shield, commercial insurance companies also entered the field, offering health insurance plans to employers and industry as part of their "life/health/retirement/disability" packages. With the rapid advances made by Blue Cross/Blue Shield and the commercial insurance carriers, the percentage of Americans covered by some form of health insurance rose from less than 20% prior to World War II to more than 70% by the early 1960s.

In the early 1960s, a major battle was fought and won by those advocating a greater societal role in the organization of health services. The battle involved the creation of government-sponsored health insurance plans for people over the age of 65 and resulted in the passage of legislation which created Medicare. Although Medicare itself was directed primarily to the needs of the country's elderly, its impact was soon felt throughout the entire health care system. The creation of the Medicare program had two immediate major social implications. First, Medicare provided financing for health care for all persons over the age of 65 simply on the basis of their reaching that age and not on the basis of their need. The American society in effect determined that there were certain things that the society should do for all of its members, regardless of individual need, since society could insure equity. The second major effect of Medicare was the assumption by the federal government of the responsibility for planning, financing, and monitoring a significant portion of the health care services in this country. The society not only wanted social insurance programs for health care, but also wanted the federal government to assume a central role in operating these programs.

A further significant change in the social organization of health care in this country occurred in the mid-1960s with the development of the Neighborhood Health Centers program of the U.S. Office of Economic Opportunity. Within the "War on Poverty," a number of health programs were funded for underserved areas of the country, each of which was required to have significant participation of consumers, often through governing boards and committees. This involvement of consumers was a substantial change from the past and soon became standard policy in new governmental programs. More recently, this philosophy was most vigorously put forward in the National Health Planning and Resources Development Act of 1974, which requires a majority of consumers on all local health planning boards.

In the late 1970s, the health care system of this country may have entered into a fourth phase of its development, an era of *resource limitation, restriction of growth, and regulation of effort.* It is significant to note government concern over the rising costs of health care and the desire of the Health Care Financing Administration, the federal agency responsible for the Medicare program, to protect Medicare resources. These developments, to be discussed in detail in the chapters of this book on health care financing and health planning and regulation, further reinforce the powerful central role of the federal government in health services in this country. The federal government now not only "controls" a significant amount of the financial support for health care in this country (approximately one-third of total health care expenditures), but also is able to set some of the rules by which all health care, governmentally funded or not, is provided.

Thus, this country started the twentieth century with a social philosophy that people should care for themselves or be satisfied with charity. It then adopted, in the middle of the century, a philosophy that society should care for those who, through no fault of their own, could no longer take care of themselves. Finally, towards the end of the century, it had moved to a philosophy that society, operating through the national government, should assume responsibility for providing the solution to certain large-scale problems of life for all of its members, even if some individual members could solve these problems for themselves.

The trend for the future seems to be that society has determined that government, particularly the federal government, will organize and coordinate large-scale programs of health care for the people of this country. The society has decided, to some extent, that "health care is a right, not a privilege," and will increasingly expect government to make that slogan a reality.

SUMMARY OF THE HISTORICAL TRENDS

The past 125 years of history have witnessed major changes in the American health care scene (Table 1–2). The predominant health problems of our people have changed from epidemics of acute infections to a different kind of "epidemic," chronic illness. The range of technology available has mushroomed from almost none in 1850 to a condition of such abundance now that the health care system has been virtually overwhelmed and captured by the technology it has created. Society's social values have changed from a *laissez-faire* approach in the 1850s that depended upon individual initiative or organized private charity to one now which assumes that health care is a right the federal government must assure everyone "enjoys" to the fullest extent possible.

TABLE 1–2. Major Trends in the Development of Health Care in the United States, 1850–Present

Trends	1850–1900	1900 to World War II	World War II to Present	Future
Predominant health problems of the American people	Epidemics of acute infections	Acute events, trauma, or infections affecting individuals, not groups	Chronic diseases such as heart disease, cancer, stroke	Chronic diseases, particularly emotional and behaviorally related conditions
Technology available to handle predominant health problems	Virtually none	Beginning and rapid growth of basic medical sciences and technology	Explosive growth of medical science; technology captures the health care system	Continued growth and expansion of technology, with attempts to repersonalize the technology
Social organization for the use of technology	None; individuals left to their own resources or charity	Beginning societal and governmental efforts to care for those who could not care for themselves	Health care as a right; governmental responsibility to organize and monitor health care for everyone	Greater centralization of responsibility and control in federal government

Source: From *The American Health Care System: Issues and Problems,* Paul R. Torrens, St. Louis, The C.V. Mosby Company, 1978.

SECTION II.
OVERVIEW OF HEALTH SERVICES IN THE UNITED STATES

When visitors from abroad come to the United States, particularly those engaged in health services in their own country, they frequently want to know about "the American health care system" and how it works. They are usually puzzled by the answer they get:

"There isn't any *single* 'American health care system.' There are many separate sub-systems serving different populations in different ways. Sometimes they overlap; sometimes they stand entirely separate from one another. Sometimes they are supported with public funds and at other times they depend solely on private funds. Sometimes several of these different sub-systems use the same facilities and personnel; other times they use facilities and personnel which are entirely separate and distinct."

It should not be surprising that there is this multiplicity of health care systems (or sub-systems) in the United States, given the historical development of health services in this country. In the earliest days, health care was entirely a private matter and people were expected to take care of themselves by obtaining services of private physicians and nurses when needed, purchasing medications from drugstores and chemist shops, and paying for all these services from their own personal funds. For those persons who could not take care of themselves, charitable institutions were established as voluntary, non-profit corporations to provide charity health care for those who otherwise could not obtain it on their own. These groups usually centered their efforts around hospitals and were usually located in the larger towns and cities of this country.

In the early part of the twentieth century, a new element was added with the development of the city/county hospitals. These were established by local governments to care for the poor in their area who could not get care either by their own efforts or from the voluntary non-profit charity hospitals. These public facilities were generally large acute-care, general hospitals, with busy clinics and emergency rooms and with close connections to local government ambulance services, police departments, and other community services. At the same time, state governments were developing mental hospitals. The cities had previously been responsible for the care of "lunatics" and the "insane," but after the turn of the century, state governments began to assume this burden. Every state soon had at least one mental hospital where the emotionally disturbed were offered what little care was available.

With the explosive growth in the size of the federal government and in the numbers of persons in the armed forces during World War II, a separate system of care developed for active duty military personnel and their dependents, retired military personnel, and veterans. These were almost entirely self-contained systems, employing salaried physicians and nurses, working entirely in military or veterans hospitals directly operated by the federal government.

As the cost of health care began to rapidly increase after World War II, the United States experienced a rather sudden and somewhat bewildering development of a wide variety of health insurance plans. The first to be operated were community-based, non-profit Blue Cross and Blue Shield plans, developed by hospital and physician associations to spread the cost of health care more widely among the population. These were followed by labor union health and welfare trust funds, established as a consequence of benefit negotiations for union members. At the same time, the private, for-profit commercial insurance companies expanded their efforts, for both individuals and large groups of employees. Finally, several large government-sponsored and publicly-supervised health insurance plans evolved, such as Medicare and Medicaid, a program to aid the medically indigent.

Private medical practitioners, voluntary non-profit hospitals, city and state government hospitals, military and veterans hospitals, and health insurance plans of a variety of forms and origins all developed in the United States at the same time, separately, and for specific purposes. The resulting picture has been described as having "a rich diversity of opportunities and approaches for meeting the health care needs of a population that has in itself a rich diversity of people and situations." It has also been described as "chaotic, uncoordinated, overlapping, unplanned, and wasteful of precious personal and financial resources." The reality probably lies somewhere in between.

If there is no single, easily described American health care system, at least some of the sub-systems that together compose the larger entity can be identified. Although an endless set of variations is possible, it seems appropriate to examine four models or sub-systems of health care in the United States, each of which serves a different group of Americans. By looking at the component parts, the system as a whole might be better understood. These systems are those serving 1) middle-class, middle-income families and individuals; 2) poor, inner-city, minority people; 3) active duty military personnel and their dependents; and 4) veterans of U.S. military service. For each of these "systems," the manner in which some basic elements of health care are provided to the people the system serves is reviewed.

MIDDLE-CLASS, MIDDLE-INCOME AMERICA (PRIVATE PRACTICE, FEE-FOR-SERVICE SYSTEM)

It is appropriate for two reasons to first consider the system of health care utilized by a "typical" middle-class, middle-income individual or family. First, this system is frequently described as *the* American health care system (all others, therefore, immediately becoming somehow secondary to it), and second, this system is frequently said to include the best medical care available in the United States and perhaps anywhere in the world.

The most striking feature of the middle-class, middle-income system of care is the absence of any *formal* system at all. Each individual or family puts together an *informal* set of services and facilities to meet their own needs. The system, therefore, has no formal structure or organization and is different for each individual or family. Indeed, each family's system may vary widely according to the particular situation in which it is used. The only constant feature of this system is the family itself; all other aspects are transient, changeable, and widely-varied.

Two other characteristics are also immediately noteworthy. First, the service aspects of the system concentrate around and are coordinated by physicians in private practice. Second, the system is financed by personal, non-governmental funds, whether paid directly out-of-pocket by consumers or through private health insurance plans. As the system is described, it will become readily apparent that these two features are not only important descriptive features; they have been important forces in shaping the system into its present form.

Public health and preventive medicine services for the middle-class, middle-income system are provided from two different sources. Those services which are aimed at the protection of large numbers of people *en masse,* such as water purification, disposal of sewage, and air-pollution control, are provided by local or state governmental agencies. Frequently those agencies are called "public health departments." These agencies usually provide their services to the entire population of a region, with no distinction between rich and poor, simple or sophisticated, interested or disinterested. Indeed, these mass public health services are common to all of the systems of health care to be discussed. Those public health and preventive medicine services which are aimed at individuals, such as well-baby examinations, cervical cancer smears, vaccinations, and family planning, are provided by individual physicians in private practice. If a middle-income family desires a vaccination in preparation for a foreign trip or wants their blood cholesterol level checked, the family physician is consulted and provides the service. If it is time for the new baby to have its first series of vaccinations, the family pediatrician is usually the one who provides them.

Ambulatory patient services, both simple and complex, are also obtained from private physicians. Many families use a physician who specializes in family practice, while others use an array of specialist physicians such as pediatricians, internists, obstetrician/gynecologists and psychiatrists who provide both primary care and specialty services. When special laboratory tests are ordered, x-ray films required, or drugs and medications prescribed, private commercial for-profit laboratories or community pharmacies are used. Many of these services, from individual preventive medicine services to complex specialist treatments, are financed by individuals through out-of-pocket payment since most health insurance plans do not provide complete coverage for these needs. When the middle-income family begins to use institutional services, such as hospital care, the source of payment shifts almost completely from the individual to third-party health insurance plans.

Inpatient hospital services are usually provided to the middle-class, middle-income family by a local community hospital that is usually voluntary and non-profit. The specific hospital to be used is determined by the institution in which the family physician has medical staff privileges. Generally, the smaller, less specialized, more local hospitals will be used for simpler problems, while the larger, more specialized, perhaps more distant hospital will be used for the more complicated problems. Many of these larger hospitals will have active physician-training programs, conduct research, and may have significant "charity" or "teaching" wards.

The middle-class, middle-income family obtains its long-term care from a variety of sources, depending on the service required. Some long-term care is provided in hospitals, and as such, is merely an extension of the complex inpatient care the patient has already been receiving. This practice was more common in the past but utilization review procedures have increased pressures on the hospital to reduce the length of time people are hospitalized. More commonly, long-term care will be obtained at home through the assistance of a visiting nurse or voluntary non-profit community-based nursing service. If institutional long-term care is needed, it will probably be obtained in a nursing home or a skilled nursing facility, usually a small (50–100 patients) facility, operated privately, for-profit, by a single proprietor or small group of investors. The middle-class, middle-income family usually pays for its long-term care with its own funds, since most health insurance plans provide relatively limited coverage for long-term care.

When middle-class families require care for emotional problems, they will again use a variety of mostly private services. However, as the illness becomes more serious, families may, for the first time, rely on governmentally-sponsored service. When emotional problems first begin to appear in the middle-class family, the patient will probably turn to the family physician who may provide simple supportive services such as tranquilizers, informal counselling, and perhaps referral for psychological testing. The physician may even arrange for the patient to be hospitalized in a general hospital for a rest, for "nervous exhaustion," or for some other non-psychiatric diagnosis. As the emotional problems become more severe, the family physician may refer the "patient" to a private psychiatrist, or to a community mental health center which most likely will be a voluntary non-profit agency, or under the sponsorship of one (such as a voluntary non-profit hospital). If hospitalization is required, the psychiatrist or the community mental health center is likely to use the psychiatric section of the local voluntary non-profit hospital if it seems that the stay in a hospital will be a short one. If the hospitalization promises to be a long one, the psychiatrist may use a psychiatric hospital, usually a private, non-governmental community facility.

In those cases in which very extended institutional care is required for an emotional problem and where the patient's financial resources are relatively limited, the middle-class family may request hospitalization in the state mental hospital. This usually represents the first use of governmental health programs by the middle income family, and as such it frequently comes as a considerable shock to patient and family alike.

In summary, the middle-class family's system of health care is an informal unstructured collection of individual services, put together by the patient and the private physician to meet the needs of the moment. The individual services themselves have little formalized relationship among themselves, and the only thread of continuity is provided by the family's physician or by the family itself. In general, all the services are provided by non-governmental sources and are paid for by private funds, either directly out-of-pocket or by privately financed health insurance plans.

For all its apparent looseness and lack of structure, the middle-class family's system of health care allows for a considerable amount of decision and control by the patient, and more than that of the other systems to be discussed. The patient is free to choose the physicians, the health insurance plan, and frequently even the hospital. If additional care is required, the patient can seek out and utilize (sometimes over-utilize) that care to the limit of the financial resources available. If the patient does not like the particular care being provided, dissatisfaction can be expressed in a most effective manner: the patient can seek care elsewhere from another provider.

On the other other hand, the middle-class family's system of care is a poorly-coordinated, unplanned collection of services which frequently have little formal integration with one another. It can be very wasteful of resources and usually has no central control or monitor to determine whether it is accomplishing what it should. Each individual service may be of very high quality, but there may be little evidence of any "linking" taking place to ensure that each service compliments each other to the maximum extent possible.

One special sub-set of the middle-class, middle-income model now involves millions of patients in this country. When people reach age 65, they are automatically eligible for Medicare, the federally sponsored and supervised health insurance plan for the elderly. A patient covered by Medicare benefits can utilize the same system of care as the middle-income family, including private practice physicians and voluntary non-governmental hospitals. The main difference now is that the bills are paid by a federal government health insurance plan, rather than the usual private plan in which the typical middle-class family is enrolled. The physicians are the same and the hospitals are the same; only the health insurance plan is different.

POOR, INNER-CITY, MINORITY AMERICA (LOCAL GOVERNMENT HEALTH CARE)

A second major system of health care in the United States serves the poor, inner-city, and generally minority population. While the specific details may vary from city to city, the general outline is well-known throughout all major cities of the country. If it was important to study the middle-class, middle-income system of care because it represented the *best* health care possible in this country, it is equally important to study the poor, inner-city system of care, since it frequently represents the *worst*.

The most striking feature of the health care system of the poor, inner-city resident is exactly the same one that was so outstanding in the middle-class system: there is no *formal* system at all. Instead, just as in the middle-class system, each individual or family must put together some *informal* set of services, from whatever source possible, to meet the health care needs of the moment. There is one significant difference, however: the poor do not have the resources to choose where and in what style they will obtain their health services. Instead, they must take what is offered to them, and try to put together a system from whatever they are told they can have.

There are two other important characteristics of the system. First, the great majority of services are provided by local government agencies such as the city or county hospital and the local health department. Second, the patients have no *real* continuity of service with any single provider, such as a middle-class family might have with a family physician. The poor family is faced with an endless stream of health care professionals who treat one specific episode of an illness and then are replaced by someone else for the next episode. While the middle-class system of health care was able to establish at least some thread of continuity by the continued presence of a family physician, the poor family is not able to maintain any thread of continuity at all.

The poor obtain their mass public health and preventive medicine services, including a pure water supply, sanitary sewage disposal, and protection of milk and food from the same local government health departments and health agencies that serve the middle-class system. In contrast to the middle-class system, however, the poor also get their individual public health and preventive medicine services from the local health department. When a poor family's newborn baby needs its vaccinations, that family goes to the district health center of the health department, not to a private physician. When a low-income woman needs a Papanicolau smear for cervical cancer testing or when a teenager from a low-income family needs a blood test for syphillis, it is most likely that the local government health department will give the test.

To obtain ambulatory patient services, the poor family cannot rely on the constant presence of a family doctor for advice and routine treatment. Instead, they must turn to neighbors, the local pharmacist, the health department's public health nurse, or the emergency room of the city or county hospital. It has often been said that the city or county hospital's emergency room is the family doctor for the poor, and the facts generally support this: when the poor need ambulatory patient care, it is quite likely that the first place they will turn is the city or county hospital emergency room.

The emergency room also serves the poor as the entry point to the rest of the health care system. The poor obtain much of their ambulatory services in the outpatient clinics of the city/county hospitals, and to gain admission to these clinics, the poor frequently must first go through the emergency room and be referred to the appropriate clinic. Once out of the emergency room, they may be cared for in two or three specialty clinics, each of which may handle one particular set of problems, but none of which will take responsibility for coordinating all the care the patient is receiving.

When the poor need inpatient hospital services, whether they be simple or complicated, they again usually turn to the city or county hospital to obtain them. Admission to the inpatient services of these hospitals is usually obtained through the emergency room or the outpatient clinics, thereby forcing the poor family to use these ambulatory patient services if they wish later admission to the inpatient services. The poor may also turn to the emergency room, the outpatient clinics, and the inpatient ward or teaching services of the larger, voluntary non-profit community hospitals. Since these hospitals are frequently teaching hospitals for the training of physicians, they often maintain special free or lower-priced wards. It is to these wards that the poor are usually admitted. Since the care in the teaching hospitals is generally as good or better than might be obtained at the local city or county hospitals, many poor are willing to become teaching cases in the voluntary non-profit hospitals in exchange for better care in better surroundings. By and large, however, the city and county hospitals carry the largest burden of inpatient care for the poor.

If the long-term care situation of middle-income people is generally inade-quate, the long-term care of the poor can only be described as terrible. In contrast with the middle-class, much of the long-term care of the poor is provided on the wards of the city and county hospitals, although not by intent or plan. The poor simply remain in hospitals longer because their social and physical conditions are more complicated and because the hospital staffs are reluctant to discharge them until they have some assurance that continuing care will be available after discharge. Since this is very often uncertain, poor patients are likely to be kept longer in the hospital so that they can complete as much of their convalescence as possible prior to discharge.

The greater bulk of the long-term care of the poor is provided in the same type of nursing homes or skilled nursing facilities that are used by the middle-class: small (50–100 patients) facilities, operated for-profit by a single proprietor or a small group of owners. One major difference between the two systems is the quality of the facility used, the middle-class generally having access to better equipped and better staffed nursing homes, and the poor having access to less expensive, less well-equipped facilities. Another important difference between the middle-class and the poor is that the middle-class, middle-income patients are more likely to pay for their own care in these institutions, while the poor have their care paid for by welfare or other public, governmental funds.

It is interesting to note that the system of health care for the middle-class utilizes entirely private, non-governmental facilities until long-term care for mental illness is required; at that point, a governmental facility, the state mental hospital, is used. By contrast, the system of health care for the poor is composed almost entirely of public, government-sponsored services until long-term care is required. This is usually provided in private, profit-making facilities, the first such use of private facilities by the poor.

The convergence of the poor and the middle-class systems of care in the small, private profit-making nursing homes is important, since it represents an important feature of our multiple sub-systems of health care. In a number of instances, several systems of health care that are otherwise quite separate and distinct will merge in their common use of personnel, equipment, or facilities. The emergency rooms of the city or county and voluntary non-profit teaching hospitals, for example, will serve as the source of emergency medical care for the middle-class family that cannot reach its own family physician. It will also serve as the family physician for the poor family that has none of its own. The private, for-profit nursing home will serve as the source of long-term care for the middle-class family, and may provide the same function for the poor. The radiology department of the voluntary non-profit teaching hospital will provide x-rays for the middle-class patient whose care is supervised by the private family physician as well as for the poor patient whose care is supervised by a hospital staff physician in training. This does not mean that there is any real, functional integration of the separate systems of care because of their common use of the same facility or personnel. Rather, the model is more like that of a busy harbor in which a variety of ships will berth side-by-side for a short period of time before going on their separate ways for their separate purposes.

In their use of services for emotional illnesses, the poor return once again to an almost totally public, local government system. Initial signs of emotional difficulties are haphazardly treated in the emergency rooms and out-patient clinics of the city or county hospital. From here patients may be referred to the crowded inpatient psychiatric wards of these same hospitals, but are just as likely to be referred to community mental health centers operated by local government or voluntary non-profit community agencies. When long-term care in an institution is required, the poor are sent to the psychiatric wards of the city or county hospital, and then from there to the large state government mental hospitals, frequently many miles away.

In the past, health services for the poor were usually free, at least to the patient. Neither the local health department, the city or county hospital, nor the state mental hospital generally charged for their services, regardless of the patient's ability to pay. In the last few years, both local health departments and city and county hospitals have been forced to initiate a system of charges for services which were previously free. They have done this to recapture third-party payments to which the poor patient might be eligible, and patients who are unable to pay are still ordinarily provided the services they need. The imposition of these charges for previously free health services has probably changed how these programs are viewed by the poor, but it is still too early to determine the implications of these changes.

As with the middle-class, middle-income system, there is a sub-set of the health care system of the poor that requires special comment. Certain persons who are poor enough by virtue of extremely low income or resources may qualify for Medicaid, the federal-state cooperative health insurance "plan" for the indigent, frequently termed "Title 19" in reference to the section of the federal legislation by which it was created (Medicare, an entirely different program, is termed "Title 18"). Under Medicaid people whose income and resources are below a level established by the individual states can utilize a state government-sponsored health insurance program to purchase health care in the private, middle-class marketplace. The purpose of this program is to move the poor out of their usual local government health care system and into the supposedly better private practice health care system of the middle-class. Unfortunately, the ability of Medicaid to move the poor into a better system of care has been limited by the reluctance of the private physicians and private hospitals to assume responsibility for many Medicaid patients. This reluctance is based on Medicaid's low rate of reimbursement for services, its incredible paperwork and red tape, and its frequently appalling system of retroactive denial of payment for services already provided.

Medicaid has succeeded to a degree in moving poor patients from local government hospitals into voluntary non-profit teaching hospitals, but its greatest effect has probably been in moving poor patients into private, profit-making nursing homes and skilled nursing facilities. In many states, for example, more than two-thirds of all patient bills in private nursing homes are now paid by the Medicaid program, providing some indication of the importance of this program in the provision of long-term care. And, for all its problems, the Medicaid program has allowed certain aspects of the middle-class, middle-income system of health care to be shared with the poor, inner-city minority system of health care, a blending, merging, or sharing of resources and services that is characteristic of the American health care system and which makes it so difficult to evaluate any one sub-system separately.

In summary, the system of health care for the poor is as unstructured and informal as that for the middle-class, but the poor have to depend upon whatever services the local government offers to them. The services are usually provided free of charge, or at low cost, but the patient has relatively little opportunity to express a choice and exercise options. Poor patients often cannot move to another set of services if they dislike the one first offered, since those first offered are usually the *only* services available.

As with the system of health care for the middle-class, the system for the poor is poorly coordinated internally and almost completely unplanned and unmonitored. It is certainly as wasteful of resources as the middle-class system, but because of the external appearances as a low-cost, poorly-financed system, the exact extent of wasted resources is difficult to document. At the same time, the great positive virtue of the health care system for the poor, its openness and accessability to all people at all times for all conditions (albeit with considerable delays), is difficult to evaluate adequately as well. An optimist would view health services for the poor in this country today as considerably better than they have ever been before. A pessimist would say that they still have a long way to go towards meeting even minimal acceptable standards for care. Both would be right!

MILITARY MEDICAL CARE SYSTEM

A person joining one of the uniformed branches of the American military sacrifices many aspects of civilian life that non-military personnel take for granted. At the same time, however, this person receives a variety of fringe benefits that those outside the military do not enjoy at all. One of the most important of these fringe benefits is a well-organized system of high quality health care provided at no direct cost to the recipient. Certain features of this military medical care system (the general term used to include the separate systems of the United States Army, Navy, and Air Force) deserve comment. First, the system is all-inclusive and omnipresent. The military medical system has the responsibility of protecting the health of all active duty military personnel wherever their military duty may take them, and of providing them with all the services that they may eventually need for any service-connected problem. The military medical system goes wherever active duty military personnel go, and assumes a responsibility for total care that is unique among American health care systems.

The second important characteristic of the military medical care system is that it goes into effect immediately whether the active duty soldier or sailor wants it or not. No initiative or action is required by the individual to start the system, and indeed, the system frequently provides certain types of health services, such as routine vaccinations or shots, that the soldier or sailor would really wish not to have. The individual has little choice regarding who will provide the treatment or where, but at the same time, the services are always there if needed, without the patient having to search them out. If a physician's services are needed, they are obtained; if a hospitalization is required, it is arranged; if emergency transportation is necessary, it is carried out. There is little that the individual can do to influence how medical care is provided, but at the same time, there is never any worry about its availability.

The third important characteristic of the military health care system is its great emphasis on keeping personnel well, on preventing illness or injury, and on finding health problems early while they are still amenable to treatment. Great stress is placed on preventive measures such as vaccination, regular physical examinations and testing, and educational efforts towards prevention of accidents and contagious diseases. In an approach that is unique among the health care systems of this country, the military medical system provides "health" care and not just "sickness" care.

In the military medical system, the same mass public health and preventive medicine services that are provided to a locality or a community by a local government health department or health agency, may also be provided to the active duty military personnel. However, whenever the personnel are actually within the boundaries of a military reservation or post, an additional set of mass public health and preventive medicine services may be provided by the military itself. Sanitary disposal of sewage, protection of food and milk, purification of water supply, and prevention of vehicular or job-related accidents may be provided for by a local government agency, but each military installation will usually have a second separate system of its own, staffed by its own public health and safety officers. Individual public health and preventive medicine services are also provided by the military medical system, according to a well-organized regularly-scheduled routine of yearly examinations, surveys of patient records, vaccinations, and other measures. The persons providing the specific preventive service (for example, a routine tetanus shot) are usually medical corpsmen or other non-physician personnel; however, their work is carried out according to carefully developed guidelines and will be monitored by well-trained supervisory medical personnel.

Routine ambulatory care is usually provided to most active duty military personnel by the same medics who provide the individual preventive services. These services are usually provided at the dispensary, sick bay, first aid station, or similar unit that is very close to the military personnel's actual place of work. These ambulatory services may also be provided by physicians or nurses at the same locations, but this is less likely. More complicated ambulatory patient care services are usually provided by physicians, frequently specialists, working at the same dispensary or medical station as the medics, or more likely, in a clinic or outpatient department of a larger facility such as a military hospital. Patients are usually referred by medics or physicians who have first cared for the patients for more simple problems; laboratory tests, x-ray examinations, and medications are obtained at the same military facility to which the patient is referred.

The most simple hospital services are provided using short-stay beds at base dispensaries, in sick bays aboard ship, or at small base hospitals on various military installations around the world. Usually the range of services that can be offered at these installations is limited, and referral to larger institutions is routinely carried out if a more complex problem is suspected. More complicated hospital services are provided to active duty military personnel in regional hospitals that possess a wide variety of specialized services and facilities. Frequently these hospitals also have large teaching and training programs, where the atmosphere and the quality of care is similar to what might be expected at a university hospital or a large community teaching hospital.

The military medical system does not pretend to offer the same extensive range of long-term care services that it provides for more acute short-term problems. The military medical system does provide care for potentially long-range problems in military hospitals, as long as there is some reasonable expectation that the patient will some day be able to return to full active duty. Whenever it is determined, however, that the problem is genuinely long-term in nature and that complete return to active duty is not possible, the patient is given a medical discharge from the service and long-term care will be provided through the Veterans Administration facilities.

If military personnel develop emotional difficulties, care is most likely to be provided initially by the medical corpsman and then by a physician assigned to that military unit. These personnel will provide short-term non-psychiatric support and counselling, and possibly prescribe certain medications, such as tranquilizers. For more severe problems, the patient is referred to the psychiatric services of larger military hospitals where the severity of the problem will be determined. If the problem is short-term and is not felt to affect the patient's work seriously, an attempt *may* be made to provide the short-term treatment at the military hospital itself, first on an inpatient basis, and later as an outpatient. More likely, if there is a significant psychiatric diagnosis, the patient will be given a medical discharge, with follow-up care to be provided through the psychiatric services of the Veterans Administration hospitals.

In general, the military medical system is closely organized and highly integrated. A single patient record is used, and the complete record moves from health care service to health care service with the patient. Once the need for health care is identified, the system itself arranges for the patient to receive the required care and usually even provides transportation to the services. The patient does not have to search out the necessary service nor determine how to utilize it. All of this is provided at no cost to the patient, requires little effort by the patient to initiate services, and generally involves a high quality product. The system is centrally planned, utilizes non-medical and non-nursing personnel to the utmost, and is entirely self-sufficient and self-contained. The services are provided by personnel who are salaried employees within facilities that are wholly-owned and operated by the system itself. The system is not generally available to persons who are not active duty military personnel or their dependents, although in cases of emergency or pressing local need they can be. Generally, the patient has little choice regarding the manner in which services will be delivered, but this is counterbalanced by the assurance that high-quality services will be available when needed.

Dependents and families of active duty military personnel are served by a special sub-system of military medicine which combines the services of both the middle-class, middle-income system and the active duty military system. The dependents and families of active duty military personnel are covered by an extensive health insurance plan, the Civilian Health and Medical Program of the Uniformed Services (CHAMPUS), provided, financed, and supervised by the military. This health insurance plan allows dependents and families of active duty military personnel to purchase medical care from private medical practitioners and from local community non-military hospitals when similar services cannot be provided at a military installation within reasonable distance. The dependents and families of active duty military personnel can also use the same military services that the active duty personnel use, provided space and resources are available and military authorities determine that this is appropriate. The resulting sub-system of care for military dependents and families generally allows them to participate to some degree in two separate systems of care: the middle-class, middle-income private practice system and the military medical system. Their participation in either is generally not as clearly focused or as active as it would be for someone firmly planted in either one system, but it still provides them with two viable options for obtaining care.

VETERANS ADMINISTRATION HEALTH CARE SYSTEM

Parallel to the system of care for active duty military personnel is another system operated within the continental United States for retired, disabled, and otherwise deserving veterans of previous U.S. military service. Although the Veterans Administration (VA) system is in many respects larger than the system of care for active duty military personnel, it is not nearly as complete, well-integrated, or extensive. At the present time, the Veterans Administration system of care is primarily hospital oriented and not really a "health care system." The VA operates 171 hospitals throughout the country which provide most VA care. In recent years, the VA has increasingly provided outpatient services and now maintains more than 200 outpatient clinics; however, the major thrust of VA health care is still focused on the hospitals.

A second important characteristic of the Veterans Administration system is the great preponderance of male patients with long-term care problems. By and large, the patients using the VA health care system are older, inactive men in whom the occurrence of multiple and chronic physical and emotional illnesses is much higher than in the general population.

A third important feature of the VA system is its existence as only one part of a much larger system of social services and benefits for veterans. Many of the people eligible to utilize the Veterans Administration health care system are also receiving other kinds of financial benefits as well, and indeed, access to the VA health care system is sometimes directly dependent upon eligibility for financial benefits. As Table 1–3 demonstrates, more than one million veterans received health care in the VA system during 1974. During this same time period, 2,500,000 veterans also received educational assistance, over 3,000,000 veterans received VA disability compensation, and 3,750,000 veterans had VA home loans outstanding. Since health care is only one of many VA programs, a vast set of social services interact with, and compete for, all available resources.

A further feature of the Veterans Administration health care system is its unique relationship with organized consumer groups. Since the VA is organized to provide care exclusively for veterans and since many of those veterans are members of local and national veterans clubs and associations, the VA health care system is constantly in direct communication with groups representing the interests of veterans. In a manner that is unparalleled in any other health care system in this country, the interests of the veterans are constantly put forward to individual VA hospitals, to the VA administration in Washington, and to the Congress of the United States. In no other health care system in this country, does organized consumer interest play such a constant, important, and influential role.

TABLE 1–3. Veterans Receiving Various Services and Benefits from Veterans Administration During 1974

Service or Benefit	Veterans Benefiting
Medical care	1,140,750
Educational assistance	2,461,000
Disability compensation	3,241,263
Home loans	3,750,000
VA supervised life-insurance plans (approximate)	8,000,000

Source: Administrator of Veteran Affairs, Annual Report, 1974, Veterans Administration, Washington, D.C., 1975.

Since the Veterans Administration system is primarily a hospital system, there are few attempts to provide general public health services or routine ambulatory care services. Veterans usually obtain these services from some other system of care, either the middle-class, middle-income system or the local government system that serves the urban poor. The VA does provide the more complicated ambulatory care services, usually through its hospital outpatient clinics. This is in preparation for possible hospital admission or as follow-up after hospitalization. Many veterans who require these services obtain them from other systems of care and come to the VA system only after a condition is apparent and hospitalization is required. Admission to VA hospitals can be gained either through the ambulatory patient care services operated by the VA itself, by direct referrals from physicians in private practice, or by referrals from hospitals in the community. The services in VA hospitals are provided by salaried, full-time medical and nursing personnel; as in the military medical system, most of the VA hospitals are self-contained, relatively self-sufficient units that require little outside support or staff.

The Veterans Administration health care system provides a tremendous quantity of long-term care for both physical and emotional illnesses. Indeed, the VA is probably the largest single provider of long-term care in the country, if not the world. In addition to providing considerable long-term care in the acute, short-term care hospitals, the VA also operates a number of domiciliaries and nursing homes. The VA has also recently begun to pay for care in local community nursing homes and skilled nursing facilities.

The VA system of care is difficult to fully describe for two important reasons. First, it is a system that does not attempt to provide a complete range of services, but instead concentrates on acute hospital services and on long-term care for physical and emotional problems. Second, eligibility for entry into the system is somewhat unclear and sometimes open to variable local interpretation. The system is designed to serve veterans with service-connected disabilities, but offers services to other veterans if they cannot obtain adequate care elsewhere and if adequate VA resources are available. In practice, the actual eligibility requirements and patient "mix" vary substantially from one VA hospital to the next.

If the system of health care for active duty military personnel focuses on preventive, ambulatory, and acute inpatient care, the Veterans Administration system of care stresses long-term, chronic inpatient care for both physical and emotional problems. Whereas the military medical system offers a complete, well-integrated, well-coordinated package of health care services, the services that the VA offers are primarily hospital-related. In contrast to the military medical system that actively seeks out and offers services to patients as part of their work environment, the VA provides its services to patients only when they come forward seeking them. If they don't seek out the care, the VA system doesn't actively pursue them. Despite these reservations about the Veterans Administration as a complete system of health care, it should be stressed that the VA serves as the primary source of inpatient hospital care for one million veterans a year, and is a potential source of inpatient care for many millions more. As such, it is the largest single provider of health care services in this country and must be considered an integral, important component of the American health care scene, both now and in the future.

HEALTH SERVICES: A SUMMARY OF PERSPECTIVES

In reviewing each of these four major systems of health care for Americans, the middle-class, private practice system, the local government system for the urban poor, the military medical system for active duty military and their dependents, and the Veterans Administration health care system, it becomes apparent that there are any number of additional systems that could have been included as well. Other systems of health care include that utilized by rural farming families and the Indian Health Service operated for native Americans by the federal government. There are also any number of variations possible within the four systems discussed here. The purpose however, is not to be exhaustive in describing the systems themselves, but rather to point out that there are multiple systems providing services to different populations with different needs. No one single system predominates in terms of persons served or benefits provided to patients. Indeed, the purpose here is to point out that there is no one single "American health care system," but rather that there is a mosaic of sub-systems, each with its own characteristics and going in its own particular direction.

Is it bad to have so many separate sub-systems? Why is it even worth pointing out the obvious fact that many such systems exist? Several pressing reasons exist for reviewing this country's compartmentalized organization of health care. The first and most important is quite simple: to improve health services to everyone in this country, an understanding of the entire situation is essential; otherwise, piece-meal solutions will be proposed to specific problems without recognizing the possible long-range potentials for the entire system. In a system that could be compared to a jigsaw puzzle, it would be foolish and perhaps even dangerous to consider each individual piece of the puzzle without first considering the puzzle as a whole.

The second reason for considering the various separate systems of health care in this country is the vigorous competition for scarce resources of money, people, and facilities. Although the four systems described stand separate and apart from one another, they all compete for the same set of resources since they are all dependent upon the same economy and the same supplies of health personnel and skills.

Whenever there is this vigorous competition for resources, two things frequently happen. First, the stronger, more vigorous, more aggressive, or better connected competitors obtain the larger portion of the resources—whether or not this is justified by their needs. In practice, this has meant that the middle-class, private-practice system, the military medical system, and the Veterans Administration system have all done relatively well, while the local government health care system has not. Indeed, the local government health care system for the poor has always been severely under-financed and understaffed in view of its mammoth task of providing health care to those who lack access elsewhere.

Second, intense competition for resources frequently results in wasteful duplication and ineffective use of resources. For example, in the same region, a city or county hospital, a private teaching hospital, a military hospital, and a VA hospital may all be operating exactly the same kind of expensive service, although only one facility might be needed and where undoubtedly, one large integrated service would provide more efficient use of resources than four smaller ones. Because each institution is part of a separate system, serves a different population, and approaches the resource pool through a different channel, no really purposeful planning or controlled allocation of resources is possible. In the past, this might have been acceptable because the resource pool seemed bottomless, but in these days of very apparent limits on resources, this is no longer acceptable.

In addition to this economic inefficiency, there are other reasons for looking with a critical eye at multiple systems of care, reasons that are related to quality and accessability of services. Unfortunately, not all of these sub-systems of care serve people in the same way with the same results. There is great inequality among the various systems of health care, with the result that different people receive different levels of care simply by accident of birth or membership in one special group or another. Since all the separate systems of health care in this country ultimately depend on public funds for their continued existence, it is imperative that the inequalities between systems be removed as rapidly as possible. This does not necessarily mean eliminating the various separate sub-systems of care, but rather requires that all the systems rise to a common high level and equitably share responsibilities and resources.

In recent years, there have been various approaches to the problem of reorganizing these separate sub-systems of care so that they function together in a more integrated and effective fashion. Although these proposals have often been limited to specific aspects, such as financing or quality of care, their overall purpose has generally been to move the various pieces of the American health care system into a better and more efficient relationship with each other. These approaches are interesting not in and of themselves, but in how they will shape health care in the future. The specific scenarios for the specific issues will undoubtedly change, but the overall effort at developing a more rationally integrated system will certainly continue unabated and will, indeed, expand as resources are stretched to the limit.

Two proposals can be mentioned briefly, not because they are unimportant but rather because the possibility of their implementation is so slight that they have relatively little practical impact. The first of these might be described as a *laissez-faire,* free-market approach which implies in effect, "Leave everyone alone, stop meddling, stop regulating and let the workings of the market place with its active competition eventually force the health care system to reorganize." The second approach, at the other political and social extreme implies, "What this country needs is a single, governmentally-controlled health care system, such as the British National Health Service, which would allow for greater centralized control and planning for all aspects of the system." For different reasons, both of these approaches have been viewed as so politically impractical for this country at this time that they have not been seriously considered.

Another approach that has been used has been the "health planning" approach. With the passage of the original Comprehensive Health Planning legislation and more important, with the passage of the National Health Planning and Resources Development Act of 1975, it has been proposed that providers, consumers, and public officials come together and mutually develop health plans for all states and localities which then become the blueprint or framework for a more rationally organized system of care.

A slightly different approach has been one centered around the financing of health care, particularly through a national health insurance plan. The more conservative supporters of this approach feel that it would allow each person to purchase care wherever and in whatever systems he or she feels may be most appropriate. This would create competition between each of the various sub-systems to perform better or lose their share of the market. The more liberal supporters of this approach would use the inherent financial power of a single, large, bill-paying agency to force organizational changes in the system. The implication is that the central "insurance agency" could withhold funds from those parts of the system which do not follow some masterplan developed by that agency. In either case, this approach uses the power of health care financing, spent either individually or collectively, to reorganize the system.

Another possible solution, which has yet to receive considerable attention, is the "public utility" approach. In this approach toward a rational system, all the component parts of the health care system, or at least the large institutional ones, would be placed under the regulatory supervision of public bodies which would have total control over licensing, financing, mode of function, packages of services offered, personnel development, and so forth. Both public and private components could continue to exist as they do at present under their own auspices (just as individual utilities do, for example), but what they would be able to do and how much they would be allowed to charge would be matters of control by the single regulatory agency. A strong argument for this approach is that all these individual regulatory efforts are conducted now, in a poorly coordinated and often conflicting fashion, by multiple regulatory agencies. Having one single body would remove much of the present jungle of regulatory efforts. A strong argument *against* such a body is that it would put immense power over the system into a single super-agency.

A final approach towards rationalization of the present system might be called "incremental tinkering" and it is one which tacitly assumes that no major, sweeping, overall reorganization is possible. The proponents of this approach try instead to do whatever they can whenever an opportunity presents itself anywhere within the system to increase rationality. A new piece of state legislation here, a new form of federal health insurance there, a new form of local cooperative planning are all added in piecemeal fashion without any great effort to relate them to each other or to some underlying master plan. The hope in this approach is that all the individual accretions to the system will provide for a more efficient and integrated end product.

These six approaches are obviously not mutually exclusive, so it is entirely possible that someone might support several of them because they work together well. Someone interested in reorganizing the health care system through health planning might also want to see a national health insurance program because it would provide the centralized financial leverage to have mandatory health planning. In the same fashion, someone might propose a mostly *laissez-faire* approach to any intentional reorganization and also support a national health insurance plan which would allow all people the ability to formulate their own individual choices in an open market.

In the future, all six approaches (and possibly more) will probably continue to be fostered and most likely no single approach will predominate. What certainly will continue however will be efforts to bring the various pieces of the sub-systems and the various sub-systems themselves into some more efficient and effective new relationship with one another and with the consumers who must use them. Indeed, this issue is so important and so central to all our other interests that the future of health care in this country will be shaped by the direction our society decides to follow.

The remaining chapters of this book describe, dissect, and analyze the health services system of the United States. Trends, issues, interrelationships, and problems are revealed and assessed. Only by thoroughly understanding the evolution, structure, attributes, and deficiencies of the system, or "systems," can the fundamental decisions facing the nation be addressed.

*Part Two
Causes
and Characteristics
of Health Services
Utilization in
the United States*

CHAPTER 2

The Physiologic and Psychologic Bases of Health, Disease, and Care Seeking

Lawrence A. May

In this chapter, the physiological bases of disease and the psychological character-istics of care-seeking behavior are explored. The concepts of illness and disease, and the complexities surrounding the exact definitions of diseases are discussed. The orderly relationship between pathologic abnormality, physiological alteration, and clinical manifestations of disease are presented, especially as they relate to care-seeking behavior. The influence of biological, pharmacological, and environ-mental factors on changing disease patterns is reviewed, and some of the effects of these changing disease patterns on the health services system are demonstrated as a prelude to the remaining chapters of the book.

DEFINING ILLNESS AND DISEASE

The distinction between illness and disease is essential for the understanding of care-seeking behavior. Illness is a lay experience that connotes both a physical and a social state (1). It is a person's reaction to a biological alteration, and is defined differently by different people according to their individual states of mind and their cultural beliefs. The term "illness," therefore, is extremely imprecise and represents a highly individual response to a specific set of physiologic and psychologic stimuli.

By contrast, "disease" is a professional construct. It is perceived as being very precise and reflecting the highest state of professional knowledge, particularly that of the physician. The definition of disease is used as the vehicle for informing the patient of the presence of pathology, as a means for deciding on a course of treatment, and as a basis for comparing the results of therapy. It becomes an essential element in the planning and organization of the health care system and in the allocation of resources within that system.

Since the accurate definition of disease is so important, it is crucial to understand the considerable imprecision that actually exists in this process. An individual physician using the best professional judgment available may define the presence of a specific disease in a particular patient, but this definition may not be shared by other physicians. And even when the definition of a particular disease is similar in different patients, the impact of the diagnosis on those patients may vary widely depending upon how the definition is applied and on the unique social and biological characteristics of individual patients.

Attempts to link "illness" (the individual's perception of loss of functional capacity) with "disease" (the professional definition of a pathological process) is even more complicated. Illness may occur in the absence of "real" disease and disease may be present in the absence of perceived illness. Since it is "illness," the individual's perception of impaired function, and not "disease" that stimulates care-seeking behavior, the relationship between these two concepts is important to understand.

The complexity of defining disease and its interaction with care-seeking behavior is well illustrated by the condition "diabetes mellitus." Both the general public and the health professional understand that diabetes results in an elevated blood sugar, but the physiological bases for this metabolic alteration can vary widely (2). In one person, the disease may result from impaired secretion of insulin by the pancreas, but in another person, it may be caused by a resistance to sufficient amounts of insulin in a patient who is obese. In one person diabetes mellitus may result from the imposition of a normal physiological condition such as pregnancy, while in yet another, it may be due to the use of exogenous drugs, such as diuretics or steroids.

Quite aside from the varying causes for an elevated blood sugar, a much more important issue is the level of hyperglycemia (elevated blood sugar) that defines a patient as diabetic. Various criteria have been suggested to define who is diabetic, using different numerical measures of elevated blood sugar, but these criteria do not necessarily separate those who are "ill" from those who feel healthy, nor does it define a level at which treatment is indicated (3). Diabetes in a 14-year-old boy, caused by inadequate supplies of circulating insulin and requiring exogenous provision of additional insulin for the rest of his life, is quite different from diabetes in a 62-year-old woman whose major physiologic reason for inadequate insulin effect is obesity.

The problem illustrated by diabetes extends to many other disease conditions that are defined by an abnormal laboratory measurement or blood test. Hypertension is a common medical problem resulting from a variety of different physiological bases, including abnormalities in hormone production and utilization, improper resetting of neurological control centers, or acquired loss of blood vessel elasticity secondary to atherosclerosis.

In view of the variety of causes of hypertension, the selection of an arbitrary number to define individuals or members of a population as having an abnormal condition is a very difficult and possibly futile effort. The blood pressure reading of 140/90 has been offered as the boundary of normality, but the meaning of this reading in different persons may be markedly different. A blood pressure of 150/ 100 in a 72-year-old woman has quite different implications from the same reading in a 26-year-old man. An elevated blood pressure after a half-hour of bed rest means something quite different from an elevated blood pressure in a person waiting anxiously for half an hour in a physician's office.

To complicate matters further, as with diabetes, there is no direct relationship between the presence of elevated blood pressure and the development of either perceived symptoms or actual pathological damage to body organs, at least at the lower ranges of hypertension. Some people with only slightly elevated hypertension will attribute a variety of functional complaints to their "blood pressure," while other individuals with dangerously elevated levels may not have any symptoms at all and perceive themselves as being well (4).

The definition of diabetes or of hypertension is relatively straightforward when compared to diseases that cannot now be numerically defined such as rheumatoid arthritis. The definition of this disease is clinical rather than numerical and is based on the presence of four or more diagnostic characteristics determined by the American Rheumatism Association to be valid criteria for the disease. Even with the use of this symptom aggregation approach, there are still many professionals who confuse rheumatoid arthritis with degenerative joint disease and with other forms of arthritis. And even with this more orderly approach to the definition of this disease, the ability to measure its impact on a population is still comparatively limited.

In summary, the definition of disease is a much more imprecise and inexact process than is usually thought. Although it is frequently associated with apparently solid objective measurements such as blood sugar levels or blood pressure, the implications of these values may vary widely. Finally, the relationship between illness, which is a personal observation on the part of patients, and disease, which is a scientific judgment on the part of professionals, needs to be understood and constantly remembered.

DISEASE PROCESSES

THE PHYSIOLOGIC BASES OF DISEASE

The major pathophysiologic processes involved in disease production are vascular, inflammatory, neoplastic, toxic, metabolic, and degenerative. These processes give rise to disease conditions, but their expression is modified by factors in the host such as age, immunologic status, medication ingestion, concurrent disease, or psychological perceptions. The combination of the initial pathophysiologic processes and the different host factors create the various disease patterns.

Vascular abnormalities may produce disease in a variety of ways in multiple organ systems. The gradual narrowing and eventual blockage of blood vessels by the deposit of fatty materials in the walls and the lumens of the vessels is a characteristic of arteriosclerotic cardiovascular disease. Other vascular disease may be produced by the more rapid occlusion of a blood vessel by an embolus, material floating in the blood stream coming from a distant site. Other disease pictures may be produced by bleeding from a ruptured blood vessel in the brain or elsewhere. In some disease conditions, such as stroke, the same clinical picture may result from any one of the three causes. Whatever the initial cause, gradual occlusion, embolus, or rupture, the result is damage to brain tissue and resultant paralysis. It is usually an easy task to determine that a cerebrovascular accident (stroke) has occurred, but it is frequently impossible to determine whether it was caused by gradual occlusion, embolus, or rupture of a blood vessel.

Inflammation is the basis of disease in many organ systems, but the physiologic basis of that inflammation may be infectious, autoimmune, traumatic, or something else. For example, presented with the clinical picture of arthritis (inflammation of a joint), the treating physician must not only consider how to alleviate the symptom of inflammation, but must also consider how to remove the underlying cause of that inflammation, if possible.

Neoplastic disease is caused by an abnormal new growth of tissue. Benign neoplasms are abnormal growths which remain localized and do not spread to distant locations in the body. Malignant neoplasms, generally called "cancer," by contrast not only grow locally, invading surrounding tissues, but also spread distantly in the body by a process called metastasis. Benign neoplasms may cause considerable damage by continued local growth and pressure on surrounding tissues, such as pressure on the brain from a "benign" growth on the surface. Malignant neoplasms, by contrast, invade the organs directly and disrupt their normal functioning by actually replacing normal tissue with diseased tissue. Neoplasms may occur spontaneously or may be caused by environmental, toxic, or host factors (5-10).

Toxic bases for disease involve the presentation to individual organs of chemical materials which are inherently damaging. These materials may originally come to the body from environmental pollutants, from the use of potentially damaging materials such as alcohol or cigarettes, or from the ingestion of medications. Alcohol, for example, is toxic to the liver under appropriate conditions, causing hepatitis, fibrosis and eventual cirrhosis. Cobalt in beer can be toxic to heart muscle cells, bee stings may damage the glomerulus of the kidney, and asbestos may contribute to the development of lung cancer. Cigarette smoking may destroy, inflame, or alter the cells of the lung producing emphysema, chronic bronchitis, or cancer. Digitalis, an ordinarily useful drug in the treatment of various heart conditions, in excess doses may produce toxicity and life-threatening arrhythmias. In a society of increasing environmental pollutants, drug use, and industrial exposure, toxins are unfortunately becoming a more common cause of disease.

Metabolic diseases are caused by chemical disorders within cells of the body, usually secondary to some excess or deficiency of a hormone or important nutrient. The excess or deficiency of thyroid, parathyroid, or adrenal cortical hormone causes clinical disease pictures easily recognized by well-trained physicians. A deficiency of insulin, secreted by glands in the pancreas, gives rise to diabetes, as mentioned earlier. Deficiency of important nutrients, caused either by a scarcity of the elements in the diet or an inability to absorb and utilize them, results in a wide variety of clinical pictures ranging from anemia to pellagra.

Degeneration is the final pathophysiologic cause of disease, and may occur as a primary idiopathic disorder or secondary to some other process such as aging. Physicians generally resist accepting degeneration as an explanation for disease, but there are many diseases that currently cannot be otherwise explained. A large number of people, for example, who have senile dementia have a pathologic process that is characterized by unexplained cellular deterioration and primary degeneration of brain cells. Degenerative joint disease is usually related to age and may be accelerated by unusual use or trauma, but remains primarily a degenerative process without specific vascular, metabolic, or inflammatory explanation.

It also should be clear that a particular disease may be caused or affected by a variety of pathophysiologic mechanisms. Peptic ulcer, for example, is a common disease with a multifactorial physiologic basis. The ulceration of the mucosal lining of the duodenum is caused by gastric acid, may occur in genetically predisposed people, and may be abetted by the toxic effect of drugs such as aspirin or corticosteroids which impair the protective barrier of the mucosa. There may be a secondary inflammation producing pain or obstruction, and the ulcer may erode a blood vessel producing bleeding. To say that any single pathophysiological process "causes" ulcers would be extremely misleading.

Once the initial pathophysiologic process has given rise to a particular disease entity, its clinical manifestations are then modified by a variety of host factors such as age, immunologic status, medication ingestion, concurrent disease, or psychological makeup. For example, in a healthy person with high tolerance for pain, a case of herpes zoster ("shingles") may be perceived as a minor discomfort, while in a person with a low threshold for pain, it may become a disabling illness for which professional attention and potent analgesics are required. Under the influence of a concurrent disease or the ingestion of drugs such as steroids which suppress the immunologic response, a usually nonpathogenic fungal infection may produce serious illness. A minor inflammation of the connective tissue such as cellulitis, for example, may become a serious life-threatening problem in a diabetic with impaired vascular, sensory, or immunologic status. In a genetically susceptible host, an infectious agent may precipitate an inflammatory response and antibody production leading to systemic lupus erythematosus, while in a genetically non-susceptible host it may not produce any effect at all.

Thus, there are a variety of pathophysiologic processes which can initiate disease, but the expression of the disease itself may be modified by a variety of factors in the host. Any review of a particular disease entity, therefore, should include consideration of both aspects, so that a complete understanding of the disease can be developed.

SYMPTOM PRODUCTION AND THE PATHOLOGIC PROCESS

A pathologic process may begin and exist silently for some time without any evidence of physiological alteration being present. Although the "disease" is present and active, it may be undiscovered for a considerable period of time. In many chronic disease situations, it is now well known that the disease condition may be present for considerable lengths of time before becoming detectable by current diagnostic procedures. Atherosclerosis, for example, has been detected in autopsy in healthy young 18-year-olds dying from accidental causes (11–13); many prostatic cancers are discovered at autopsy which were never known or recognized during life.

After a pathological process has been present for a time, it not only may begin to produce physiological alterations which can be discovered by appropriate diagnostic tests, but may also begin to produce clinical symptoms which are, for the first time, recognized by the patient or the physician. There can be a significant time lag, however, between the onset of physiological alteration and the production of symptoms just as there was between the onset of the pathological process and the physiological alteration. A pathological process may be present and discoverable by diagnostic tests long before it produces sufficient symptoms for a patient to feel its presence.

Atherosclerosis and atherosclerotic vascular disease illustrate very well this continuum of pathologic process, physiologic alteration, and symptom production, and are reviewed to provide further insight into the disease process.

Atherosclerosis is a pathologic process characterized by focal accumulation of lipids and complex carbohydrates, producing a secondary narrowing of the arteries. The process affects arterial vessels of the body in the cerebral, coronary, peripheral, and abdominal circulation and is now the leading cause of death in the United States.

As was mentioned previously, atherosclerosis without physiologic alteration has been documented to be present in 18-year-olds. At this stage, it is a subclinical or presymptomatic process and can only be identified by direct examination of the blood vessels.

Coronary artery disease is a specific manifestation of atherosclerosis in the arteries which provide blood to the muscle of the heart. As it becomes progressively more serious, it interferes with arterial capability for providing sufficient oxygen to meet the heart muscles' metabolic demands. As the reduction in oxygen supply worsens, ischemia of the heart muscle may occur. As it progresses still further, any increased demand on the cardiac muscle, as in any kind of exertion, may produce angina pectoris or chest pain, the cardinal symptom of coronary artery disease.

Long before the angina is present, coronary artery disease may be identified by an abnormal electrocardiogram (EKG). If an electrocardiogram with the patient at rest does not produce evidence of disease, frequently an electrocardiogram during carefully controlled exercise will yield the necessary evidence. In these cases, the coronary artery disease may not be sufficiently serious to produce EKG changes during normal demands on the heart, but the increased cardiac demands associated with exercise will produce the necessary diagnostic evidence.

None of this may yet evoke any symptoms in the patient, but eventually the patient may experience intermittent chest pain on exertion and seek medical care. At this time, the chances of obtaining an abnormal EKG and confirming the presence of coronary artery disease become much greater, but even at this stage a patient may have typical angina pain with an apparently normal EKG.

If the atherosclerosis continues, it may eventually completely occlude a coronary artery, causing the heart muscles supplied by the artery to die. This clinical event is known as myocardial infarction, commonly called a "heart attack," and is accompanied by prolonged chest pain, nausea, sweating, shortness of breath, and weakness. However, the arterial occlusion and subsequent tissue death may occur silently and without symptom and only be discovered by EKG at some later date.

Following the pathologic process a step further, loss of heart muscle function secondary to coronary artery disease may affect the heart's ability to maintain adequate circulation to the rest of the body and may produce a range of secondary signs and symptoms in other organs of the body. As the heart becomes weaker, there may be progressive difficulty breathing, swelling of the legs and feet, inability to maintain blood supply to the brain and subsequent faintness, and impairment of kidney function and reduction of urinary output. These events are sometimes described by the single clinical description of "heart failure."

Since atherosclerosis is usually a generalized disease and not just limited to the coronary arteries, as this process is taking place in the heart a similar series of events may be occurring in the blood vessels of the other organs. This may produce primary effects in a wide-ranging assortment of organs throughout the body that are not related in any way to the secondary effects of heart failure as described above. Abdominal pain, bowel necrosis, neurological deficits, strokes, renal failure, calf pain, or aortic aneurysms all may be produced by the damage to the arteries of the various organs. The combination of this primary damage to the organs themselves and the secondary effects of heart failure are complicated and serious, and strikingly illustrate why atherosclerosis is such a major cause of morbidity and mortality.

THE PHYSIOLOGICAL BASES OF CHANGING DISEASE PATTERNS

Over the years, the pattern of diseases affecting the people of this country has changed profoundly, generally as a result of changes in the environment, in the population's demographic composition, and in medical practice. Infectious diseases have been replaced as the major cause of mortality by those chronic diseases associated with aging. At the turn of the century, these diseases struck the young and healthy, and moved with rapidity, often resulting in death. The confluence of improved sanitation, a higher standard of living, antibiotics, and vaccines reduced death and disability from infectious diseases so markedly that they are now a comparatively minor cause of death as discussed in Chapter 1.

The treatability of syphilis, for example, has reduced its incidence and impact markedly, and it is now increasingly rare for physicians to have to treat cases with the secondary or tertiary manifestations of this potentially devastating disorder. Smallpox, polio, mumps, diphtheria, measles, pertussis, rubella, tetanus, typhoid, and cholera, all once highly prevalent, have now all but disappeared. Bacterial infections of childhood and infantile diarrheas of all kinds are now effectively treated with antibiotics and intravenous feedings, and as a result do not present anything like the threat they did at the turn of the century.

While these disease entities have been diminishing or disappearing entirely, new disease patterns have been emerging to take their place as the most important threat to life and health. Some of these have been the result of the removal of the causes of death in early life (e.g., childhood infections) which has allowed time for the diseases of later life (e.g. atherosclerosis) to appear. Other disease patterns, however, are comparatively new, did not exist previously to the extent they exist today, and are the result of new forces in modern life and environment.

Changes in the incidence and prevalence of some cancers, for example, provide dramatic evidence of these patterns. In the early part of the century, cancer of the lung was not a major cause of death, but began to increase in men as the rate of cigarette smoking in men increased. The incidence of lung cancer in women lagged behind that of men until recent years when it began to rise to levels paralleling that of men, probably secondary to the increase in cigarette smoking among women.

In the same vein, there has been a rise in endometrial carcinoma in women, attributed at least in part to the increased use of estrogens by post-menopausal women (14). Pancreatic cancer has increased in recent years and is occurring in people at a younger age than previously, but no clear explanation of this changed disease pattern has been forthcoming. It may possibly be due to changes in dietary patterns in this country or to the increased ingestion of certain medications (10, 15). Again, recent years have seen a marked rise in mesothelioma, a previously rare type of lung cancer, probably secondary to the markedly increased use of asbestos in manufacturing and construction.

In the same fashion, improvement in our medical technology has changed the patterns of disease, not just by wiping out previously existing scourges, but also by creating new ones (See Chapter 8). The morbidity and mortality of common diseases such as pneumonia and wound infections have been replaced by serious infections with once non-pathogenic bacteria that are now resistant to antibiotics. Patients whose own defense mechanisms have been compromised by corticosteroids, immunosuppressive agents, and cancer chemotherapy are now susceptible to serious infections with fungi, yeast, protozoa, or bacteria which are not normally harmful (16).

A substantial percentage of hospitalizations now are attributable to drug toxicity and the secondary effects of new surgical procedures such as ileojejunal bypass for morbid obesity or the complications of kidney dialysis for chronic renal disease. Cardiac pacemakers prolong life but also produce a new spectrum of morbidity as do other new prosthetic devices such as cardiac valves, artificial joints, or silicone implants.

The increased effectiveness of medical intervention is also having a considerable effect on the patterns of disease by changing the gene pool controlling the incidence of certain diseases. Improvements in prenatal and high risk obstetrical care allow completion of pregnancies in diabetic women who otherwise may not have reproduced. This may increase the prevalence of an already common disease such as diabetes. The successful introduction of vigorous physical therapy and prophylactic antibiotic use have increased the survival of patients with cystic fibrosis and a few have successfully reproduced. The impact of the longer term survival on the gene pool for this disease remains to be seen, but is a good example of some of the potential hazards caused by new technology.

An additional powerful influence affecting our patterns of disease is environmental change. Vehicle accidents are an increasingly important cause of morbidity and mortality, and directly reflect our increasing use of the automobile for transportation. Pollution of air and water has already been suggested as at least partially causative in a number of conditions, and toxic aspects of industrial work environments have been suggested as the cause of many more. Indeed, it has been argued that as many as three-fourths of all cancers are at least in part environmentally determined, but this is still unproven.

Dietary habits have also been suggested as contributing to changes in disease patterns in recent years. The most obvious result of dietary change is obesity which is associated with hypertension, heart disease, and diabetes. Burkitt and associates have suggested that diverticulosis, hemorrhoids, appendicitis, and even cancer of the colon may be a consequence of changes in the amount of fiber in the Western diet (15). Epidemiologists have implicated the increased ingestion of certain foods as possibly causing increased atherosclerosis. Increased salt intake has already been indicted in certain aspects of hypertension and increased ingestion of refined sugars has definitely been associated with increased incidence of dental caries and possibly with several other conditions.

In summary, not only is there a wide variety of causes of disease in individuals and a wide variety of responses in individual hosts, the overall patterns of diseases in a society can change markedly over time as well. In this country, the pattern of disease has moved from one of acute infectious disease several generations ago to one of chronic disease today. Further, the pattern of disease has been influenced by our ability to wipe out certain diseases, thereby allowing others to express themselves. Finally, many aspects of modern life such as improved medical technology and environmental pollution, have caused new disease patterns which have never existed before.

SOCIAL AND CULTURAL INFLUENCES ON DISEASE AND BEHAVIOR

It has been estimated that 70 to 90% of all self-recognized illness is not generally treated within the conventional medical care delivery system (17). Conversely, it is reported that over half the visits to physicians are related to patient-identified problems for which no ascertainable biologic basis can be determined. It is clear from this that seeking medical care may or may not be associated with actual pathologic processes, and that social and cultural values greatly influence whether an attempt will be made to obtain professional care (18).

A large number of physician visits are for complaints in which the physiological function is well within normal limits, but for which the individual patient feels that some abnormality exists. Many people seek medical attention for constipation, for example, when bowel function is basically normal and no serious pathology can be documented. For some reason, either internally generated or imposed by the prevailing culture, these patients feel things are not quite right and they seek medical attention. They have somehow been led to expect bowel function which is different from that which they are experiencing, and a medical remedy is sought.

Symptoms of fatigue may be attributed to a "non" disease such as hypoglycemia by the patient (19). Conversely, a disease with a well-defined physiologic basis may not produce care seeking at all, since it may not be interpreted as a disease at all. The teenager with acne, for example, has a problem with a well-understood physiologic basis and an obvious clinical manifestation. The potential patient, however, may interpret it as a normal consequence of adolescence that will eventually resolve and for which treatment is either ineffective or unavailable (20). Seeking care for serious conditions is often delayed because of fear or uncertainty (21).

Disease and the perception of illness are not the only reasons people seek medical care. Normal physiologic processes frequently are the occasion for seeking care as well. Pregnancy or contraception are certainly not pathologic or "disease" processes, but they usually require professional attention of some sort. Heavy menstrual flow, missed or irregular periods, and menopause are usually the result of basically normal physiologic processes, and yet medical attention is frequently sought concerning them.

Indeed, in many cases, medical care is sought because the patient is healthy and wants to remain that way. Parents bring infants and small children to the pediatrician for routine evaluations, in order to ensure that the child is developing normally. Adults visit their physician periodically for an examination, a chest x-ray, a Papanicolaou smear, and possibly other tests because they have been told it is important to do so. Indeed, the entire pattern of care-seeking behavior is carried out in a framework that is intensely affected by current social, cultural, and political values, regardless of the type or severity of the pathologic process. Cultural influences frequently determine what society considers to be a medical problem, while economic or political realities determine whether medical care is sought or not.

As social and cultural values change, the understanding of what is "disease" and the subsequent care-seeking patterns may change as well (22, 23). The transference of marital adjustment and child rearing problems from the category of family problems best handled by a member of the clergy, to psychologic problems best handled by a physician or psychologist, is one example of this. The recent shift towards description of alcoholism as a disease requiring medical treatment is another. The equally recent court decision changing abortion from a criminal act to a recognized medical service is yet another. The numerous manifestations of psychological problems, discussed further in Chapter 7, represent many examples of difficult to define "illness" with a substantial political and value-laden component.

It should be noted in all of these examples that the underlying pathologic process has not changed at all; rather, it is the perception of these processes as "disease" or not which has been altered. In other circumstances, even our perception of certain conditions as illness doesn't change; instead, external social values change how we react to them.

For example, the increased mobility and weakened family structure of modern American life has made it more difficult to care for elderly and infirm family members at home. Smaller housing units, increased numbers of families in which both adults are employed, and a variety of other social pressures have altered the ability to handle the health problems of the elderly in the fashion of the past. Instead, society has created a new network of health institutions, nursing homes, to provide professional care for pathologic processes which previously were handled at home. The underlying pathologic processes have remained the same. It is the societal response to them that has changed.

THE INFLUENCE OF SUPPLY

Within the total spectrum of pathologic processes that affect the health of people in this country, it is important to note that some processes receive much more interest and attention from the health care system than others. It is also important to speculate about why this occurs.

The structure and availability of health services contributes significantly to the amount and nature of the care that will be sought. The patient makes the initial decision to seek professional attention, but once that decision has been made, much of the additional medical care is a derived demand, resulting directly from the decisions of the physician (24). The physician usually decides what laboratory tests, x-rays, treatment procedures, and hospitalizations are necessary, and in so doing, shapes a particular pattern of care for each patient. In some ways, these decisions on the part of the physician also shape the health care system itself by creating a demand for certain services. As long as the demand is there, the institutions, programs, and services will expand to fill the need.

But does the process work in that direction or is the reverse true? Do pathologic processes occur stimulating patients to seek care from physicians, who in turn generate a demand for certain services as a result of their decisions? Or, do the specialized services become available to physicians, thereby influencing the manner in which they approach disease, and do physicians then shape patients' perceptions and demands on the basis of what physicians know is available (25)? There is some evidence to suggest that the latter is true, at least in part, and is becoming progressively more important.

Physicians generally take the greater part of their training in hospitals and are introduced early to the use and benefits of sophisticated procedures and tests. The availability of these tests and treatments then influence the physicians' view of disease, since they now make possible the treatment of conditions that were previously beyond consideration. The surgical treatment of degenerative processes such as hip replacement for osteoarthritis, laser treatment for diabetic retinopathy, and replacement of diseased heart valves with prosthetic devices have all created many new options for the physician. They have also created many new reasons for patients to seek care.

Unfortunately, the development of these new approaches are not always in keeping with the real need for care among patients, as determined by the pathological processes which are actually damaging their lives. Just because a particular pathologic process such as arthritis or alcoholism, for example, has a major impact on the health of the public does not necessarily mean that sophisticated technology will then be developed to attack that problem. Instead, the more sophisticated technologies frequently develop in areas of lesser importance, leaving the more serious problems relatively less well-attended. Patients' perceptions of illness and importance are then shaped more by areas where major technology is available than by areas of perhaps greater need.

It is unclear whether the development of the pathologic processes or the availability of services to treat them creates the demand for health care. It is clear, however, that the utilization of services is the result of a unique interaction involving the pathologic processes themselves, the patient and the physician's perceptions of them, and the availability of services to care for them (26). Each element is important to consider if the utilization of health services is to be better understood by all concerned.

REFERENCES

1.   Apple D: How laymen define illness. *J Health Hum Behav* 1:219–225, 1960.
2.   Siperstein MD: The glucose tolerance test: a pitfall in the diagnosis of diabetes mellitus. *Adv Intern Med* 20:297–323, 1976.
3.   O'Sullivan JB, Mahan CM: Prospective study of 352 young patients with chemical diabetes. *N Engl J Med* 278:1038–1041, 1968.
4.   Mabry J: Lay concepts of etiology. *J Chronic Dis* 17:371–386, 1964.
5.   Lowenfels AB: Alcoholism and the risk of cancer. *Ann NY Acad Sci* 252:366–373, 1975.
6.   Merliss RR: Talc-treated rice and Japanese stomach cancer. *Science* 173:1141–1142, 1971
7.   Selikoff IJ, Churg J, Hammond EC: Asbestos exposure and neoplasia. *JAMA* 188:22–26, 1964.
8.   Poskanzer DC, Herbst AL: Epidemiology of vaginal adenosis and adenocarcinoma associated with exposure to stilbestrol in utero. *Cancer* (supplement) 39:1892–1895, 1977.
9.   Dungal N: The special problem of stomach cancer in Iceland with particular reference to dietary factors. *JAMA* 178:789–798, 1961.
10. Lowenfels AB, Anderson ME: Diet and cancer. *Cancer* (supplement) 39:1809–1814, 1977.
11. Enos WF, Beyer JC, Holmes RH: Pathogenesis of coronary disease in American soldiers killed in Korea. *JAMA* 158:912–194, 1958.
12. Enos WF, Holmes RH, Beyer JC: Coronary disease among United States soldiers killed in action in Korea. *JAMA* 152:1090–1093, 1953.
13. McNamara JJ, Molot MA, Stremple JF, et al: Coronary artery disease in combat casualties in Vietnam. *JAMA* 216:1185–1187, 1971.
14. Jick H, Watkins RN, Hunter JR, et al: Replacement estrogens and endometrial cancer. *N Engl J Med* 300:218–223, 1978.
15. Burkitt DP, Walker ARP, Painter NS: Dietary fiber and disease. *JAMA* 229:1068–1074, 197.
16. Schafner W: The ongoing problems of hospital infections. *Adv Intern Med* 21:175–187, 1977.
17. Dingle JH, Badger GF, Jordan WS: Illness in the home: a study of 25,000 illnesses in a group of Cleveland families. Cleveland: Western Reserve University, 1964.

18. Zola IK: Culture and symptoms: an analysis of patients' presenting complaints. *Am Sociol Rev.* 31:615–630, 1966.
19. Meador CK: Art and science of nondisease. *N Engl J Med* 272:92–95, 1965.
20. Ludwig EG, Gibson G: Self perception of sickness and the seeking of medical care. *J of Health and Soc Behav* 10:125–133, 1969.
21. Battistella RM: Factors associated with delay in the initiation of physicians care among late adulthood persons. *Am J of Public Health* 61:1348–1361, 1971.
22. Parsons T, Fox R: Illness therapy in the modern urban American family. *J of Soc Issues* 13:31–44, 1952.
23. Parsons T: Definitions of health and illness in the light of American values and social structure. In *Patients, Physicians and Illness.* Jaco EG, (ed): Free Press, Glenco, Illinois, 1958.
24. Fuchs V: *Who Shall Live.* Basic Books, New York, 1974.
25. Stoeckle JD, Zola IK, Davidson GE: On going to see the doctor, the contributions of the patient to the decision to seek medical aid: a selective review. *J Chronic Diseases* 16:975–989, 1963.
26. Rosenstock IM: Why people use health services. *Milbank Memorial Fund Quarterly* (Part 2), 44:94–127, 1966.

CHAPTER 3

Factors Associated with the Utilization of Health Services

Stephen M. Shortell

The biological and medical bases for health care needs were presented in Chapter 2. This chapter examines the translation of these needs into actual use of services. Overall trends and explanations of differences in utilization among various population groups are presented. Some of the implications of these trends and differences for health care professionals are also discussed. In addition, selected issues related to long-term care, self-care, primary and rural health care, child health, and mental health services utilization are described. Many of these issues are elaborated further in subsequent chapters of the book.

The ability to provide accessible and cost-effective health services to patients depends on a thorough understanding of those factors associated with the use of health services, and especially those factors which can be "manipulated" to improve the provision of care. The analysis of utilization patterns aids the understanding of such issues as the analysis of the distribution of health resources across the population to determine which groups have limited access to care, the relationship between utilization of services and health status, and the relationship between volume and patterns of use and strategies for controlling health care costs.

All health professionals need to understand health services utilization patterns. For health administrators, such information is essential for forecasting demand for care and planning services. Physicians, nurses, and other providers of care benefit from a knowledge of those utilization patterns which offer insight into such issues as delays in seeking or receiving care, comprehensiveness of services, continuity of care, and compliance with provider advice. Health planners use the data for many of the reasons identified above and are especially interested in the relationships among different types of utilization at an aggregate level (for example, in a county or geographic region). Health policy analysts require utilization data to examine the cost-effectiveness of alternative means of providing care. For example, for some individuals home care may be less expensive and just as effective as nursing home care. Policy analysts and researchers also require utilization data to analyze the potential impact of changes in national health policies related to such issues as financing and personnel. Finally, it is increasingly important for all health professionals to plan, provide, analyze, and evaluate services from an epidemiological perspective based on defined populations. Increased regulatory pressures and demands for greater public accountability underscore the importance of analyzing users and nonusers of services.

The next section presents analytical categories and descriptive trends pertaining to the use of personal health services. Subsequent sections discuss differences in utilization, important findings and practical implications from research studies, and the need for broader frameworks for analyzing utilization. The concluding sections highlight specific topics in health services utilization which are especially relevant to public policy.

ANALYTICAL CATEGORIES AND CONCEPTUAL DISTINCTIONS

There are many approaches to describing utilization of personal health services, but the three principal categories are the type and purpose of utilization, and the organizational setting in which care is provided. Principal types of utilization include hospital admissions, total hospital inpatient-days, physician and dental visits, admissions to long-term care facilities and total inpatient days in long-term care facilities. Utilization can also include visits to nurses, nurse practitioners, physician assistants, social workers, physical therapists, optometrists and any other type of health professional. Still other types of utilization include admissions to mental hospitals, outpatient visits to community mental health centers, drug prescriptions, and use of medical appliances. Each type of utilization can also be categorized by the purpose of the visit. Examples include preventive examinations, diagnosis, treatment, and rehabilitation.

Utilization can also be differentiated by the organizational setting in which it occurs. Examples include hospital inpatient units, outpatient departments and emergency rooms, physician offices, neighborhood health centers, nursing homes, and the patient's home.

For each of the above categories of utilization (type, purpose, and organizational setting), measures of contact and volume of services can be examined. Contact measures might include the percent of a population hospitalized in a specified year or the percent seeing a physician in a year. Volume measures might include the total number of hospital inpatient days in a specified time interval or the total number of physician visits in a year. Patterns of utilization can be described from the sequential flow of providers seen and resources used during an episode of illness. Continuity of care and other system characteristics can be determined from these patterns using various summary indexes (1, 2). The different categories for describing and analyzing health services utilization are summarized in Figure 3–1.

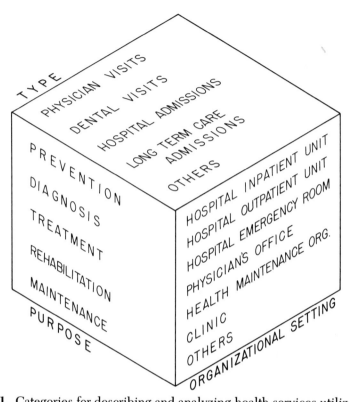

Figure 3–1. Categories for describing and analyzing health services utilization. Each of the above can be further characterized by measures of *contact* with the system, *volume* of services received, and the *pattern* or sequential flow of services received.

In analyzing utilization patterns, it is important to distinguish between the concepts of health needs and wants, and the demand for health services (3). A population's *need* for services may be determined by either normative medical judgments or individual perceived need. *Wants* refer to the quantity of health services which individuals feel they ought to consume, based on their own perceptions of their health needs. *Demand* is the quantity of health services which individuals wish to consume at specified prices, using available financial resources, and considering preferences for all other goods and services. *Utilization* is the actual quantity of services that is consumed when demand is translated into care-seeking behavior. Individuals' wants may be more or less than their needs or demands for care.

These distinctions are important because they underly notions of equity in, and relative "shortages" of, health services. Equity assumes that services are provided to meet everyone's needs for care, as determined by either professional medical judgment or the self-perceptions of patients. Failure to achieve equity may be the result of "shortages" in personnel, facilities, and other resources. However, this is a value judgment that does not conform to the economist's notion of "market shortage," which is defined as the excess of demand over supply at existing prices. Analysis of utilization and related data can reveal trends that influence public policy related to access, equity, and cost issues.

DESCRIPTIVE TRENDS

Using the framework in Figure 3–1, Tables 3–1 through 3–12 and Figures 3–2 through 3–5 indicate the major trends in health services utilization in the United States over the past 20 years. Some of the utilization data is based on national survey results from a variety of sources. Where available, for more detailed comparisons, the data are presented by age, sex, race, family size, income, education of household head, and residence.

Table 3–1 provides an overview of the utilization of selected health resources in the United States during the year 1976. Heavily utilized facilities include practitioners' offices, short-stay general hospitals, and nursing homes. These settings reflect the major organizational settings in which care is provided.

Table 3–2 and Figures 3–2 and 3–3 summarize changes over time in the percent

TABLE 3–1. Use of Health Care Resources: United States, 1976

Resource	Utilization of Resources		
	Units of Measure	Estimated Number	Estimated Number of Persons Served
Practitioners' offices	Visits	1,264,565,000	NA*
Hospital outpatient facilities	Visits	272,317,000	41,506,000
Freestanding clinics	Visits	58,553,000	13,199,000
Short-stay general hospitals	Discharges	35,919,600	22,445,300
	Days of care	290,090,800	NA
Short-stay specialty hospitals	Discharges	667,000	NA
	Days of care	7,738,600	458,100
Long-stay specialty hospitals	Discharges	592,600	829,100
	Days of care	143,856,500	NA
Nursing homes	Residents	1,286,200	2,412,900
	Days of care	405,332,000	NA
Mental health facilities other than hospitals	Residents	358,000	510,500
Home	Visits	181,079,000	37,054,000

*NA: Not available.

Source: U.S. Department of Health, Education, and Welfare: *Excerpts of Health Resources and Utilization Statistics, 1976.* Public Health Service, DHEW Publication No. (PHS) 79–1245, Hyattsville, Maryland, October, 1978.

TABLE 3–2. Estimated Percent of Population Seeing a Physician, by Sociodemographic Characteristics: United States, Selected Years

Sociodemographic Characteristic	Percent of Population Seeing a Physician			
	1958	1963	1970	1976
Sex				
Male	62	62	65	71
Female	70	68	71	80
Age				
1– 5	73	75	75	87
6–17	64	58	62	69
18–34	68	67	70	77
35–54	64	65	67	75
55–64	66	68	73	79
65 and over	68	68	76	79
Family income				
Low	NA*	56	65	73
Middle	NA	64	67	75
High	NA	71	71	79
Race				
White	NA	68	70	76
Non-white	NA	49	58	74
Education of head				
8 years or less	NA	56	62	NA
9–11 years	NA	63	66	NA
12 years	NA	69	69	NA
13 years or more	NA	76	76	NA
Residence				
SMSA, central city	NA	NA	65	79
SMSA, other urban	NA	66	72	78
Urban, non-SMSA	NA	NA	71	73
Rural, nonfarm	NA	57	68	75
Rural, farm	NA	NA	62	68
Total	66	65	68	76

*NA: Not available.

Sources: Reprinted with permission from Andersen R, Lion J, Anderson OW: *Two Decades of Health Services*. Cambridge, Massachusetts, Ballinger Publishing Company, copyright 1976, p. 44; and Aday L, Andersen R, Fleming GV: *Health Care in the United States: Equitable for Whom?* Sage Publications, Beverly Hills, California, 1980.

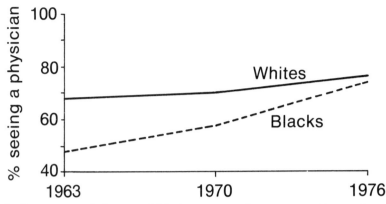

Figure 3–2. Percentage of whites and blacks seeing a physician in a 12-Month period. (*Source: America's Health System: A Portrait,* special report. The Robert Wood Johnson Foundation, No. 1, 1978, p. 7.)

of individuals seeing a physician during selected years. Overall, they indicate a steady increase in the percentage of the population seeing a physician over the past twenty years. Increases have been especially substantial for children (aged 1–5), for low income families, for non-whites and for people residing in standard metropolitan statistical areas (SMSA), and central cities. Figure 3–2 illustrates the closing of the gap between whites and blacks in the percentage of each population group seeing a physician in a 12-month-period. Figure 3–3 demonstrates the narrowing of the difference in the percentage seeing a physician annually for selected income groups. Although not shown, individuals in the age groups 1–17 and 65 and over, and those with low family incomes living in SMSA and central city areas, were less likely than other groups to have seen a physician during a given year. This was also true for individuals aged 1–17 with low family incomes in rural areas.

Differences in utilization are sometimes dependent on the type of care obtained. Figure 3–4 indicates that the ratio of preventive care visits to diagnosis and treatment

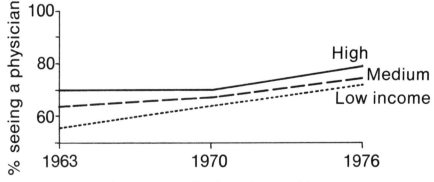

Figure 3–3. Estimated percentage of high, medium, and low income groups seeing a physician in a 12-Month period. (*Source: America's Health System: A Portrait,* special report. The Robert Wood Johnson Foundation No. 1, 1978, p. 8.)

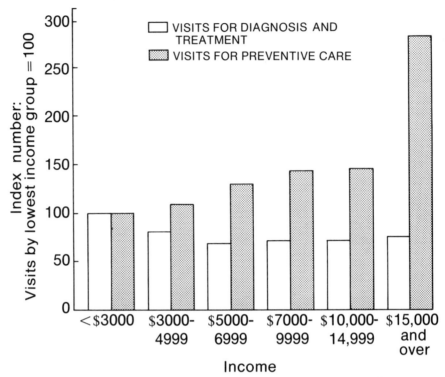

Figure 3–4. Relative number of physician visits per person per year by income and types of visits, United States, 1971. (*Source:* Reprinted from *Medical Care Chart Book,* ed. 6, Department of Medical Care Organization, School of Public Health, The University of Michigan, 1976.)

visits increased with family income in 1971. Differences were particularly significant for families with incomes of $15,000 and over. Similar differentials have continued throughout the 1970s.

There have also been substantial changes in the location of care over the years. During the period 1928–1931, 40% of all physician visits occurred in the home; by 1971 less than two percent of visits were in the home. During the same period, office visits increased from 50% to 70% of all visits (4). Approximately 43% of these visits were to general and family practitioners, although this increased to 65% in nonmetropolitan areas and decreased to 35% in metropolitan areas (5). In 1970, 14% of visits by the poor and 19% of visits by non-whites were to hospital outpatient departments, as compared to seven percent for the total population (6). Ambulatory care utilization is discussed further in Chapter 4.

Table 3–3 summarizes trends in physician visits per person. In 1963, those with high family incomes had more physician visits per person annually than those with low family incomes, but since 1970 the differential has reversed. In 1976 the low income group experienced 4.6, and the high income 3.8, physician visits per person annually. However, when considering "need" for medical services, as measured by the ratio of visits to days of disability, the poor have a lower ratio

TABLE 3–3. Estimated Mean Number of Physician Visits per Person-Year, by Sociodemographic Characteristics: United States, Selected Years

Sociodemographic Characteristic	Mean Number of Physician Visits			
	1958	1963	1970	1976
Sex				
Male	3.5	3.8	3.6	3.4
Female	5.3	5.0	4.5	4.6
Age				
0– 5	4.6	3.9	4.2	4.6
6–17	2.7	2.5	2.2	2.4
18–34	4.1	5.0	4.2	4.3
35–54	4.7	4.9	4.0	4.3
55–64	5.1	5.7	6.3	4.9
65 and over	7.4	6.8	6.4	6.0
Family income				
Low	NA*	4.4	4.9	4.6
Middle	NA	4.3	3.9	4.0
High	NA	4.6	3.6	3.8
Race				
White	NA	4.7	4.1	4.1
Non-white	NA	3.2	3.6	4.2
Education of head				
8 years or less	NA	3.9	4.2	NA
9–11 years	NA	4.7	3.6	NA
12 years	NA	4.7	3.6	NA
13 years or more	NA	5.3	4.5	NA
Residence				
SMSA, central city	NA	NA	4.2	4.6
SMSA, other urban	NA	4.6	4.2	4.1
Urban, non-SMSA	NA	NA	4.4	3.9
Rural, nonfarm	NA	4.4	3.7	3.8
Rural, farm	NA	3.6	3.4	2.7
Total	4.4	4.4	4.0	4.1

*NA: Not available.

Sources: Adapted and reprinted by permission from Andersen R, Lion J, Anderson OW: *Two Decades of Health Services.* Cambridge, Massachusetts, Ballinger Publishing Company, copyright 1976, p. 48; and Aday L, Andersen R, Fleming GV: *Health Care in the United States: Equitable for Whom?* Sage Publications, Beverly Hills, California, 1980.

than those with incomes above the poverty line (10.3 versus 16.4 visits per 100 disability days) (7). Table 3–3 also indicates that rural farm residents continue to experience a lower number of annual physician visits per person relative to other residential groups (2.7 versus 4.6 for those in the SMSA, central city area in 1976). However, by 1976 there was essentially no difference in the number of physician visits by race. When including only people who have experienced at least one visit, low income groups still have more visits per person than middle and high income groups (7.3 versus 5.7 and 5.1). However, among those who have made at least one visit, there is virtually no difference between whites and non-whites (5.8 versus 6.0) (8).

Tables 3–4 and 3–5 summarize ambulatory visits to selected outpatient facilities and to community mental health centers. The highest rate of visits to these institutional sources of care was in the health department clinics, schools, and insurance offices. Table 3–5 indicates that ambulatory visits to community mental health centers are age dependent but are almost identical for males and females. However, as discussed in Chapter 7, utilization data such as these are difficult to assess.

Tables 3–6 through 3–8 summarize the historical trends in hospital inpatient utilization. Table 3–6 reflects increasing hospital admission rates over time for the older age categories (55–64, and 65 and over) and higher admission rates for lower income families and for whites. Table 3–7 indicates generally declining lenths-of-stay for hospital admissions in the United States among those aged 0–53 and a slightly increased number of days per admission at ages 54 and above. More recent

TABLE 3–4. Number and Rate of Visits to Selected Freestanding Outpatient Facilities: United States, 1973–74

	Visits	
Type of Outpatient Facility	Number	Rate per 1,000 U.S. Population
Health department clinic, school, insurance office, etc.	47,079,000	228.8
Company or industry health unit	8,605,000	41.8
Family planning clinics	5,453,800	97.6
Community mental health centers	5,202,000	25.0
Freestanding psychiatric clinics	NA*	NA
Public Health Service clinics	694,100	NA

*NA: Not available.

Source: Adapted from Division of Health Interview Statistics, National Center for Health Statistics, unpublished data from the 1973 Health Interview Survey and related sources.

TABLE 3–5. Number and Rate of Outpatient Care Episodes for Community Mental Health Centers by Selected Patient Characteristics: United States, 1971

Characteristic	Patient Care Episodes	
	Number	Rate per 100,000 U.S. Population
Total	622,900	305.0
Age		
Under 18 years	194,900	280.3
18–24 years	92,600	384.5
25–44 years	221,800	463.9
45–64 years	95,400	225.3
65 years and over	18,200	88.8
Sex		
Male	299,000	303.5
Female	323,900	306.3
Diagnoses		
Mental retardation	23,600	11.6
Organic brain syndromes	12,900	6.3
Schizophrenia	62,900	30.8
Depressive disorders	80,100	39.2
Other psychoses	7,400	3.6
Alcohol and drug disorders	61,100	29.9
All other diagnoses, and undiagnosed	374,900	183.5

Source: National Institute of Mental Health: *Utilization of Mental Health Facilities, 1971.* Analytical and Special Study Reports. Series B., No. 5. DHEW Publication No. (NIH) 74–657. National Institutes of Health. Washington, D.C. U.S. Government Printing Office, 1973.

data are virtually identical to 1970. Although not shown, there is little variability in the mean number of in-hospital surgical procedures, except for those patients under age 6, for which the rate doubled between 1963 and 1970 (from 3 to 6 surgical procedures per 100-person years).

Table 3-8 summarizes the number and rate of patient care episodes in state and county mental hospitals during 1971. The rates increase linearly with age, are higher for males than for females, and are higher for schizophrenia and alcohol disorders than for any other diagnostic categories. The data are similar for private mental hospitals as well. These patterns are discussed further in Chapter 7.

The most prominent provider for long term care services is the nursing home. Admission rates to nursing homes increase with age, are higher for females than for males, and are higher for whites than for non-whites. The primary "diagnoses"

TABLE 3–6. Estimated Hospital Admissions by Sociodemographic Characteristics: United States, Selected Years

Sociodemographic Characteristic	Hospital Admissions per 100 Person-Years				
	1953	1958	1963	1970	1975*
Sex					
Male	9	9	10	11	13
Female	15	15	15	16	19
Age					
0– 5	8	10	8	11	NA†
6–17	8	6	6	6	NA
18–34	16	20	19	19	NA
35–54	12	11	14	12	NA
55–64	12	10	17	19	NA
65 and over	13	18	18	21	NA
Family income					
Under $2,000	12	14	16	19	NA
$2,000–3,499	12	12	12	15	NA
$3,500–4,999	12	14	12	17	NA
$5,000–7,499	12	12	14	16	NA
$7,500–9,999	⎰11	⎰10	14	16	NA
$10,000–12,499	⎱	⎱	11	12	NA
$12,500–14,999			⎰10	11	NA
$15,000 and over			⎱	9	NA
Race					
White	NA	NA	NA	15	NA
Non-white	NA	NA	NA	11	NA
Residence					
Large urban	10	11	10	12	NA
Other urban	11	14	13	14	NA
Rural, nonfarm	14	14	15	15	NA
Rural, farm	12	13	11	13	NA
Total	12	12	13	14	16

*Based on hospital records.

†NA: Not available.

Source: Adapted and reprinted with permission from Andersen R, Lion J, Anderson OW: *Two Decades of Health Services*. Cambridge, Massachusetts, Ballinger Publishing Company, copyright 1976, p. 51. 1974 data from Department of Health, Education, and Welfare: *Health—United States: 1978*. Washington, D.C., U.S. Government Printing Office, December 1978, p. 308.

TABLE 3–7. Estimated Mean Length of Stay and Hospital Days by Age and Sex: United States, Selected Years

Age and Sex	Mean Number of Days per Admission				Hospital Days per 100 Person-Years			
	1953	1963	1970	1975*	1953	1963	1970	1975*
Age								
0–17	5.3	4.9	4.2	NA†	41	30	32	NA
18–53	6.8	6.6	6.1	NA	96	108	94	NA
54 and over	11.9	11.9	12.3	NA	148	208	242	NA
Sex								
Male	8.3	8.0	8.1	8.2	71	83	83	110
Female	7.0	7.1	7.1	7.4	101	108	117	138
Total	7.4	7.4	7.5	7.7	87	96	100	125

*Based on hospital records.

†NA: Not available.

Source: Adapted and reprinted with permission from Andersen R, Lion J, Anderson OW: *Two Decades of Health Services.* Cambridge, Massachusetts, Ballinger Publishing Company, copyright 1976, p. 52. 1974 data from Department of Health, Education, and Welfare: *Health—United States: 1978.* Hyattsville, Maryland, U.S. Government Printing Office, 1978, p. 309.

include hardening of arteries, stroke, mental disorders, senility, and old age. These patterns are discussed in detail in Chapter 6.

Tables 3–9 and 3–10 summarize the historical trends in the use of selected preventive care services. Table 3–9 indicates that over half of the population had a physical exam in each of the years studied. The percentage is highest for children aged 1–5, due to well-child examinations, is higher for females than for males, is markedly lower for rural farm residents, and has increased markedly for low income families. Of course, these utilization data do not consider the efficacy of such examinations.

Table 3–10 indicates that the percentage of women having live births who initiated physician care during the first trimester of pregnancy increased overall from 65 to 83% between 1953 and 1970, with marked increases among low and middle income families and among people with lower levels of education. Although not shown, the median number of prenatal visits per pregnancy has increased from 8.4 in 1953 to 10.9 in 1970. This increase has been especially marked for low income families and for women with less education. These data suggest increased access to preventive and "elective" care.

Table 3–11 indicates the major historical trends in the estimated percentage of individuals visiting a dentist, using data for selected years. Overall, this percentage increased from 34% to 45% of the population between 1953 and 1970. The increase has been most marked among the very young, the very old, and those living in rural farm areas. The percentage seeing a dentist is positively related to family income. Figure 3–5 indicates that these income differences have not

TABLE 3–8. Number and Rate of Patient Care Episodes in State and County Mental Hospitals by Selected Patient Characteristics: United States, 1971

Characteristic	Patient Care Episodes	
	Number*	Rate per 100,000 Population†
Total	745,300	364.9
Age		
Under 18 years	39,200	56.4
18–24 years	97,300	404.0
25–44	236,300	494.2
45–64	238,700	563.7
65 years and over	133,700	652.6
Sex		
Male	411,900	418.1
Female	333,400	315.3
Diagnoses		
Mental retardation	40,200	19.7
Organic brain syndromes	104,000	50.9
Schizophrenia	283,500	138.8
Depressive disorders	65,400	32.0
Other psychoses	7,800	3.8
Alcohol disorders	125,000	61.2
Drug disorders	28,500	14.0
Other and undiagnosed	90,800	44.5

*Figures may not add to total due to rounding.

†Denominator for rates is civilian population, July 1, 1971.

Source: National Institute of Mental Health: *Utilization of Mental Health Facilities, 1971.* Analytical and Special Study Reports. Series B., No. 5 DHEW Pub. No. (NIH) 74–657. National Institute of Health, Washington, U.S. Government Printing Office, 1973.

narrowed over the years. Furthermore, within every age category people with high family incomes are more likely to see a dentist than lower income groups. Table 3–12 indicates that while there are race, income, and education differences in overall dental visits per-person-year, there are virtually no differences in total annual visits for those who visit a dentist at least once.

These descriptive data provide an overview of the utilization of health services in the United States. Over the years, a larger percentage of the population seems to have gained increased financial access to medical care, which appears to be associated with a significant narrowing of differences by income and race in the percentage seeing a physician annually. Significant improvements have also been achieved in the percentage of pregnant women seeing a physician in the first trimester, especially for low income women. There is considerable variability in

**TABLE 3–9. Estimated Percent of
Population with Physical Exam by Selected
Sociodemographic Characteristics: United
States, Selected Years**

Sociodemographic Characteristic	Percent with Exam within the Year		
	1963	1970	1976
Age			
1– 5 years	65	72	72
6–17	49	53	47
18–34	56	57	47
35–54	50	48	50
55–64	50	54	55
65 years or more	53	52	55
Sex			
Male	52	52	47
Female	54	57	56
Residence			
SMSA central city		57	55
SMSA other urban	56	56	53
Non-SMSA urban		53	50
Rural nonfarm	50	52	50
Rural farm	38	49	42
Family Income			
Low	45	51	50
Medium	51	54	52
High	59	57	54
Education of Head			
8 years or less	46	50	45
9–11	52	52	48
12	55	53	53
13 years or more	62	63	56
Total	53	55	52

Source: Aday L, Andersen R, Fleming G: *Health Care in
the United States: Equitable for Whom?* Sage
Publications, Beverly Hills, California, 1980.

the annual percentage of Americans visiting a dentist, which is positively associated
with income and education. But for those who make contact with a dentist, there
is little difference in the mean number of annual dental visits. The data also
indicate several groups in the population for whom utilization of, and probably
access to, health services is apparently a problem. These include children living in
central cities and rural areas; the rural farm population, regardless of age; and, for

TABLE 3–10. Estimated Percent of Women Having Live Births Seeing a Physician in the First Trimester of Pregnancy by Family Characteristics of Mother: United States, Selected Years

| Characteristic | Percent Seeing Physician by End of First Trimester | | | |
	1953	1958	1963	1970
Family Income				
Low	42	67	58	66
Middle	66	77	86	92
High	89	86	88	85
Education				
8 years or less	42	57	68	71
9–11 years	58	75	88	81
12 years	72	79	80	88
13 years or more	90	88	88	81
Race				
White	NA*	NA	NA	86
Non-white	NA	NA	NA	65
Residence				
SMSA, central city	NA	NA	NA	72
SMSA, other urban	NA	NA	NA	84
Urban, non-SMSA	NA	NA	NA	96
Rural, nonfarm	NA	NA	NA	90
Rural, farm	NA	NA	NA	NA
Total	65	77	80	83

*NA: Not Available.

Source: Adapted and reprinted by permission from Andersen R, Lion J, Anderson OW: *Two Decades of Health Services*, copyright 1976, Ballinger Publishing Company, Cambridge, Massachusetts, p. 57.

certain preventive services and dental care, non-white, low income, and less educated individuals.

ANALYTICAL MODELS AND KEY FINDINGS

The descriptive trends presented above provide necessary background information. But from policy, planning, and administrative perspectives, factors associated with the differences in utilization must be examined to facilitate the design of effective intervention strategies for improving the health services system. A number of different models have been developed for this purpose.

TABLE 3–11. Estimated Percent of Population Seeing a Dentist by Sociodemographic Characteristics: United States, Selected Years

Sociodemographic Characteristics	Percent Seeing a Dentist		
	1953	1963	1970
Sex			
Male	31	36	44
Female	36	40	46
Age			
1– 5	10	12	21
6–17	44	47	56
18–34	44	46	52
35–54	39	43	46
55–64	25	32	34
65 and over	13	19	26
Family Income			
Under $2,000	17	16	23
$2,000–3,499	23	} 25	23
$3,500–4,999	33		33
$5,000–7,499	} 44	} 40	35
$7,500–9,999			44
$10,000–12,499			51
$12,500–14,999	} 56	} 58	50
$15,000–17,499			53
$17,500 and over			67
Race			
White	NA*	43	47
Non-white	NA	20	24
Education of Head			
8 years or less	NA	25	27
8–11 years	NA	35	39
12 years	NA	48	49
13 years or more	NA	55	61
Residence			
SMSA, central city	NA		41
SMSA, other urban	NA	} 42	54
Urban, non-SMSA	NA		45
Rural, nonfarm	NA	37	41
Rural, farm	NA	27	40
Total	34	38	45

*NA: Not Available.

Source: Adapted and reprinted by permission from Andersen R, Lion J, Anderson OW: *Two Decades of Health Services,* copyright 1976, Ballinger Publishing Company, Cambridge, Massachusetts, p. 60.

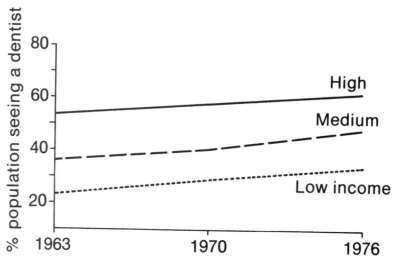

Figure 3–5. Percentage of high, medium, and low income groups seeing a dentist in a 12-Month period. (*Source: America's Health System: A Portrait*, special report. The Robert Wood Johnson Foundation. No. 1, 1978, p. 8.)

DESCRIPTION OF MODELS

Six distinctive types of models have been developed to explain differences in health services utilization (9). These models are typically described as: 1) demographic; 2) social structural; 3) social-psychological; 4) economic; 5) organizational; and 6) the systems model.

Demographic models of health services utilization primarily emphasize variables such as age, sex, marital status and family size. The rationale of the demographic approach is that such variables represent physiological states of individuals, and stages of the family life cycle, which might be associated with differences in health status and the use of health services. There has been relatively little research which relies solely on demographic variables to explain differences in health services utilization, although these variables have been used extensively in more comprehensive models.

The social-structural approach primarily emphasizes variables such as education, occupation, social class, and ethnicity. These factors reflect not only an individual's life style, which may predispose to certain types of health services utilization, but also reflect the general physical and social environment in which people live. For example, economists have suggested that education may affect the ability of individuals to combine their financial knowledge and other resources to more intelligently use health services and thus maximize their health status (10).

The social-psychological approach emphasizes the influence of values, attitudes, norms, and culture in explaining the utilization of health services. An example of the social-psychological approach is the "Health Belief Model" developed by Irving Rosenstock (11). The Health Belief Model suggests that four concepts influence

TABLE 3–12. Mean Number of Dentist Visits by Sociodemographic Characteristics: United States, 1970

Sociodemographic Characteristic	Visits per Person per Year	Visits per Person Seeing a Dentist at Least Once
Sex		
Male	1.3	3.0
Female	1.5	3.4
Age		
1– 5	0.5	2.2
6–17	1.7	3.1
18–34	1.6	3.2
35–54	1.6	3.5
55–64	1.1	3.4
65 and over	0.8	3.3
Race		
White	1.5	3.2
Non-white	0.8	3.5
Family Income		
Low	0.9	3.2
Middle	1.2	3.0
High	1.9	3.3
Education of head		
8 years or less	0.5	3.3
9–11 years	1.0	3.3
12 years	1.2	3.0
13 years or more	1.7	3.3
Residence		
SMSA, central city	1.4	3.4
SMSA, other urban	1.8	3.5
Urban, non-SMSA	1.3	3.0
Rural, nonfarm	1.1	2.8
Rural, farm	1.1	2.7
Total	1.4	3.2

Source: Adapted and reprinted by permission from Andersen R, Lion J, Anderson OW: *Two Decades of Health Services,* copyright 1976, Ballinger Publishing Company, Cambridge, Massachusetts, p. 62.

whether or not a person will seek preventive health care services: perceived susceptibility to the disease, perceived severity of the disease, the expected benefits of seeking care weighed against the costs involved, and a "cue," such as a media campaign, to trigger action. A number of small-scale studies have indicated support for some components of this model, and the model is discussed further in a later section of this chapter.

The economic approach considers the factors influencing an individual's demand for services as well as the supply of services. Demand factors include an individual's income and health insurance coverage. Supply factors include the number of health facilities, such as hospital beds, and providers, such as physicians or nurses, per population in a community. The economic approach argues that the interaction of the demand and supply factors determines the volume of services consumed.

The organizational approach is primarily based on factors that influence utilization once patients have gained entry into a health care system. Variables include the organization of physicians' practices, such as group practice versus solo practice, use of ancillary personnel, and professional referral patterns.

The systems approach argues that factors in all of the above models must be considered in explaining differences in health services utilization. The approach considers the nature of the "inputs" into providing medical care services, the transformation of these inputs into services to patients, and the resulting "outputs" or outcomes of the transformation process. While this approach is probably the most realistic, since it considers many of the complex interrelationships that shape health services utilization, systems models also present difficult measurement problems. However, a number of studies (12, 13, 14) are beginning to indicate the potential utility of the systems approach.

In each of these models, it is important to identify those variables which can be directly affected by planners, providers and administrators through health policy or direct intervention (Table 3–13). Variables in the demographic and social-structural models cannot be directly influenced. Rather, these factors represent target group variables that aid the identification of subgroups in the population that have limitations in access to health services. In contrast, variables in the economic and organizational approaches are more susceptible to changes in health policy and direct administrative intervention. Examples include changes in third party insurance coverage, changes in provider and facility ratios, and changes in the organization of services. Planners and policy analysts can influence the economic variables while providers and administrators are more likely to influence the organizational factors. The variables contained in the social-psychological approach represent an intermediate degree of intervention potential. Such factors as values, attitudes, norms, and culture cannot be changed in the short-term period but may be influenced eventually through health education and related efforts. The advantage of the systems approach is its consideration of the relationships among the many variables contained in the other approaches. It suggests the need for a more coordinated effort among policy makers, planners, providers, and administrators in the attempt to change the system.

The distinction between variables which are potentially susceptible to intervention and those that comprise target group variables is not intended to suggest that the latter are unimportant. Realistically, both types of variables must be considered in any interventions in a health services system and in local planning. It is the interaction of the target group variables and the other variables which will ultimately determine the success of specific programmatic efforts. For example, having a regular source of care may be more important for some age groups than for others. The distinction between "manipulable" variables and "target group" factors, as well as the relationship between them, needs to be considered in reviewing the empirical findings from the literature.

TABLE 3–13. Classification of Health Services Utilization Models by Degree to Which They Can Be Influenced by Changes in Public Policy or Administrative Intervention

Model	Variables	Subject to Direct Policy or Administrative Intervention	Useful in Identifying Groups in "Need"	Health Professionals Who Can Exert the Most Influence
Demographic	Age, sex, marital status, family size, residence	No	Yes	Not Relevant
Social Structure	Social class, ethnicity, education, occupation	No	Yes	Not Relevant
Social Psychological	Health beliefs, values, attitudes, norms, culture	No—Short run Possibly—long run	No	Health educators, Providers, Administrators
Economic	Family income, insurance coverage, price of services, provider/ population ratios, regular source of care	Yes	Yes	Planners, Policymakers
Organizational	Organization of practice, referral patterns, etc.	Yes	No	Providers, Administrators
Systems	Most of above considered as complex set of interrelationships	Yes	Yes	At the level of the overall system—planners and policymakers; At the level of individual organizations—providers and administrators

THE "BEHAVIORAL MODEL"—RESEARCH FINDINGS

One model which incorporates a number of the variables contained in the demographic, social-structural, economic, and social-psychological approaches was developed by Ronald Andersen and is known as the "behavioral model" of health services utilization (15). The model (Table 3–14) proposes three sets of factors which influence differences in initial contact with the health services system and in volume of utilization by those who achieve access: predisposing, enabling, and medical need variables. Predisposing variables include age, sex, marital status, family size, education, ethnicity, personal beliefs about the value of health services, and attitudes toward physicians. Enabling variables include family income, insurance coverage, the availability of a regular source of care, and facility and provider per capita ratios. Medical need variables include disability days, symptoms, perceived health status, and physician-evaluated severity of diagnosis and symptoms.

Some of the variation in utilization may be explained by such predisposing characteristics as age, sex, education levels, ethnicity, and personal beliefs about medical care. For example, age is highly correlated with levels of illness in the population. Variables such as ethnicity, education, and occupation suggest the possible importance of life-styles and the physical and social environments of individuals in relation to the use of health services. Personal beliefs about medical care, physicians, and disease can also influence care-seeking behavior. For example, people who believe strongly in the efficacy of health care treatment might be more likely to seek services sooner than those without such beliefs.

The predisposing variables alone are inadequate to explain differences in utilization. Individuals must also have the necessary means to seek and receive care. Thus, such demand factors as family income, level of health insurance coverage, and the availability of a regular souce of care, and supply factors such as the number of health facilities and professionals in the community, can be expected to influence utilization. Region of residence, particularly rural versus urban, may influence utilization as a result of the geographic distance to a source of care as well as local attitudes toward medical care.

The level of illness in the population, as perceived by consumers or as evaluated by physicians, is also an important correlate of utilization. Illness levels can be measured by the number of disability days or symptoms experienced by individuals, self-perceived health status, and ratings by physicians or other providers of the severity of reported conditions and symptoms in terms of the relative need for care.

In an equitable system of health care, the primary determinants of access, measured by initial contact and volume of services utilized, should be need for care and not factors such as income, health insurance coverage, education, and occupation. Thus, to the extent that differences in utilization are explained primarily by medical need variables and demographic correlates of need, the distribution of services would be relatively equitable. However, to the extent that enabling or predisposing variables explain differences in utilization, there would be some inequity in the use of health services.

Effect of Predisposing Variables.   Among the empirical tests of this model is a 1970 nationwide survey of 3,880 families comprising 11,882 individuals (16). Information was collected from household interviews, health providers and insurers, and employers. Age was significantly and positively related to length of hospital stay and to initial contact with, and number of visits to, a dentist, even adjusting for the other factors that were correlated with age. Age was not related to number of physician visits after adjusting for other age-related factors such as medical need. Sex had no impact on the rate of physician visits, hospital admissions, or dental visits. Individuals, especially children, in larger families had fewer physician visits than those in smaller families.

Race (white versus non-white) was significantly and positively related to number of physician and dental visits; non-whites had significantly lower utilization than whites even considering all other variables in the model. High income blacks were less likely to seek physician care for discretionary services (elective and preventive care) than high income whites. Furthermore, low income whites were even more likely than high income blacks to have seen a dentist during the survey year.

Personal beliefs about physicians and the efficacy of medical care were generally not related to health services utilization. However, beliefs explained more of the differences in use of dentists than any other variable, probably because dental care is highly discretionary. Among high income blacks, a favorable attitude toward health care was associated with increased discretionary dental care utilization. None of the other predisposing variables was consistently related to differences in utilization.

Effect of Enabling Variables.   A regular source of health care was positively related to having some contact with a physician, and, for individuals with major illness episodes (five or more annual visits or $100 or more in annual expenditures), a regular source of care was an important predictor of differences in the number of visits. Income, even independent of education, was an important variable in explaining differences in the rate of dental visits, but was not related to the frequency of physician visits or of hospital admissions. Although previous analyses in a 1963 study had indicated that income was an important determinant of the physician visit rate, the introduction of Medicare and Medicaid in 1966 and the expansion of major medical insurance coverage essentially eliminated these effects. Insurance coverage in 1971 was important only as a predictor of the number of physician visits for individuals with major illness episodes. As might be expected, people with comprehensive insurance coverage tended to be higher utilizers of physician and hospital services. Finally, the physician to population ratio in the community showed a positive correlation to number of physician visits.

Effect of Medical Need Variables.   The number of disability days and individual concern about health status were the best predictors of hospital care; severity of diagnosis was the best predictor of the physician visit rate. The number of dental symptoms was the best predictor of whether or not dental care was sought.

TABLE 3–14. Overview of the Behavioral Model of Health Services Utilization

Predisposing Component	Enabling Component	Medical Need Component	Types of Utilization to be Explained
A. Demographic	A. Family Resources and Related Factors	A. Perceived Illness	A. Hospital
			Contact
			Volume
Age	Family income	Disability days	B. Physician
Sex	Insurance	Symptoms	Contact
Marital status	Coverage	Perceived health	Volume
Family size	Group enrollment	Worry about health	C. Dentist
Birth order	Physician office	Pain frequency	Contact
Past hospitalizations	Coverage	Dental symptoms	Volume
Neighborhood tenure	Dental coverage		
	Regular source of care		
	Group practice		
	Appointment		
	Time		
	Travel time		
	Waiting time		

B. Social Structure

Education
Social class
Occupation
Ethnicity
Religion

C. Beliefs

Value of health
services
Value of physicians
Knowledge of disease
Response threshold

B. Community
Resources

Residence
Region
Physician to
population ratio
Hospital bed to
population ratio

B. Physician Evaluated

Diagnosis
Symptoms

Source: Adapted from Andersen R, Kravits J, Anderson OW: *Equity in Health Services: Empirical Analysis in Social Policy*, Ballinger Publishing Company, Cambridge, Massachusetts, copyright 1975, pp. 14,15.

The results of all aspects of the model indicate that measures of illness and demographic factors, such as age, are the primary predictors of hospital utilization, suggesting that these services are approximately equitably distributed among population groups. To an extent, physician services also appear to be somewhat equitably distributed since diagnostic severity is the principal predictor of differences in physician visits. However, other factors are also important, including the availability of a regular source of care, insurance coverage, and the number of providers in the community. In addition, some population groups, such as non-whites, used a lower number of services than other groups, controlling for the other variables in the model.

Dental care was more highly related to predisposing and enabling variables than hospital and physician services, and was less related to need. Dental care is poorly distributed among population groups. Whites who have a higher education, live in a higher social class, and enjoy a better than average income are more likely to obtain dental services than people in other social, economic or racial groups.

These results can be evaluated as to their potential for public policy or administrative intervention (Table 3–15). Of the 19 most important relationships, seven are related to predisposing variables which cannot be manipulated, five are related to enabling factors which can be manipulated, and the remaining seven concern medical need. The predisposing variables suggest target groups for which public policies might be developed. Among the enabling variable relationships, family income, insurance coverage, and physician to population ratios are of relevance to policy makers. The availability of a regular source of care can be affected by federal health personnel policies and by the actions of administrators and providers. It is also of interest to note that most of the significant relationships are related to volume of services, rather than to contact with providers, suggesting that somewhat more is known about total volume of use than about those factors associated with initial contact.

The findings outlined above are also supported by other studies. For example, a study of 2,168 households in five New York and Pennsylvania counties indicated that need for care, insurance coverage, age, and average cost of a visit strongly affected the volume of physician visits utilized (17). A recent analysis of national data by Berki and Kobashigawa suggests that medical need variables such as chronic disability days and education were positively, and family size was negatively, related to the volume of ambulatory visits utilized (18). Chronic disability also had indirect effects through its association with increased incidence of acute conditions. Another study of a rural area in Northern California found that health status and usual source of care measures were most strongly related to utilization (19). There was also a strong relationship between income and elective visits, including routine physical examinations.

Strong relationships between utilization and number of disability days, usual source of care, insurance coverage, and price for services have also been demonstrated by Bice and associates in their study of a low income population (20). The importance of insurance is especially evident from the effect of coinsurance or copayment by the patient, discussed further in Chapter 10. In a study by Scitovsky and Snyder, a 25% coinsurance rate resulted in a 24% decrease in the per capita number of physician visits (21). In another study, Richardson showed that utilization

TABLE 3–15. Summary of Strongest Predictors of Health Services Utilization Using the Behavioral Model

Variable	Directly Manipulable	Hospital Utilization		Physician Utilization		Dental Utilization	
		Contact	Volume	Contact	Volume	Contact	Volume
Predisposing							
Age	No		X*			X	X
Race	No						X
Beliefs	No (short run)						X
Family size	No				X		
Enabling							
Regular source of care	Yes			X	X		
Family income	Yes						X
Insurance coverage	Yes				X		
Physician to population ratio	Yes					X	
Medical need							
Disability days	No		X		X		
Worry about health	No (short run)		X		X		
Diagnostic severity	No					X	
Symptoms	No				X		X

*X = Strongest Predictors.

of services by a low income population was affected by race (less use by blacks), but there was a more moderate relationship between insurance coverage and physician visits (22). Other reviews of the literature generally support these research results (23).

THE "HEALTH BELIEF MODEL"—RESEARCH FINDINGS

The research described above does not deal in a central way with the role of health beliefs in explaining utilization of services. This section examines a widely used model which incorporates health belief concepts. First, however, it is important to differentiate health behavior, illness behavior, and sick role behavior.

Health behavior has been defined as "any activity undertaken by a person who believes himself (herself) to be healthy, for the purpose of preventing disease or detecting disease in an asymptomatic stage" (24). *Illness behavior* is "any activity undertaken by a person who feels ill, for the purpose of defining the state of his (her) health and of discovering a suitable remedy." In contrast, *sick role behavior* is "the activity undertaken by those who consider themselves ill, for the purpose of getting well." Examples of health behavior include visits to health care providers for which individuals do not perceive symptoms, but are seeking to prevent disease or to detect disease in the absence of symptoms (for example, general physical examinations). The concept could also be extended to include such health "promoting" activities as exercise, proper nutrition, and attention to hygiene. Illness behavior includes visits to health care providers for the purpose of defining the state of one's health in the presence of symptoms. Sick role behavior includes actions in response to the care-seeking process, such as compliance with medical regimens.

The Health Belief Model was originally developed to explain differences in health and illness behavior (25), but it has also been used to explain differences in sick role behavior, particularly in regard to patient compliance with medical advice. In addition to the previously noted concepts of perceived susceptibility, perceived severity, benefit versus cost of action, and a "cue," various demographic, socio-psychological, and structural variables have recently been incorporated into the model (Fig. 3–6).

Empirical investigations over the past twenty years have indicated consistent support for several of the variables contained in the model, but the associations with health services utilization have generally indicated that perceived susceptibility and perceived benefits are related to preventive health behavior, while the role of perceived severity has been less strongly supported (26). More recent studies have examined the relationship between the Health Belief Model and different kinds of preventive health behavior, while at the same time testing such "social network" variables as socio-economic status and frequency of interaction with friends. Results indicate that individuals who belong to a high socio-economic status group with frequent interaction among friends are more likely than other groups to follow preventive health behaviors such as seat belt use, exercise, and immunizations (27).

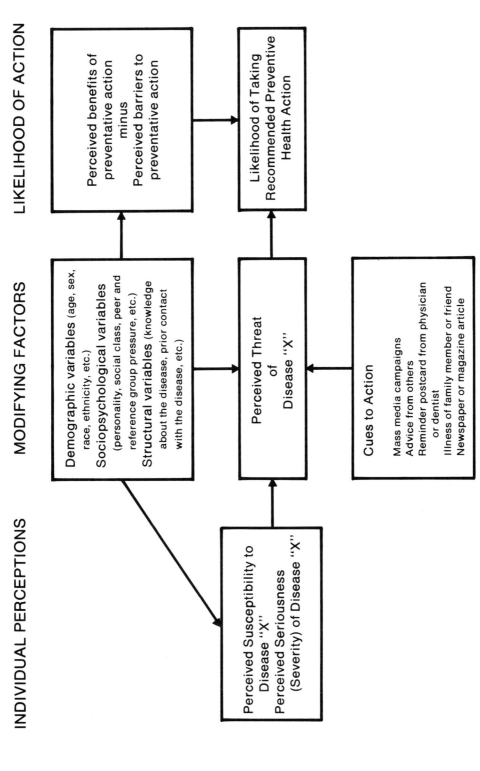

Figure 3–6. Expanded health belief model. (*Source:* Rosenstock IM: Historical origins of the health belief model. *Health Education Monographs* **2**:344, 1974. Adapted from Becker MH, et al: A new approach to explaining sick role behavior in low income populations. *American Journal of Public Health* **64**:205–216, 1974. Reprinted by permission.)

However, social network variables had little effect on other behaviors such as safe driving and avoidance of smoking.

In regard to illness behavior, such as physician visits, most of the studies indicate some relationship between perceived benefits and utilization (28). The evidence is somewhat less clear concerning the impact of perceived susceptibility. None of the results indicate that the combination of the variables in the model have an additional effect on explaining differences in utilization.

In regard to sick role behavior, and specifically with regard to adherence to medication taking, a number of studies have indicated positive relationships between perceived susceptibility, perceived severity, and perceived benefits and costs (29). Most of these associations are relatively weak, but they tend to be consistent across studies.

Other factors that have been found to be related to compliance or adherence with medical advice include the patterns of communication between providers and patients (30), continuity of physician care (31), and age (32). In general, existing evidence indicates no relationship between compliance and sex, intelligence, education, or marital status.

Since experimental studies utilizing the Health Belief Model variables are only beginning to be conducted, it is not possible to draw any inferences concerning the possible causal relationships involving these factors and actual health services utilization. Thus, while the current findings have little predictive value for health professionals, the relationships found thus far suggest approaches to influencing health care seeking behavior. Particularly relevant is the importance of demonstrating the possible benefits and costs of certain health behaviors, factors that are more easily affected by health professionals than are perceived susceptibility and perceived seriousness.

THE IMPACT OF ORGANIZATIONALLY RELATED VARIABLES

Most of the utilization literature ignores the impact of different forms of organization on the volume of services and the patterns of use. Recent studies, however, have begun to examine these issues, especially by comparing prepaid group practices with other organizational forms. These results are important because many of these organization factors can be influenced by managers, planners, policymakers and providers.

A number of studies have indicated that enrollees in prepaid plans have significantly lower hospital utilization than people receiving care under fee-for-service arrangements (33, 34, 35), as discussed further in Chapters 4 and 10. However, differences in benefit packages, consumer characteristics, and financial arrangements for paying for care have limited many analyses. For example, most studies of ambulatory care utilization have not simultaneously considered differences in enrollee characteristics, benefit packages, and financing mechanisms. Results have not conclusively demonstrated that any one organizational arrangement, such as prepaid practice, is associated with lower use (36, 37, 38, 39, 40, 41).

A recent study in Seattle offered an unusual opportunity to examine differences in utilization between two systems for providing services for patients with comprehensive care at no cost to the enrollee and with geographic access to care (42). In this four year experiment involving over 8,500 people, low income residents of the Seattle Model City area had the choice of receiving care from a well-established, consumer-operated, prepaid group practice or from a plan comprising most independent office-based private practitioners in the community. Approximately one-third of the residents chose the group practice plan. The findings indicated that hospitalization was significantly lower among the group practice enrollees, as compared to those enrolled in the private practice plan (110 versus 140 admissions per 1,000 enrollees annually). These results confirm other research findings that utilization patterns can be affected by different organizational systems even when enrollee characteristics, benefit packages, financing arrangements, and geographic access are not factors.

In the Seattle study, there were also no significant differences in ambulatory care utilization, as measured by overall visit rates between the two systems of care. However, the number of visits per user was greater in the private practice plan, while the percentage of people having any contact with a provider was significantly higher in the group plan. Despite the absence of financial barriers, whites experienced more physician visits than blacks in both plans, especially among younger enrollees. Among enrollees in poorer health, those in the private practice plan had significantly more provider visits than those in the group plan, suggesting that in prepaid group practices economic barriers may be replaced by other barriers, such as long waiting times for an appointment. Interestingly, there was no relationship between enrollee perceived access to care and the volume of services utilized, although significant relationships did exist between perceived access and patient satisfaction, particularly in the group plan (13).

A study by Riedel and associates of the Federal Employees Health Benefits Program compared hospital and ambulatory care utilization for employees under a Blue Cross/Blue Shield insurance plan and a prepaid group practice plan (43). Substantial differences in hospital admission rates (121 versus 69 admissions annually per 1,000 memberships) remained even after correcting for demographic differences between the two groups. The Blue Cross/Blue Shield admission rate was also significantly higher in 39 of 46 diagnostic categories examined in detail.

Controlling for race, there was virtually no difference in ambulatory visits between the two plans (44). However, as in the Seattle study, the volume of visits for whites was higher under both plans than for blacks. Nearly all younger people in smaller families with high incomes had at least one annual visit. In large, low income families, only 14% of Blue Cross/Blue Shield and 44% of the group plan enrollees had at least one visit. Interestingly, among families with four or more persons, children and young teenagers used significantly more health services if only one parent was working full time. As in previous studies, the need for care explained most of the difference in physician visits. High users were more likely to be Jewish, white, female, in a family that was large or where adults have high levels of income and formal education, were knowledgeable about plan coverage, and believed in preventive care. They were also more likely to have a personal physician, be very young or very old, be separated, divorced, or widowed if an adult, and have been members of the plan for a long time. There was no evidence for any substitution of ambulatory care for inpatient services.

Another study, by Gaus and associates, compared utilization in ten Health Maintenance Organizations (HMO) and a fee-for-service plan for a Medicaid population (45). The only important difference between the plans was significantly lower hospital utilization in the HMOs that were organized as group practices; however, foundation model HMOs (discussed in Chapter 10) did not have lower utilization than the fee-for-service plans. These findings suggest that capitation payments to HMOs alone does not appear to be associated with changes in use. Rather, the organized, multi-specialty group practice arrangement with largely salaried group physicians may be a more significant factor.

Finally, a recent study of Medicare enrollees in several prepaid group practices and fee-for-service plans indicated that prepaid enrollees incurred higher physician services costs, including care provided by practitioners outside the plans, and lower costs for provider-initiated services, such as in-hospital care and extended care, but excluding home health care. Inpatient hospital services did not reduce the use of extended care or home care services. Group practices which were relatively small and hospital based appeared to provide care at the least cost among the plans studied (46).

All of these studies suggest that enrollees in prepaid group practices experience significantly lower hospital admission rates than people who receive care in fee-for-service and other settings. There is little evidence for the substitution of ambulatory care for inpatient care, although this issue has not been fully tested. Beyond the organizational factors, medical need is the most dominant factor in explaining differences in use of services, although socio-demographic characteristics, such as race and family size, also explain some percentage of the variation.

More research is needed on the relative performance of different organizational forms for providing care. The available results raise some interesting questions as to what organizational forms should be encouraged. What are the comparative advantages of independent fee-for-service practice plans, free standing groups, hospital sponsored groups, HMOs, and other organizational forms? Some of the answers to these and related questions will be forthcoming from research currently in progress, but others will become apparent only as further innovations are undertaken and evaluated.

CRITIQUE OF EXISTING MODELS OF HEALTH SERVICES UTILIZATION

Existing models of utilization have been useful for thinking about health services, and have suggested possible avenues for intervention in the health services system. But these models explain relatively little of the variation in use (generally 15–25%). The inability of the models to explain a greater amount of variation may be due to measurement error, specification error, and dependent variables which are too aggregate and too heterogeneous. For example, "race and ethnicity" may not allow for heterogeneity within ethnic subgroups (47); income may not represent social structure or purchasing power; poor health may lead to low income, as well as low income leading to poor health; and insurance variables may not adequately reflect the comprehensiveness of coverage. Traditional measures of utilization, such as hospital admissions and number of physician visits, may also be too heterogeneous or aggregate (48). For example, physician visits include prevention, diagnosis, treatment, and rehabilitation, may be initiated by the patient or another family member, and may be a first visit or a return visit.

Models of utilization need to be developed which use more refined variables and are specific to the different types of interaction that people experience in health services. One way of capturing such interactions is to analyze episodes of illness from symptom perception to subsequent care and outcomes. Models also need to be developed which consider other aspects of community and organizational environments related to health care behavior. A further understanding and modeling of decision processes related to care-seeking behavior and the use of resources would be valuable. Anthropological (49), socio-psychological, organizational, and decision-theory approaches can be developed to supplement current predisposing, enabling, and need factors related to health services utilization.

BROADER FRAMEWORKS FOR THE STUDY OF HEALTH SERVICES UTILIZATION

Health services utilization is of interest primarily in relation to issues of equity and access to care, and the relationships between utilization and costs of care and health status. As a result, utilization must be analyzed within a broader context which includes not only patient and provider characteristics, but also the issues of access, costs, continuity, quality, and outcomes of care. There have been few efforts thus far to develop models of the health services system which examine the interrelationships among these factors. This would involve examining relationships among socio-psychological (patient's beliefs, perceptions, and attitudes toward care), structural (types of providers and organizational characteristics), and behavioral (utilization of services and technical quality of care) variables.

An example of a more complete model of utilization is presented in Figure 3–7 (13). In this model, patient and provider characteristics are considered as exogenous (predetermined by external factors not included in the model), while the remaining variables are considered endogenous (determined by the other variables in the model). The model includes structural variables (patient and provider characteristics), process variables (access to care, utilization of services, continuity of care, and physician performance), and outcome variables (costs, technical quality of care, and patient satisfaction). Arrows indicate those variables hypothesized to affect other variables. For example, costs are directly affected by patient characteristics, provider characteristics, utilization of services, and continuity of care; but there is no assumed direct effect of perceived access on costs because this relationship is predicted to be indirect through the utilization of services. Access to care is determined by patient and provider characteristics, and all three in turn determine utilization of services. For example, older patients should have more visits because they are sicker, regardless of the degree of access to care. In

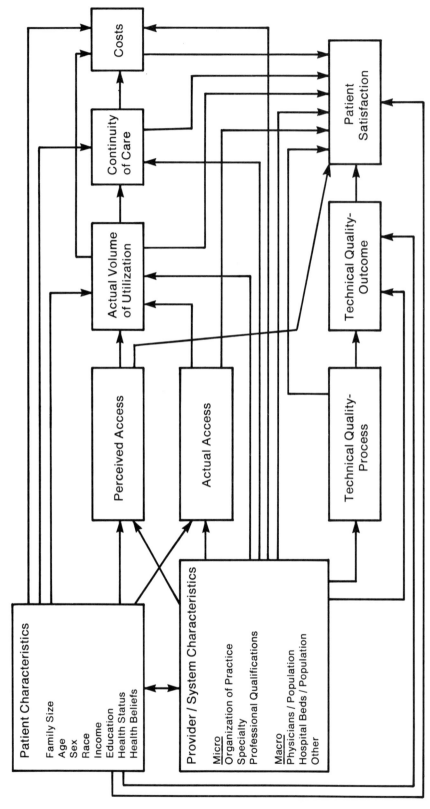

Figure 3–7. Causal model of dimensions of health services provision. (*Source:* Expanded from Shortell SM, Richardson WC, LoGerfo JP, et al: The relationships among dimensions of health services in two provider systems: a causal model approach. *Journal of Health and Social Behavior* **18:**139–159, 1977. Reprinted by permission.)

this model, perceived access refers to the patient's perception of the ease with which services can be obtained when needed while actual access refers to organizational, financial, and geographic realities facing the patient in seeking care.

Continuity of care is an intermediate outcome of utilization and is affected by patient and provider characteristics. Costs depend on continuity (poor continuity contributes to higher costs), utilization, and patient and provider characteristics. Technical quality (provider skill) is determined by the provider's characteristics, while technical outcome of care depends in turn on technical quality, provider characteristics, and, in some instances, the patient's initial health status. Finally, patient satisfaction is determined by provider and patient characteristics, access to care, and the quality, costs, and continuity of care.

This model is intended only as an example of possible relationships between structural, process, and outcome variables and is not the only model which might be constructed. For example, an alternative model would be to suggest direct effects of utilization and continuity of care on the technical outcome of care, assuming that greater use of physician services corresponds to closer monitoring of the patient's condition and thus might result in an improved outcome. A single contact point for care might lead to improvement in coordination of services, adherence with medical regimen and, thus, better outcomes of care (31, 50, 51).

While the model in Figure 3–7 appears complex, it is actually oversimplified, and feedback loops should be drawn between some variables, reflecting the dynamic nature of human behavior. For example, patient satisfaction might change over time and would affect subsequent utilization and compliance behavior, which might in turn affect future outcomes of care. The development and testing of such non-recursive two-way causation models involving feedback loops represents an important avenue for future research.

A version of the model in Figure 3–7 has been tested on hypertension (13) and diabetes patients (14), and the results indicated modest support for several of the hypothesized relationships, especially between patient characteristics and satisfaction, perceived access and satisfaction, and provider characteristics and utilization of services. Alternative models need to be further tested to provide more systematic knowledge of the health services system. Such knowledge can provide a foundation for more realistic changes in public policy and administrative and provider practices.

SPECIAL ISSUES IN HEALTH SERVICES UTILIZATION

A number of special issues concerning the utilization of health services require further discussion. These are use by the elderly and by children, primary care services and self care, mental health services, and rural health care. Many of these topics are further elaborated in later chapters.

LONG TERM CARE

Utilization of health services among the elderly will continue to expand over the next 25 years as people live longer and as the number of older Americans increases. For example, life expectancy increased from 68.2 years to over 71 years between 1950 and 1975. By the year 2000, it is estimated that 20% of the population will be over 65 years of age (52), and individuals 75 years old and older (the "old-old," while those aged 65–75 are "young-old") will represent 45% of the elderly population (53). The elderly, particularly those 75 and over, suffer from more diseases, have higher rates of hospital admission and longer lengths-of-stay, and have per capita health expenditures which are three times higher than those of adults under age 65. Perhaps 15% of the elderly over age 65, and 30% over age 80, need treatment for some form of mental illness (54); and Medicare now pays less than half of the total health care costs for those over age 65.

As discussed in Chapter 6, a complex web of genetic, biomedical, mental, social, organizational, and financial issues are involved in providing services to the increasing number of elderly people. This interplay of forces requires that administrators, planners, policymakers and providers think across organizational and institutional lines, using a "systems" perspective. Those individuals who can play effective brokerage and coordinative roles will likely assume increased power and influence, as opposed to those who manage or plan for single institutions.

CHILD HEALTH CARE

Young children in low income families are less likely to have contact with a physician than those in higher income families, and they also use fewer services. Non-white children, regardless of family income, have fewer physician visits than white children. These utilization data suggest target groups in particular need of services and illustrate the value of health services utilization data for assessing patterns of care.

There are other potentially alarming data. In 1971, an estimated 28% of the child population under age 16 (60,000,000 children) had no contact with the health services system (55). Children in families with incomes of less than $6,000 were nearly eight times as likely to be without a regular source of care as those in families with incomes above $11,000 (56). Furthermore, only 44% of children in these lower income families reported a physician as a regular source of care, as compared to 75% in higher income families; 15% of all child care, and 33% in poor urban areas, is obtained from hospital emergency rooms and outpatient departments.

As of 1974, 22% of children aged 6–12 had not seen a dentist in the previous two years. For children in families earning less than $7,000, 21% had never seen a dentist (57). When children reach shcool age, they have an average of three decayed teeth and about 50% of all school age children suffer from periodontal disease (58). In 1975, one-third of all children were not adequately immunized against polio, and nearly 40% were not vaccinated against rubella (59). Preventive medical care is also more likely to occur among children from wealthier families (60, 61).

The substantial variation in child health indicators in different areas of the country (62) suggests a need for more preventive and health promoting services, such as prenatal care and immunizations, particularly for the poor and for non-whites. Given past experience, however, it is unlikely that extending financial coverage alone will have much of an impact unless attention is also directed toward the design of effective health services systems.

There are also other related problems in health care for children that have received relatively little attention. These have been labeled the "new morbidity" (63) and include learning difficulties, behavioral disturbances, allergies, speech difficulties, child abuse, and societal adjustment problems. Although these problems may not constitute traditional illnesses and labeling them as such may increase the "medicalization" of social deviance, many parents and teachers seek solutions and help from the health services system, as discussed in Chapter 7. Since these problems encompass social and health services, the ability to manage and plan across institutional and organizational boundaries is essential.

EXPANSION OF PRIMARY CARE

Primary care includes first contact and continuous care for routine health needs. There has been renewed interest in primary care as a substitute for more expensive inpatient care, and as the most appropriate approach to meeting many health needs, especially in "underserved" areas where resources are scarce (64, 65, 66, 67). However, there is little evidence that the provision of a higher volume of ambulatory services substitutes for hospital inpatient care. Primary care also raises issues related to composition of providers, new role relationships involving nurse practitioners and physician assistants, inadequate third party coverage for ambulatory care, the need for different management and medical information systems from those that presently exist in hospitals, and the need to develop quality assurance systems. These and related issues are discussed in many of the chapters that follow.

SELF-CARE

Increasing costs, barriers to access, attention to consumer participation, increased interest in the nursing field to new approaches to patient care, interest in behavior modification, and other factors have resulted in a new "self-care" movement. Self-care is a "process whereby a lay person can function effectively on his (her) own behalf in health promotion and prevention, and in disease detection and treatment at the level of the primary health resource in the health care system" (68). The impact of self-care on health services utilization, costs, quality, and related issues is largely unknown. However, it is important for health professionals to anticipate the potential impact of this trend. For example, research on health beliefs suggests that interest in self-care may be highest among young educated whites and low among blacks, suggesting that health programs serving minority groups would find it difficult to "sell" a self-care program (69).

Increased emphasis on self-care may result in decreased health services utilization and costs. However, there is no evidence yet to support this possibility. Further, any decreased utilization would likely be in routine visits and not in expensive, high technology inpatient care.

Available evidence indicates that there is a definite trend, of unknown magnitude, in consumer health education toward self-diagnosis and self-care, with consumers increasingly assuming responsibility for tasks previously performed by health providers, including diagnosis, screening, and treatment (70). While it is difficult to predict the exact implications of this trend, a number of general issues can be suggested. First, to what degree can consumers be trained to diagnose and treat themselves, versus acquiring enough knowledge and judgment to recognize when they need to contact health care providers? Second, what is the utility of consumer algorithms (diagrams that aid consumer decision making)? Third, if higher income, better educated groups are more likely to adopt self-care, what is the potential for generalizing health education and self-care education strategies for other population groups that could also benefit from such knowledge? Fourth, to what degree can self-care be integrated into the existing health care delivery system? Finally, and perhaps most significantly, what impact will self-care have on the self image and professional identity of health care professionals themselves; that is, how will they adjust to a change in their role from "healer" to "educator"?

MENTAL HEALTH SERVICES

From 1955 to 1971, the number of individuals under treatment for mental illness in hospitals and outpatient psychiatric services in the United States more than doubled to 4,038,000 (71). Social problems related to drug addiction, alcoholism, and deaths from suicide and homicide are also rising. For example, the number of new narcotics addicts reported to the Drug Enforcement Administration by police authorities rose from 6,012 in 1965 to 24,692 in 1972 (72). Death rates from cirrhosis of the liver have increased from 9.2 to 15.7 per 100,000 population from 1950 to 1972 (73). The suicide rate was 10.2 deaths per 100,000 population in 1955, and it rose to 11.7 per 100,000 population in 1972. The suicide rate for white males aged 15–24 and that for non-whites doubled between 1950 and 1970. The suicide rate for females has risen somewhat since 1950, but it has remained far below that of males (74). There was an 84% increase in homicides between 1964 and 1973 (75).

These forms of "social deviance" are increasingly included under the umbrella of the "medical model." However, there is considerable uncertainty in both how to treat these forms of "deviance" and the potential outcomes of treatment. Experts disagree on the nature, character, nosology, and etiology of mental disorders and on the efficacy of various forms of intervention (76). In spite of these concerns, administrators and planners can expect increasing demands for care. Research suggests that users of mental health services also tend to be high users of other health services (77). This and the social nature of mental illness further emphasize the importance of a "systems" orientation which considers linkages to social agencies. The many complex issues involved in the provision of mental health services are discussed in Chapter 7.

RURAL HEALTH CARE

The deficiency of health resources in rural areas is widely known. For example, 25% of the nation's population resides in rural areas, but only 13% of the nation's physicians practice in rural areas. Rural areas also include a higher proportion of people living in poverty (21%—twice that in urban areas), a higher concentration of children and elderly people (nine dependents for every ten working-age adults, compared to seven in urban areas), and notable environmental and social health hazards, such as impure water supplies, inadequate sewage treatment, and considerable substandard housing (78).

Rural health care is complicated by Medicare reimbursement rates that are 30% lower than in urban areas; lack of payment for nonphysician services provided without the presence of a physician, which discourages the use of other types of practitioners; and noncoverage for preventive care, nutrition, and transportation services. As a result of these and other constraints, the average Medicaid expenditure in 1973 per poor child was $76 in metropolitan areas and only $5 in nonmetropolitan areas. The availability of services is further limited by restrictive income eligibility requirements in such rural states as Alabama, Arkansas, Louisiana, Mississippi and South Carolina, where only one of every 10 poor children is covered by Medicaid. In most states, Medicaid also fails to cover two-parent families and families with an employed head of household. As a result, less than one-half of the rural poor are eligible for Medicaid. A number of new programs, such as the National Health Service Corps, Health to Underserved Rural Areas, and Rural Health Initiative, as well as a number of foundation programs, have been established to attempt to deal with some of these issues.

AN ASSESSMENT OF UTILIZATION

This chapter has presented a descriptive and analytical approach to the determinants of health services utilization. The existing data suggest that there have been improvements in access to care which have resulted in increased utilization of services and higher total health care costs. Many of the improvements have been among low income and minority groups. However, some evidence indicates that when "medical need" is considered, the number of visits is less among lower income groups than among higher income groups. There are also differences in utilization among population groups, such that children aged 0–5 in low income families, rural residents, and blacks experience comparatively less utilization of medical and dental services than other groups. Other descriptive data on the utilization of services is available elsewhere (4, 5, 6, 23, 79, 80, 81, 82, 83).

Models that explain some of the differences in utilization and selected results from these models were presented. Generally, need for care is the best predictor of differences in utilization, although the availability of a regular source of care, insurance coverage, and socio-demographic characteristics such as age are also associated with various patterns of use. Some variables in the Health Belief Model, such as perceived susceptibility and concern about one's health, have been associated with certain forms of preventive health care utilization, particularly compliance with medical regimens. Studies of organizational influences on utilization indicate that enrollees in prepaid group practices consistently experience lower hospitalization rates than those in fee-for-service plans, possibly as a result of employing salaried physicians in the groups. Broader models which incorporate continuity of care, costs, quality, and patient satisfaction in an integrative and more comprehensive framework are needed.

Finally, a number of special issues related to use of services were discussed. These issues are of increasing concern to providers, planners, policymakers, and managers, and suggest the need for health professionals to think about systems of care and to provide linkages among primary, secondary, and tertiary levels of care, not only within the "health care" system, but within the larger human services system, as well. A number of the issues and challenges raised in this chapter are discussed further in the chapters which follow.

REFERENCES

1. Shortell SM: Continuity of medical care: conceptualization and measurement. *Medical Care* 14:377–391, 1976.
2. Bice TW, Boxerman SB: A quantitative measure of continuity of care. *Medical Care* 15:347–349, 1977.
3. Jeffers JR, Bognanno MF, Bartlett JC: On the demand versus need for medical services and the concept of "shortage." *American Journal of Public Health* 61:46–63, 1971.
4. Axelrod S, Donabedian A, Gentry DW: *Medical Care Chartbook.* 6th Edition, Ann Arbor, University of Michigan, School of Public Health, Department of Medical Care Organization, September, 1976.
5. U.S. Department of Health, Education, and Welfare: Provisional Data from the National Ambulatory Medical Care Survey. Division of Health Resources Utilization Statistics, National Center for Health Statistics, 1976.
6. Andersen R, Lion J, Anderson O: *Two Decades of Health Services.* Cambridge, Massachusetts, Ballinger Publishing Company, 1976, p. 47.
7. Aday L: Economic and noneconomic barriers to the use of needed medical services. *Medical Care* 13:447–456, 1975.
8. Andersen R, Lion J, Anderson O: *Two Decades of Health Services, op cit.,* p. 47.
9. Andersen R, Anderson OW: Trends in the use of health services. In Freeman HE, Levine S, Reeder LG, (eds): *Handbook of Medical Sociology.* Third ed., Englewood Cliffs, Prentice-Hall, 1979, p. 385.
10. Grossman M: *The Demand for Health: A Theoretical and Empirical Investigation.* National

Bureau of Economic Research Occasional Paper No. 119. New York, Columbia University Press, 1972.

11. Rosenstock I: Prevention of illness and maintenance of health. In Kosa J, Antonovsky A, Zola I, editors: *Poverty and Health: A Sociological Analysis.* Cambridge, Massachusetts, Harvard University Press, 1969, pp. 168–190.

12. Anderson JG: Causal model of a health service system. *Health Services Research* 7:23–42, 1972.

13. Shortell SM, Richardson WC, LoGerfo JP, *et al.:* The relationships among dimensions of health services in two provider systems: A causal model approach. *Journal of Health and Social Behavior* 18:139–159, 1977.

14. Williams S, Shortell SM, LoGerfo J, *et al.:* A causal model of health services for diabetic patients. Medical Care 16:313–326, 1978.

15. Andersen R: *Behavioral Model of Families' Use of Health Services,* Research Series 25. Chicago, Center for Health Administration Studies, University of Chicago, 1968.

16. Andersen R, Kravits J, Anderson OW: *Equity in Health Services: Empirical Analysis in Social Policy.* Cambridge, Ballinger Publishing Company, 1975.

17. Wan TH, Soifer SJ: Determinants of physician utilization: A causal analysis. *Journal of Health and Social Behavior* 15:100–108, 1974.

18. Berki SE, Kobashigawa B: Socioeconomic need determinants of ambulatory care use: Path analysis of the 1970 health interview survey data. *Medical Care* 14:405–421, 1976.

19. Hershey JC, Luft HS, Gianaris JM: Making sense out of utilization data. *Medical Care* 13:838–854, 1975.

20. Bice TW, Eichhorn RL, and Fox PD: Socio-economic status and use of physician services: A reconsideration. *Medical Care* 10:261–271, 1972.

21. Scitovsky AA, Snyder NM: Effect of co-insurance on use of physician services. *Social Security Bulletin* 35(6):3–19, 1972.

22. Richardson WC: Measuring the urban poor's use of physicians' services in response to illness episodes. *Medical Care* 8:132–142, 1970.

23. Aday L, Eichhorn R: *The Utilization of Health Services: Indices and Correlates.* Rockville, National Center for Health Services Research and Development, Publication No. (HSM) 73–3003, 1972.

24. Kasl SV, Cobb S: Health Behavior, illness behavior, and sick role behavior. *Archives of Environmental Health* (Part I) 12:246–266, 1966; (Part II) 12:534–541, 1966.

25. Rosenstock IM: Why people use health services. *Milbank Memorial Fund Quarterly* 44:94–127, 1966.

26. Rosenstock IM: The health belief model and preventive health behavior. *Health Education Monographs* 2:354–386, 1974.

27. Langlie JK: Social networks, health beliefs, and preventive health behavior. *Journal of Health and Social Behavior* 18:244–260, 1977.

28. Kirscht JP: The health belief model and illness behavior. *Health Education Monographs* 2:387–408, 1974.

29. Becker MH: The health belief model and sick role behavior. *Health Education Monographs* 2:409–432, 1974.

30. Svarstad B: Physician-patient communication and patient conformity with medical advice. In Mechanic D (ed): *The Growth of Bureaucratic Medicine.* New York, John Wiley and Sons, Inc., 1976, pp. 220–238.

31. Becker MH, Drachman RH, Kirscht JP: A field experiment to evaluate various outcomes of continuity of physician care. *American Journal of Public Health* 64:1062–1070, 1974.

32. Blackwell B: Drug therapy: Patient compliance. *New England Journal of Medicine* 289:249–252, 1973.

33. Donabedian A: An evaluation of prepaid group practice. *Inquiry* 6:3–27, 1969.
34. Klarman H: Economic research in group practice. In *New Horizons in Health Care,* Proceedings of First International Congress on Group Medicine, Winnipeg, 1970, pp. 178–193.
35. Roemer M, Shonick W: HMO performance: The recent evidence. *Milbank Memorial Fund Quarterly* 51:271–317, 1973.
36. Anderson OW, Sheatsley P: *Comprehensive Medical Insurance—A study of Cost, Use, and Attitudes Under Two Plans.* New York, Health Information Foundation, Research Series No. 9, 1959.
37. Hastings J, Mott FD, Barclay A, *et al.:* Prepaid group practice in Sault Ste. Marie, Ontario: Part I: Analysis of utilization records. *Medical Care* 11:91–103, 1973.
38. Hetherington RW, Hopkins C, Roemer M, *et al.: Health Insurance Plans: Promise and Performance.* New York, John Wiley and Sons, Inc., 1975.
39. Robertson RL: Comparative medical care use under prepaid group practice and free choice plans: A case study. *Inquiry* 9(3):70–76, 1972.
40. Shapiro S, Williams JJ, Yerby AS, *et al.:* Patterns of medical use by the indigent aged under two systems of medical care. *American Jouranl of Public Health* 57:784–790, 1967.
41. Williams J: *Family Medical Care Under Three Types of Health Insurance.* New York, Foundation on Employee Health, Medical Care, and Welfare, 1962.
42. Richardson W, Boscha M, Diehr P, *et al.: The Seattle Prepaid Health Care Project: Comparison of Health Services Delivery.* Seattle, University of Washington, 1976.
43. Riedel DC, Walden DC, Singsen AG, *et al.: Federal Employees Health Benefits Program: Utilization Study.* Rockville, National Center for Health Services Research, Health Resources Administration, U.S. Public Health Service, 1975.
44. Meyers SM, Hirshfeld SB, Walden DC, *et al.:* Ambulatory and medical use by federal employees: Experience of members in a service benefit plan and in a prepaid group practice plan. Paper presented at the 105th annual meeting of the American Public Health Association, Washington D.C., November 1, 1977.
45. Gaus CR, Cooper BS, Hirschman CG: Contrast in HMO and fee-for-service performance. *Social Security Bulletin* 3(5):3–14, 1976.
46. Weil PA: Comparative costs to the Medicare program of seven prepaid group practices and controls. *Milbank Memorial Fund Quarterly* 54:339–365, 1976.
47. Geertsen R, Kane RL, Klauber MR, *et al.:* A re-examination of Suchman's views on social factors in health care utilization. *Journal of Health and Social Behavior* 16:225–237, 1975.
48. Ware J: *A Cross-Sectional Study of Patient Perceptions in Use of Health Care Services.* Rand Paper P-5691, Rand Corporation, Santa Monica, 1977.
49. Chrisman N: The health seeking process: an approach to the natural history of illness. *Culture, Medicine, and Psychiatry* 1:351–377, 1977.
50. Becker MH, Drachman, RH, Kirscht, JP: Continuity of pediatrician: New support for an old shibboleth. *Journal of Pediatrics* 84:599–605, 1974.
51. Starfield B, Simborg DW, Horn SD, *et al.:* Continuity and coordination in primary care: Their achievement and utility. *Medical Care* 14:625–636, 1976.
52. Cambridge Research Institute: *Trends Affecting the U.S. Health Care System.* DHEW Publication No. (HRA) 76–14503, Washington, D.C., July, 1976.
53. Neugarten B: Age groups in American society and the rise of the young-old. In Eisele F, (ed): Political Consequences of Aging. *Annals of the American Academy of Political and Social Science* 415:187–198, 1970.
54. Butler, RN: Questions on health care for the aged. *Conditions for Change in the Health Care System.* Health Resources Administration, DHEW Publication No. (HRA) 78–642, Washington, D.C., September, 1977, pp. 98–106.

55. Lowe D, Alexander D: Health of poor children. In Schorr A, editor: *Children are Decent People.* New York, Basic Books, 1974, p. 81.

56. Butler JA, Baxter ED: Current structure of the health care delivery system for children, in Harvard Child Health Care Project, Vol. III. In *Developing a Better Health Care System for Children.* Cambridge, Ballinger Publishing Company, 1977, p. 42.

57. U.S. Department of Health, Education, and Welfare, National Center for Health Statistics: Unpublished Data from Health Interview Survey. Hyattsville, Maryland, 1974.

58. *Dentistry and National Health Programs.* American Dental Association, Chicago, 1971.

59. *Immunization Surveillance Report.* Center for Disease Control, Atlanta, 1977.

60. Richardson WC: Poverty, illness, and use of health services in the United States. *Hospitals* 43(13):34–40, 1969.

61. Richardson WC: Measuring the urban poor's use of physician services in response to illness episodes. *Medical Care* 8:132–142, 1970.

62. U.S. Department of Health, Education, and Welfare: Conditions of health and health care. In *Baselines for Setting Health Goals and Standards.* DHEW Publication No. (HRA) 77–640, U.S. Government Printing Office, Washington, D.C.

63. Haggerty R, Roghmann K, Pless J: *Child Health and the Community.* New York, John Wiley and Sons, Inc., 1975.

64. Ullman R, Kotok D, Tobin JR: Hospital-based group practice and comprehensive care for children of indigent families. *Pediatrics* 60:873–880, 1977.

65. Blendon RJ: The reform of ambulatory care: a financial paradox. *Medical Care* 14:526–534, 1976.

66. Kane RL: Primary care: contradictions and questions. *New England Journal of Medicine* 296:1410–1411, 1977.

67. Lewis CR, Fein R, Mechanic D: *A Right to Health: The Problem of Access to Primary Medical Care.* New York, John Wiley and Sons, Inc., 1976.

68. Levin L: The lay person as the primary health care practitioner. Paper adapted from an address to the *Patient Education Symposium,* sponsored by the Department of Social Perspectives in Medicine, University of Arizona, 1975.

69. Fleming GB, Andersen R: *Health Beliefs of the U.S. Population: Implications for Self-Care.* Perspectives Series A-11, Chicago, Center for Health Administration Studies, University of Chicago, 1975.

70. Green LW, Werlin SH, Schauffler HH, et al.: Research and demonstration issues in self-care: Measuring the decline of mediocentrism. *Health Education Monographs* 5(2):161–189, 1977.

71. U.S. Department of Commerce: *Statistical Abstract of the United States,* Table 128. Washington, D.C., U.S. Government Printing Office, 1974.

72. U.S. Department of Commerce: *Statistical Abstract of the United States,* Table 139. Washington, D.C., U.S. Government Printing Office, 1974.

73. U.S. Department of Commerce: *Statistical Abstract of the United States,* Tables 86 and 87. Washington, D.C., U.S. Government Printing Office, 1974.

74. U.S. Department of Commerce: *Statistical Abstract of the United States,* Tables 86 and 90. Washington, D.C., U.S. Government Printing Office, 1974.

75. Klebba AJ: Homicide trends in the U.S., 1900–1974. *Public Health Reports* 90:195–207, 1975.

76. Mechanic D: *Medical Sociology,* 2nd Edition. New York, The Free Press, 1978.

77. Williams SJ, Diehr P, Shortell SM, *et al.:* The relationship between utilization of mental health and somatic health services by low income enrollees in two provider plans. *Medical Care,* in press.

78. Davis K: Health Care Financing: A Rural Perspective. Paper presented at the American Public Health Association Meeting, New York, Fall, 1977.

79. U.S. Department of Health, Education, and Welfare: *The Nation's Use of Health Resources.* Public Health Service, Health Resources Administration, National Center for Health Statistics, Division of Health Resources Utilization Statistics, DHEW Publication No. (HRA) 77–1240, 1976.

80. U.S. Department of Health Education, and Welfare: *Health Interview Survey: United States—1975.* Vital and Health Statistics, Series 10, No. 115, Health Resources Administration, National Center for Health Statistics, Rockville, Maryland, March, 1977.

81. Robert Wood Johnson Foundation: America's health care system: A comprehensive portrait. *The Robert Wood Johnson Foundation Special Report,* No. 1, Princeton, New Jersey, 1978.

82. U.S. Department of Health, Education, and Welfare: *Health, United States, 1976–1977.* Public Health Service, Health Resources Administration, Hyattsville, Maryland, 1977.

83. U.S. Department of Health, Education, and Welfare: *Health, United States, 1978.* Public Health Service, Health Resources Administration, Hyattsville, Maryland, 1978.

Part Three
Providers of Health
Services

CHAPTER 4

Ambulatory and Community Health Services

Stephen J. Williams

Most of the contact that people have with the health services system occurs in practitioners' offices and hospital clinics. Although there are few systematic definitions of ambulatory care, it can be defined as that care provided outside of inpatient institutional settings. Since so many types of organizations, providers, and services are included in this category of health care, the broad designation of ambulatory and community health services is used here to denote care that involves the non-institutionalized patient. These services are the backbone of the health services system and are integral to providing effective and comprehensive care.

Table 4–1 reflects the diversity of services, providers, and facilities that are involved in ambulatory and community health services. Many of these services and organizations will be discussed in this chapter. Particular attention is directed toward rapidly expanding and innovative settings such as group practice. The huge range of ambulatory care services, however, precludes a detailed discussion of all providers.

DEFINITIONS OF AMBULATORY AND COMMUNITY HEALTH SERVICES

Ambulatory and community health services can be differentiated into a number of distinct categories. Primary prevention seeks to reduce the risks of illness or morbidity by removing disease-causing agents from our society. These activities include, for example, efforts to eliminate environmental pollutants which are suspected to cause diseases such as cancer and emphysema. Other examples of primary prevention include encouraging people to use seat belts, treatment of

TABLE 4–1. Providers of Ambulatory and Community Health Services[*]

Providers	Principal Practitioners	Services
Private office-based solo and group practice	Physicians, Dentists, Nurses, MEDEX, Therapists	Primary and secondary care
Hospital clinics	Physicians, Dentists, Nurses, MEDEX, Therapists	Primary and secondary care
Hospital emergency rooms	Physicians, Nurses	Primary and urgent care
Ambulatory surgery centers	Surgeons, Nurses, Anesthesiologists,	Surgical secondary care
Community-wide emergency medical systems	Technicians, Nurses, Drivers	Emergency transportation, communications, and immediate care
Poison control centers, community hotlines	Physicians, Technicians, Nurses	Emergency advice
Neighborhood health centers, migrant health centers	Physicians, Dentists, Nurses	Primary and secondary care
Community mental health centers	Psychologists, Social Workers	Mental health services
Free clinics	Physicians, Nurses	Primary care
Federal systems—Veterans Administration, Indian Health Service, Public Health Service, Military	All types	All types
Home health services	Nurses	Primary care
School health services	Nurses	Primary and preventive care
Prison health services	All types	Primary and secondary care
Public health services and clinics	Physicians, Nurses	Targeted programs (e.g., family planning, immunization), inspections, screening programs, health education)
Family planning and other specialized clinics (non-governmental)	Physicians, Nurses, Aides	Specialized services
Industrial clinics	Physicians, Nurses, Environmental Health Specialists	Preventive, primary, and emergency care
Pharmacies	Pharmacists	Drugs and health education
Optical shops	Optometrists, Opticians	Vision care
Medical laboratories	Technicians	Specialized laboratory services
Indigenous	Chiropractors, Medicine Men, Naturopaths	Primary and supportive care

[*]Partial list only.

94

water and sewage, and sanitation inspections in restaurants. Preventive health services are more direct interventions to detect and prevent disease. Examples of these services include hypertension, diabetes, and cancer screening clinics and immunization programs. The combination of primary prevention and preventive services is our first line of defense against disease (1).

Medical care that is oriented toward the daily, routine needs of patients, such as initial diagnosis and continuing treatment of common illnesses, is termed primary care (2). This care is not highly complex and generally does not require sophisticated technology and personnel. The vision of the general practitioner of bygone days traveling from house to house ministering to the sick is the traditional role of primary care, replaced in today's society by more skilled practitioners in fancier facilities.

In addition to providing services directly, the primary care professional should serve the role of patient advisor and advocate. In this coordinating role, the provider refers patients to sources of specialized care, advises regarding various diagnoses and therapies, and provides continuing care for chronic conditions.

The evolution of technology and medicine's increasing ability to intervene in illness has led to more specialization of medical services. These more specialized services are termed secondary and tertiary care and include both ambulatory and inpatient services. The content of secondary and tertiary care practices is usually more narrowly defined than is that of the primary care provider. Specialists also often require more complex equipment and more highly trained support personnel than do primary care providers.

There are no clear dividing lines between primary and secondary and secondary and tertiary care. Secondary services include routine hospitalization and specialized outpatient care such as some diagnostic testing and more complex therapies. Tertiary care includes the most complex services, such as open heart surgery, and usually is provided in inpatient sectors of hospitals. Most of the care discussed in this chapter involves primary care and those secondary services which can be provided in office-based practice, hospital outpatient departments, or community clinics.

The differences between the types of services provided within the ambulatory care sector are an important concern throughout this chapter since one objective of improving or rationalizing the health services system is to match the capabilities of providers with the needs of consumers. As different settings for providing ambulatory care are presented, consider the advantages and disadvantages of each to patient care needs and the optimal relationships that should be developed between the different levels of care.

CHAPTER ORGANIZATION

There are numerous typologies that could be used to present a discussion of ambulatory and community health services. Often these services are divided into the private and public sectors. Other common dichotomies include fee-for-service versus prepayment and solo versus group practice. This chapter is divided into sections on private and public services. Within private services, solo practice, group practice, and institutionally based settings are discussed. Within public services, governmental direct care programs and public health programs are discussed. Since the private and public sectors are not independent of each other, a matrix of relationships would be needed to identify the interrelationships between all providers of ambulatory and community health services. For example, private practitioners refer patients to public health programs for certain services and many public institutions are developing group practices that are similar to private practice groups. Trends in the use and funding of services in the private and public sectors are discussed in Chapters 3 and 10.

The concluding sections of the chapter discuss how ambulatory services can be organized. Characteristics of "systems for care" that are responsive to both consumer and provider needs are outlined based on our developing knowledge about the organization and management of ambulatory care services.

PRIVATE OFFICE-BASED PRACTICE: SOLO PRACTICE

Most ambulatory care services have traditionally been provided by physicians in solo office-based practice. Although solo practice still accounts for more health services than any other setting (Table 4–2), group practice and hospital-based

TABLE 4–2.   Estimated Distribution of Ambulatory Care Visits By Type of Service

Type of Service	Estimated Number and Percentage of Total Visits (Mid-1970s)	
	Number (Thousands)	Percentage
Private solo medical practice	545,000	49.5
Hospital outpatient departments	200,000	18.2
Private group practice	185,000	16.8
School health services	55,000	5.0
Industrial health units	40,000	3.6
Public health clinics	30,000	2.7
Special governmental programs (e.g., Neighborhood Health Centers)	25,000	2.3
Special voluntary agencies (e.g., Free Clinics)	20,000	1.8

Source: Roemer MI: From poor beginnings, the growth of primary care. *Hospitals* **49**:38–43, 1975.

services have expanded dramatically (3). Changing lifestyles, the cost of establishing a practice, external pressures on practitioners, and governmental programs have also adversely affected the traditional dominance of solo practice. But solo practice remains an important setting for ambulatory services and one that will continue to have a major role in the nation's health services system.

Solo practitioners are difficult to characterize for a number of reasons. First, there is little data available on the practice patterns and activities of solo practitioners. Although a few studies have been conducted, they tend to focus on specific questions such as referral patterns or quality of care and do not provide a comprehensive picture of what the solo practitioner does (4,5). The studies that do contribute to a more complete understanding of the activities of solo practitioners are based on physicians in one geographic area or a particular specialty and the results of these studies, while interesting and useful, may not be generalizable to other practices or areas. The second problem in attempting to characterize solo practitioners is their heterogeneity; solo practitioners include many types of health care professionals and they provide an immense array of services.

The available evidence indicates that physicians in private solo practice generally work hard although they earn less, on average, than their counterparts in group practice. Many solo practitioners are specialists who provide secondary care only, often on referral from primary care practitioners. These practitioners include, for example, allergists, dermatologists, and surgeons. Some specialists provide both primary and secondary care since they have insufficient work in their own specialty to achieve desired income levels. Many solo practitioners, including those trained in general and family practice, internal medicine, pediatrics, and obstetrics and gynecology, provide primary care services. There is some controversy and competition among practitioners concerning which specialists should be providing primary care. The emerging specialty of family practice, in particular, represents a challenge to the role of internal medicine in providing adult primary care and to pediatrics in child care (6).

Little detailed information exists on how the individual practitioner's time during the workday is allocated between various activities. Most solo practitioners perform a number of functions in the office including patient care, consultations, and administration and supervision. Exactly how much time each of these activities requires is difficult to assess, but the requirements for administration and the supervision of personnel have been increasing in recent years.

Solo practice is often associated with a greater feeling that the provider cares about the welfare of the patient, possibly resulting in a stronger patient-provider relationship, than other settings. There is some evidence that this effect, where it occurs, is a result of the lower level of bureaucracy or organizational complexity in solo practice (7). Since there is also some evidence that the relationship between the patient and physician is related to patient compliance with medical regimens, patients who perceive that they are receiving more personalized care may respond to the care process more positively (8). Solo practitioners are also not as restricted in referrals to specialists as are providers in some other settings, such as group practice, where organizational loyalties intervene. Finally, the solo practitioner may feel a greater identification with the community served since there is a more direct relationship between patient and provider.

From the provider's perspective, solo practice offers an opportunity to avoid organizational dependence and to be self-employed. Philosophically, solo practice is most closely aligned with the traditional economic orientations that have characterized medicine and there is also no need to share resources or income. On the other hand, all the increasingly complex problems of administering a practice must be dealt with unless a professional manager is hired. Thus, solo practice offers distinct opportunities and has philosophical and emotional appeal, but is far from devoid of problems and constraints.

OFFICE-BASED PRACTICE

Although there is little information available on the practice patterns of solo practitioners, an ongoing national study of all private office-based physicians, the National Ambulatory Medical Care Survey (NAMCS), has been initiated by the federal government. While many of the participants in the study are solo practitioners, the study reflects the nature of office-based practice for physicians in all settings.

The NAMCS involves a random selection of the nation's office based non-federal physicians who are asked to complete a data collection form for each patient treated during a one week interval (9). Table 4–3 lists the most common complaints or symptoms among the patients included in the study. Among the complaints in Table 4–3 are many that are not serious and for which relatively little but supportive care can be offered. These data are for both primary and secondary care. Other studies have indicated that the majority of visits to primary care practitioners are for non-urgent problems and often for social and emotional complaints. The most frequently assigned diagnoses for the NAMCS visits were medical examination, hypertension, prenatal care, upper respiratory infections, heart disease, neurosis, ear infections, and skin conditions. Very serious acute conditions often do not appear very high on such lists because of their relative rarity and the likelihood that the patient will seek care in an emergency room. Over eighteen percent of all visits for 1976 were for non-sickness, such as well-person examinations and immunizations. In 1977, less than twenty percent of the visits were classified as serious and only 2.0% resulted in hospitalization immediately following the visit (10) while 53.6% of the physician visits resulted in the prescription of a drug (Table 4–4). Counseling was moderately frequent (27.5% of visits). Diagnostic services included a limited history or examination in just over 56% of visits and a clinical laboratory test in 21.4% of visits. About 16.9% of the visits required five minutes or less of provider time and another 56.8% took from five to 15 minutes. At least 20.5% of visits required from 16 to 30 minutes and only 5.8% of visits lasted more than 30 minutes. Although more extensive analyses of these results will be required to expand our understanding of office-based patient care, the NAMCS aids our understanding of the nature of physician office visits by providing useful descriptive data.

TABLE 4–3. Number and Percent of Office Visits, by Most Common Complaints Or Symptoms, United States, 1976

Most Common Symptom or Complaint Expressed by Patient	Number of Office Visits in Thousands	Percent of Visits
1. Pain, swelling, injury—lower extremity	21,178	3.6
2. Pain, swelling, injury—back region	16,932	2.9
3. Sore throat	16,168	2.8
4. Pain, swelling, injury—upper extremity	15,902	2.7
5. Abdominal pain	14,590	2.5
6. Cough	13,099	2.2
7. Cold	10,844	1.8
8. Allergic skin reactions	10,679	1.8
9. Headache	9,908	1.7
10. Pain in chest	9,564	1.6
11. Fatigue	9,468	1.6
12. Pain, swelling, injury—face and neck	9,122	1.6
13. Vision dysfunction, except blindness	8,569	1.5
14. Fever	8,535	1.5
15. Wounds of the skin	8,492	1.4
16. Abnormally high blood pressure	7,518	1.3
17. Earache	7,487	1.3
18. Weight gain	6,956	1.2
19. Vertigo	6,703	1.1
20. Nasal congestion	6,488	1.1

Source: U.S. Department of Health, Education, and Welfare: 1976 Summary: National Ambulatory Medical Care Survey. Advance Data, Number 30, National Center for Health Statistics, July 13, 1978.

PRIVATE OFFICE-BASED PRACTICE: GROUP PRACTICE

Private office-based practice includes, in addition to solo practitioners, group practice. This form of practice has been growing in popularity in recent years, especially as the increasing pressures of practice have led many providers to seek alternative settings in which to work.

Group practice is an affiliation of providers, usually physicians, who share income, expenses, facilities, equipment, medical records, and support personnel in the provision of services through a formal, legally constituted, organization (11).

TABLE 4–4. Number and Percent of Office Visits, by Diagnostic and Therapeutic Services Provided, United States, 1977

Diagnostic and Therapeutic Services Provided	Number of Visits in Thousands	Percent of Visits
Diagnostic services:		
None	68,301	12.0
Limited history or examination	321,040	56.3
General history or examination	127,515	22.4
Clinical lab test	122,013	21.4
Pap Test	30,620	5.4
X-ray	44,662	7.8
Blood pressure check	193,889	34.0
Electrocardiogram	17,333	3.0
Vision test	23,045	4.0
Endoscopy	6,945	1.2
Other	25,010	4.4
Therapeutic services:		
None	109,077	19.1
Drug (prescription or non-prescription)	305,607	53.6
Immunization or desensitization	37,576	6.6
Office surgery	45,029	7.9
Physiotherapy	18,584	3.3
Medical counseling	117,157	20.6
Diet Counseling	39,197	6.9
Psychotherapy and therapeutic listening	30,589	5.4
Family planning	8,372	1.5
Other	15,624	2.7

Source: U.S. Department of Health, Education, and Welfare: 1976 Summary: National Ambulatory Medical Care Survey. Advance Data, Number 48, National Center for Health Statistics, April 13, 1979.

While definitions of a group practice vary somewhat, the essential elements are formal sharing of resources and distribution of income.

Traditionally, group practice has meant participation, and ownership, by physicians. In the future, however, as new and more diversified models for the provision of services are developed, other practitioners will participate in group practices. In some communities, for example, group practices of nurse-practitioners may be the only sources of health services. Dentists, optometrists, and other specialized personnel are also increasingly developing group practices.

HISTORY OF GROUP PRACTICE

Some of the earliest group practices in the United States were started by industries that needed to provide care to employees in rural sites where medical care was unobtainable. For example, the Northern Pacific Railroad organized a practice in 1883 to provide care to employees building the transcontinental railroad. This industrial clinic was one of a number of such clinics founded in the nineteenth century. Even more significant, however, was the establishment of the Mayo Clinic in Rochester, Minnesota, the first successful non-industrial group practice. The Mayo Clinic, originally organized as a single specialty group practice in 1887 and later broadened into a multispecialty group, demonstrated that group practice was feasible in the private sector. Mayo Clinic also represented a reputable model for group practice in a national atmosphere of fierce independence where group practice was viewed with skepticism and distrust. By the early 1930s there were about 150 medical groups throughout the country, with many located in the Midwest. Most included or were started by someone who had practiced or trained at the Mayo Clinic.

In 1932, a national committee established to assess medical care needs for the nation issued a report that suggested a major role for group practice in the provision of medical care. The committee recommended that these groups be associated with hospitals to provide comprehensive care and that there be prepayment for all services (12).

Other constituencies, including some unions, also developed group practices. After World War II, especially, a number of pioneering groups were established. In New York City, the Health Insurance Plan of New York was organized to provide prepaid medical care to the employees of the city, an idea promoted by Mayor Fiorello LaGuardia. In the West, the Kaiser Foundation Health Plans were established to provide health care to employees of Kaiser Industries; Kaiser is an affiliation of plans and providers that is now serving millions of Americans. In Seattle, a revolutionary development was the establishment of Group Health Cooperative of Puget Sound, a consumer-owned cooperative prepaid group practice, now providing comprehensive care to over 200,000 people, which was founded by progressive individuals who were dissatisfied with the private medical care available to them in the late 1940s. It is probably a measure of how far group practice has developed that many of these early groups are now huge organizations, viewed by some as establishment medicine but by others as still radical concepts.

Developments in medical practice also spurred on the group practice movement. Perhaps most notable was the increasing specialization of medicine and the rapid expansion of technology. This increasing sophistication meant that no individual practitioner could provide all the expertise that patients would require. It also meant that more complex, and expensive, facilities, equipment, and personnel were needed to care for patients. Group practice provided a formal structure for sharing these costs among providers. Many people felt that resources would be used more efficiently in groups. In addition, multi-specialty groups, encompassing more than one specialty, could provide patients with more of their health care under one roof and thus reduce problems of physical access to care.

Group practice was also thought to promote higher quality care since most of the different specialists that a person required would be practicing together, and would thus have the opportunity to discuss patient problems among themselves, share a common medical record, and be more able to assure the quality and continuity of care. Thus, group practice was seen by many as offering opportunities to the physician, such as easily developed referral arrangements, sharing of after-hours coverage, more flexibility in working hours, and less financial risk, while also benefiting the patient.

Opposition to group practice has been mostly for political and philosophical reasons. The American Medical Association and local medical societies have at times opposed group practice. Many early group practices had difficulties when physicians were denied privileges in local hospitals. There have been many legal constraints on group practice in medicine. Community-based specialists sometimes refused to treat patients referred by group physicians. Some people still believe that group practice is antithecal to capitalistic entrepreneurism. In more recent years, however, opposition to group practice has somewhat lessened and laws have been changed; where there is still strong opposition, fears of competition and socialized medicine are common. The federal government has also had a role in the development of group practice through reimbursement policy and the development of new programs in ambulatory care.

The most recent survey of group practice was conducted in 1975 (13). Almost 8,500 group practices were studied, incorporating many, but not all, of the medical groups in the country. Of the groups for which there were responses to the survey, fewer than twenty percent were more than sixteen years old. These groups employed over 66,500 of the approximately 300,000 physicians in patient care in the United States. About 4,600 of the groups were single specialty, 900 were general and family practice, and almost 3,000 were multispecialty. Multispecialty groups employed approximately 58 percent of all of the physicians in group practice. Most group practices, especially single specialty groups, included relatively few physicians as illustrated in Table 4–5. Very few groups were larger than fifteen physicians although in the aggregate these larger groups employed over forty percent of all group physicians. Although group practice was originally predominantly a midwest and western phenomenon, they are now found throughout the nation as Figure 4–1 demonstrates.

ORGANIZATION OF GROUP PRACTICES

There are many possible organizational affiliations for group practice. Some groups are independent or free-standing while others may be affiliated or owned by a hospital or health plan. Many hospitals have been developing affiliated group practices which may be hospital owned or under contract to provide specific services such as emergency, radiology, and pathology services. Some group practices are fee-for-service while others are associated with prepayment plans in which enrollees pay a predetermined monthly fee for all health care. Thus, the legal and organizational arrangements for the establishment of group practice are numerous and depend on group philosophies and objectives, and state and local regulations.

TABLE 4–5. Number and Percentage Distribution of Medical Practice Groups and Group Physicians, by Type of Group and Size, 1975

Type of Group	3–7	8–15	16–25	26–59	60–99	100+
			Number of groups			
All types	6,721	1,148	326	187	66	35
Single specialty	4,079	465	43	7	3	4
General/family practice	875	41	6	2	0	0
Multispecialty	1,785	642	277	178	63	31
			Percent of groups*			
All types	79.2	13.5	3.8	2.2	0.8	0.4
Single specialty	88.6	10.1	0.9	0.2	0.1	0.1
General/family practice	94.6	4.5	0.7	0.2	0.0	0.0
Multispecialty	60.0	21.6	9.3	6.0	2.1	1.0
			Number of physicians			
All types	28,398	11,828	6,363	6,463	4,364	9,428
Single specialty	6,918	4,554	807	206	156	931
General/family practice	3,364	385	113	97	0	0
Multispecialty	7,306	6,889	5,443	6,160	4,208	8,495
			Percent of physicians*			
All types	42.4	17.7	9.5	9.7	6.5	14.1
Single specialty	71.7	19.3	3.4	0.9	0.7	3.9
General/family practice	85.0	9.7	2.9	2.5	0.0	0.0
Multispecialty	20.5	17.5	13.8	15.7	10.7	21.6

*Some horizontal lines of percentages do not add to 100.0 because of rounding.

Source: Goodman L, Bennett E, Odem R: Current status of group medical practice in the United States. *Public Health Reports* 92:430–443, 1977.

A group practice can be legally organized as a sole proprietorship, in which one individual is the owner and all other providers are employees; as a partnership in which a group of individuals share ownership and liability; as a professional corporation in which stock is issued and the stockholders, who are usually the providers, own the corporation; or as one of a number of other legal forms including associations and foundations. Approximately 88 percent of all groups are partnerships and professional corporations. The tax and personal liability arrangements are most advantageous for corporations, especially in moderate and larger sized groups. There has been a dramatic shift to corporations from partnerships in

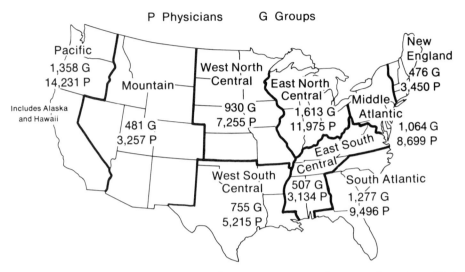

Figure 4–1. Geographic distribution of group practices and group physicians, United States, 1975. (*Source:* Goodman L, Bennett E, Odem R: Current status of group medical practice in the United States. *Public Health Reports* **92:**430–443, 1977. Reprinted by permission.)

recent years as most states have relaxed requirements for professionals to incorporate. In some instances, however, the group may not have a separate legal identity, but rather be within the structure of a larger organization such as a hospital.

The governance of the group practice depends on the legal form of organization. A corporation requires a board of directors. In many larger groups, an executive committee may be elected to conduct most of the administrative business of the group without requiring that all partners or members of the board be frequently convened. In many groups, committees composed of group members with specifically designated responsibilities are appointed or elected. Examples include the building committee to oversee new construction and a credentials committee to approve new members of the group. Larger groups often evolve into highly complex organizations.

The organizational structure of groups can vary tremendously. Larger groups are divided into departments, often based on clinical specialties. Many groups have professional managers with overall responsibility for the administration of the group and its facilities. Larger groups may have administrators for each department or may divide responsibilities along functional lines such as finance and patient care. In most groups, however, the professional manager only recommends major policy to the owners and thus does not have ultimate authority for all decision making.

Larger group practices will usually have a medical director. The medical director and the administrator share authority and responsibility to an extent that varies from group to group. However, unlike the dual lines of authority in community hospitals, the providers often own the group and are the ultimate authority to whom the administrator reports. The medical director is usually responsible for policies related to clinical services including quality of care, scope of services, and productivity of practitioners. The administrator is usually responsible for personnel practices involving most non-physician employees, patient flow and scheduling, financial management, and daily administrative matters.

AN ASSESSMENT OF GROUP PRACTICE

A critical assessment of group practice yields distinct advantages and disadvantages for both patients and providers as compared to other modalities for providing ambulatory services (14). Some of these are summarized in Table 4–6. Specific advantages and disadvantages vary from group to group and Table 4–6 is intended to list the major considerations generally associated with group practice. Some of the topics listed under the patient or provider perspectives could readily pertain to both.

The advantages of group practice from the perspective of the provider include shared operation of the practice, joint ownership of facilities and equipment, centralized administrative functions, and, in larger groups, a professional manager. The professional manager can provide expertise in areas often lacking among the providers such as billing, personnel management, patient scheduling, and supplies ordering.

Financially, the group relieves the provider from the heavy initial investment often required to establish a practice. However, in most groups, co-ownership requires that new members buy into the group through purchases of a share of the group's capital over a long period of time.

The burden of operating costs is also lessened for any individual member of a group. Rather than having to absorb the ups and downs of a practice alone, the sharing of income and expenses within the group allows for some fluctuations in individual practices. For example, a solo practitioner who becomes ill may have no practice income while a group member's income may continue during short periods of illness since other providers are generating revenue. However, the provisions of income distribution plans vary substantially between groups.

Patient care responsibilities are also shared in group practice. Sharing of patient care responsibilities results in more flexibility in working hours for the provider as well as more time for vacation and continuing education without sacrificing the quality of care for the patient. For example, providers cover for each other during vacations and after normal working hours. And although most practitioners in solo practice arrange for patient care coverage, the continuity of care and the extent of coverage is probably greater in group practice since the patient's medical records and the full resources of the group are always available even if a specific provider is not working.

Sharing of patient care has some other potential benefits. These include more peer interaction as a result of informal discussions and referral of patients between providers. The inclusion of more providers also results in the availability, by necessity, of a wider range of specialists and ancillary services, a convenience for both providers and patients and a source of added revenue for the group.

Do the sharing of administrative and patient care activities within group

TABLE 4–6. Some Advantages and Disadvantages of Group Practice*

Advantages	Disadvantages

A. From the Perspective of the Health Services Provider:

Advantages	Disadvantages
1. Availability of professional manager	1. Less individual freedom
2. Organizational responsibility for patient	2. May lead to excess use of specialists
3. Less physician administrative time	3. Fewer outside consultants
4. Shared capital expense	4. Possible reduced identity with patient and community
5. Shared financial risk	5. Group rather than individual decision making
6. Better coverage and shared on-call	6. Share all problems
7. More flexible working hours	7. Must work with others
8. More peer interaction	8. Less individual incentive and more security oriented
9. Increased access to specialists	9. Income limitations
10. Broader array of ancillary services	10. Income distribution arguments
11. Stable income for providers	
12. No direct financial concerns with patient	
13. Lower initial investment	
14. More time for continuing education	
15. More flexible vacation time	
16. Generally excellent benefits	
17. Possible efficiencies of scale	
18. Use of non-physician practitioners	

B. From the Perspective of the Group Practice Patient:

Advantages	Disadvantages
1. Care under one roof	1. Less freedom of choice of provider
2. Availability of specialists, lab, etc.	2. Possible lessening of provider-patient relationship
3. Improved coverage and emergency care	3. Possible overuse of ancillary services
4. Medical and administrative records centrally located	4. Possible high provider turnover
5. Referrals simplified	5. Heavy patient loads and waiting times may be increased
6. Peer interaction among providers	6. Less provider incentive for care
7. Better administration of group	7. More bureaucracy
8. Efficiency may be promoted in patient care	
9. Possibly better knowledge of medical care costs	

*Some advantages and disadvantages could be included under both provider and patient categories.

practice produce better care at lower cost? Although many people believed that group practice, through shared facilities, equipment, and personnel, and more effective management would use resources more efficiently than solo practice, the empirical evidence is mixed. The early evidence tended to refute these beliefs, but more recent research indicates some economies of scale, or efficiencies, attributable to the grouping of resources for smaller groups but not for larger and more bureaucratic groups (15). In addition, there is some question as to whether any savings that are achieved will be returned to consumers or represent higher income for providers. There may be other savings in the costs of providing services in group practice through bulk purchasing of supplies, centralized administrative functions, and more efficient patient care activities such as scheduling, but there is currently little empirical evidence to support these assertions.

The utilization of personnel may be more advantageous in group rather than solo practice. Receptionists, medical records specialists, laboratory and radiology technicians, nurses, and other types of personnel may be used more efficiently and in the specialized areas of their training in many medium and larger sized groups. There is some controversy over whether group practices utilize new health care professionals, such as nurse practitioners, more efficiently than solo practices. Empirical research has produced conflicting results although some evidence suggests that solo practitioners and smaller groups use these personnel more efficiently than larger groups (16). The efficient use of such personnel depends on provider practice patterns in each situation.

The effect of grouping on patient care, and especially on the quality of care, has rarely been investigated in the fee-for-service setting. Most studies examine prepaid group practices in which the incentives are substantially different since providers are paid a salary and consumers pay in advance for all care. Sharing of medical records, peer interaction, easy referrals and consultations with specialists, more sophisticated and accessible ancillary services, and more skilled and diversified support personnel are all arguments suggested in support of higher levels of the quality of care in group practice. Convincing comparative studies of quality of care in solo and group practice remain to be performed.

Group practice also offers advantages to patients and their communities. For the patient, the group offers a wide range of services under one roof so that travel between providers is reduced and access is increased. A unified medical record can contribute to continuity of care and less duplication in diagnosis and treatment. Some groups also own or operate hospitals and thus further extend the integration and scope of the services that they provide.

Group practices usually offer more accessible care after normal working hours. Some groups also offer emergency services through their own emergency room or clinic. Groups with a broader community perspective may even be involved in programs such as school health services and community immunization efforts.

The use of a professional manager should benefit the patient through more efficient scheduling and patient flow, and improved overall management of the practice. Billing is simplified since all care received can be included on one statement.

Whether group practice is, overall and on balance, more efficient than solo practice remains an unanswered question at the present time. Furthermore, issues of productivity and efficiency must be related to the quality of care and the contribution, if any, to the patient's health status.

On a community-wide basis, group practice may offer a means of attracting providers to areas with inadequate numbers of medical care personnel. By offering peer interaction, support services, and other advantages, groups may increase the appeal of practicing in rural areas or inadequately served urban centers (17).

There are also distinct disadvantages to group practice for providers, patients, and communities. From the perspective of the provider, practicing in a group implies less individual freedom with a variety of restrictions imposed through the sharing of a practice. Ideologically, the limitations of a group in this regard may be difficult for some people to accept since medicine has traditionally been an individualistic enterprise. In addition to reduced freedom, group practice means sharing responsibilities and problems with others. The interpersonal requirements for working out these responsibilities may not appeal to all practitioners. Older individuals who have been working in solo practice, especially, may be unlikely to readily adapt to group practice.

The financial advantages of group practice are a tradeoff against some imposed restrictions in income and the necessity of complying with the group's income distribution and practice pattern requirements. Thus, there often is more security and less risk, but also less incentive and reward for individual initiative and production.

The shift of some patient care responsibilities from the individual practitioner to the group also may adversely affect the patient-provider relationship by introducing a degree of impersonalization. If a group has high turnover, the patient may have to frequently change providers. Groups that have too few providers for the number of patients that they serve, common when excess capacity is being avoided, will also have waiting times for appointments and in the office which the patient may feel are excessive. The group may result in more restrictions on referral practices and limit the practitioner's willingness to utilize the expertise of other specialists in the community.

From a community-wide perspective, grouping may reduce the geographic dispersion of providers and thus increase difficulties of physical access to care. In addition, groups may reduce the competition of the health care marketplace by consolidating what would otherwise be "competing" providers.

Many of the hypothesized advantages of group practice remain to be empirically verified and there are some distinct disadvantages to both consumers and providers. However, group practice is an increasingly popular and, on balance, attractive modality for providing health services.

PREPAID GROUP PRACTICE AND HEALTH MAINTENANCE ORGANIZATIONS

Group practice that is reimbursed on a prepaid rather than fee-for-service basis is a widely publicized but as yet relatively unusual avenue for providing care. Under prepayment an enrollee pays a predetermined monthly fee which covers all health care subsequently needed, provided the services are included in the prepayment contract. Chapter 10 discusses this in further detail, but some discussion is appropriate in the context of group practice.

Prepayment within group practice alters the incentive system for the provider organization and for the professionals delivering care. Although most of these plans, such as the Kaiser Foundation Health Plan, incorporate many of the principles of group practice, physicians and other providers are on salary, sometimes supplemented by an incentive reimbursement program. Since the plan itself is reimbursed prospectively through a monthly fee for all health care provided, there is an incentive to avoid "unnecessary" utilization. This assures that the plan's prospective budget is not exceeded and that the plan can maintain its competitiveness in the health services marketplace.

Most prepayment plans have achieved lower costs for all care through rates of hospitalization that are lower than those in the fee-for-service sector. Ambulatory care use has generally been at least as high and often higher in prepaid plans as compared to fee-for-service insurance programs. The prepaid group practices attempt to ration the availability of both ambulatory and inpatient services through a number of mechanisms. Ambulatory visits initiated by the patient can be constrained by limiting the availability of care. This is achieved through longer waiting times for appointments than patients desire, for example, although the plan must do so in such a manner that only low priority care is discouraged while patients with more serious or urgent problems are assured access. Other use can be moderated by changing practice patterns to encourage outpatient care and by limiting the availability of inpatient beds. There is also little evidence that for any specific service, such as an office visit, prepaid groups can provide care at lower cost than fee-for-service groups or solo practitioners. Thus, their primary cost advantage is in reducing hospitalization rather than in achieving economies for individual services.

Prepaid group practices can assume many organizational forms. Figure 4–2 presents a simplified organizational structure of a typical health plan. The fundamental components include the plan itself, which administers the health program, recruits enrollees, and arranges all contractual relationships. The hospitals and the medical group practices are often organizationally separate from the plan administration and are the direct providers of all care. The medical groups are composed of physicians who contract with the plan to provide care and who use facilities administered by the plan. The hospitals may be owned by the plan but in many smaller prepaid groups, community hospitals are used through contractual arrangements.

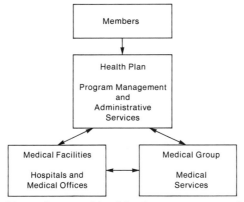

Figure 4–2. Typical prepaid health plan organizational relationships.

Another type of prepaid practice is the foundation plan in which community physicians remain in private practice using their own offices but contract individually with a central plan which, in turn, contracts with prepaid enrollees (18). The physicians in this situation are reimbursed by the plan on a fee-for-service basis. This arrangement provides for prepaid services to enrollee populations without requiring that physicians either practice together or be paid on a salaried basis. Foundation type plans were started as an alternative for preserving private fee-for-service practice within a prepayment framework. One of the earliest and best known foundations is the San Joaquin Foundation in California.

The Health Maintenance Organization (HMO) program was instituted in 1973 to promote prepayment plans and incorporates both the group practice and foundation models. The concept was originally proposed by President Richard M. Nixon, as a means of promoting private sector medicine through self regulation while at the same time incorporating some incentives for containment of health care costs (19). The HMO law provides grants and loans for the planning and establishment of HMOs and requires that certain services, including those listed in Table 4–7, be provided.

The HMO program and prepaid group practices have succeeded in providing comprehensive and acceptable quality health services at lower total costs than the fee-for-service sector (20). However, many HMOs have had difficulties attaining financial viability. This may be partially the result of program requirements which include offering a full range of services and having a period of open enrollment during which time anyone can join. Some provisions of the program, however, have helped developing HMOs. These include the dual choice requirement under which certain employers must offer the HMO as a health care option to employees in competition with other insurance plans. The most successful prepaid groups have generally been the larger plans or those serving populations with high levels of insurance coverage. Poor management and lack of commitment on the part of organizers and providers have been identified as major reasons for the failure of some HMOs (21).

TABLE 4–7. Health Services Required Under the Health Maintenance Organization Act of 1973*

Physician professional services
Outpatient services
Short-term mental health services
Short-term rehabilitative services
Certain services for substance abuse
Laboratory and radiology services
Home health services
Family planning services
Certain social services
Immunizations and preventive health services
Health education
Arrangements for emergency care
Arrangements for out-of-area coverage

*Exact services that must be provided depends on current legislation.

INSTITUTIONALLY BASED AMBULATORY SERVICES

In addition to solo and group practice in the private sector, many institutions are expanding their involvement in ambulatory care. These institutionally based settings, especially those associated with hospitals, are discussed next.

The hospital has evolved from an institution for poor people who could not be cared for at home to a provider of a full range of health services from primary to tertiary care. As technological advances have brought more services into the hospital and expanded the scope of care provided, the hospital has assumed an especially important role in the provision of highly complex health services. At the same time, more and more people have sought primary care from hospitals, sometimes due to a lack of access to other sources of care.

OUTPATIENT CLINICS

The increased demands placed on hospitals for care have taxed the abilities of many facilities to respond with appropriate and adequate resources. The result has sometimes been overcrowded facilities, the wrong mix of services, equipment, and personnel to respond to patient needs, and high levels of dissatisfaction on the part of consumers and providers. Some hospitals have successfully responded to these demands by expanding outpatient services and hiring full time providers to staff redesigned hospital ambulatory facilities (22).

Traditional hospital outpatient services have been provided in clinics and emergency rooms. In many hospitals, clinics have had second class status as compared to the complex and expensive inpatient services. However, as hospitals increasingly recognize the important role of primary care and seek to expand the base of patients that are potential utilizers of inpatient and ancillary services, more attention is being directed toward improving clinic operations and services.

Hospital clinics include both primary care and specialty clinics. Many hospitals differentiate between clinics for walk-in patients without appointments and those for scheduled visits. Specialty clinics are usually organized by clinical departments and provide services such as ophthalmology, neurology, and allergy care. In teaching hospitals, clinics serve as important opportunities for house staff to provide ongoing care to patients and to follow up after hospitalizations. Increasingly, the clinics also provide an opportunity to expose medical students and house staff to ambulatory care services to complement the traditionally more extensive experience with inpatient care. In teaching hospitals, there may be over 100 different clinics reflecting the diversity of subspecialties. In non-teaching hospitals there are fewer specialty clinics and may be more emphasis on primary care.

Many hospital primary care clinics evolved from an orientation of service to the poor and were staffed by physicians who served without reimbursement in exchange for staff privileges. The level of commitment to the patient under such circumstances was, not surprisingly, less than might be desired. Hospitals are now increasingly employing physicians and other practitioners as full time clinic staff.

Some hospitals are also establishing primary care group practices to complement other outpatient services and to assume the burden of providing primary care to patients who seek most of their care from the hospital. The development of a group practice has advantages for both consumers and the hospital by providing comprehensive and accessible care and removing primary care patients from facilities that are not designed to serve their needs, such as emergency rooms. The development of these group practices also has the potential of increasing use of the hospital's inpatient and ancillary services, an advantage if occupancy is low (23).

AMBULATORY SURGERY CENTERS

A further innovation in hospital-based care has been the development of ambulatory surgery centers. Originated in hospitals in Washington, D.C. and Los Angeles, these organized hospital units provide one-day surgical care. Patients are usually screened for acceptability by their personal surgeon and then report at an assigned date and time for surgery. The surgeon is supported by the unit's facilities, equipment, and personnel, and the patient is discharged one to three hours after surgery when recovery from anesthesia is sufficiently complete.

In the early 1970s free-standing ambulatory surgery centers were opened, one of the first of which was in Phoenix. These are independent of hospitals and usually provide a full range of services for the types of surgery that can be performed on an outpatient basis. Community surgeons are granted operating privileges and can perform surgery in these facilities in instances where the patient agrees and there are no medical contraindications.

Other facilities are also used for ambulatory or outpatient surgery. Many physicians traditionally performed surgery in their offices although this practice has declined due to malpractice concerns and the increasing availability of better equipped and staffed alternative facilities.

Free-standing emergency centers have also opened in many cities paralleling the success of ambulatory surgery centers. These emergency centers sometimes provide a wide range of primary care in addition to responding to urgent problems. The future of specialized ambulatory centers both in hospitals and as free-standing facilities will probably include further expansion into other areas of health care.

EMERGENCY MEDICAL SERVICES

The emergency room has, like other hospital departments, undergone transformation in recent years. The emergency room has expanded in scope of services and complexity. An especially important trend has been the increasing use of the emergency room for primary care. Since the emergency room requires sophisticated facilities and highly trained personnel and must be accessible 24 hours a day, costs are high and services are not designed for non-urgent care. To reduce the burdens on the emergency room and to better meet patient needs, many hospitals triage patients. This is a process, often performed by a nurse, where patient health care needs are determined and the patient is referred to a more appropriate source of care within the hospital. The misuse of the emergency room has received considerable attention and is compounded by third party insurers who have often reimbursed for primary care only if provided in the emergency room.

Emergency medical services have also been increasingly integrated with other community resources. These include drug and alcohol treatment programs, mental health centers, and voluntary agencies. Many communities are developing formal emergency medical systems which incorporate all hospital emergency rooms and transportation and communication systems. In these communities, people needing emergency care either transport themselves or call an emergency number and an ambulance is dispatched by a central communications center which also identifies and alerts the most appropriately equipped and located hospital. In some communities, regional hospital-based trauma centers have been built with extremely sophisticated capabilities. Specialized ambulance services, including mobile coronary care units and shock-trauma vans, are also increasingly prevalent. The Red Cross and other voluntary agencies have also administered programs for many years to train people to respond to accidents, drownings, and other emergencies. In Seattle a program was initiated, now expanding to other cities, to augment emergency capabilities by teaching as many people as possible to respond to heart attacks by administering cardiopulmonary resuscitation. Since accidents and heart attacks are major sources of mortality, these programs have the potential of contributing to reductions in deaths.

GOVERNMENTAL PROGRAMS: HEALTH CENTERS

In addition to private sector and institutionally initiated efforts, governmental programs have been designed to increase the availability of health care resources in many communities. These programs have adapted some of the concepts of the private institutional settings, and especially of group practice.

Neighborhood health centers have been funded since 1965. Originally intended to serve approximately 25,000,000 people, this federal program never reached its initial objectives and now serves about 1,300,000 people in over 130 centers. The program was designed to provide primary medical care with a family orientation, targeted for population groups in severe need of services as reflected by such indicators as disease prevalence and income levels. At the same time, the centers were intended to employ people from the communities they serve in positions which would offer opportunities for training and advancement. Responsiveness to community needs was to be assured through a community board or advisory panel. The centers were to be committed to the recognition that the broad attributes of a community, such as housing and employment, contributed to health and illness.

Most of the neighborhood health centers are free-standing group practices although some are organizationally affiliated with other institutions such as hospitals, medical schools, or community associations. The majority of centers are located in urban areas. There is considerable diversity in the types of services provided by the centers but all provide primary care and most offer pharmacy, laboratory, radiology, and to a lesser extent, dental services. Some centers also provide transportation for patients and social services to address broader health needs. Originally intended to serve the poor, changes in federal policy which encouraged the centers to collect fees from patients and from third party insurers have broadened the socioeconomic mixture of patients obtaining care. However, the centers still predominantly serve the poor and medically indigent.

Neighborhood health centers have been subjected to considerable criticism, especially from traditional medicine. Some of the criticisms include low productivity and substandard care as compared to the private sector, unwarranted federal intervention in the provision of health services, and high administrative costs. Although it is not possible to generalize across all of the centers, some probably have had high costs and low productivity. This is partially attributable to their goals of employing and training local residents, and to sometimes inexperienced management, constraints imposed by the federal government, and local politics (24). Neighborhood health centers have also had difficulties in finding adequate facilities, problems in physician recruitment, and high staff turnover. There have been practical problems in designing family-oriented comprehensive care for clients used to receiving few services and episodic care. Studies to measure the quality of the care provided in these centers have generally concluded that they meet acceptable standards of care and, in some instances, provide a higher quality of care than other community practitioners (25). The neighborhood health centers have succeeded in increasing access to care under difficult circumstances and have served as an interesting experimental model for the provision of ambulatory care.

Other community health centers now funded by the federal government include migrant health centers serving transient farm workers in agricultural areas and rural health centers. The National Health Service Corps supports practitioners who are placed in urban and rural areas with shortages of medical resources. Other innovations, such as mobile health vans in rural areas, have also been utilized to expand the scope of services.

COMMUNITY MENTAL HEALTH CENTERS AND MENTAL HEALTH PROGRAMS

The Community Mental Health Center program was established to provide ambulatory mental health services in underserved areas. This program has suffered from limitations in federal funding and has not been as extensive as originally envisioned. Community mental health centers were intended to provide outpatient services and emergency care and to work with other community agencies to foster action and concern for mental health. Problems of inadequate management have also been faced by this program. However, the centers have succeeded in providing mental health services, primarily through non-physician professionals, to many individuals who would otherwise not obtain such care. These centers are discussed further in Chapter 7.

OTHER FEDERAL GOVERNMENT PROGRAMS

The federal government, in addition to supporting a variety of community-based health services organizations, directly operates many health care facilities. The Veterans Administration includes the largest health services system under a unified management structure in the United States with over 170 hospitals and clinics. This system provides needed care to millions of veterans throughout the nation. The military services also provide health care to millions of individuals in the armed forces and have developed extensive facilities throughout the world as discussed in Chapter 1.

The government has a special responsibility for providing health care to a number of groups within the country. The Indian Health Service is charged with assuring access to medical care on Indian reservations and in certain other locations. Although the difficulties of operating a largely rural system are immense, the Indian Health Service has succeeded in bringing modern medicine to many people.

The U. S. Public Health Service operates eight hospitals. Originally intended to serve seamen, eligibility has been expanded and the scope of care now includes a wide range of both ambulatory and inpatient services. Faced with frequent threats of closure by past Presidents, the Public Health Service hospitals have had difficulty obtaining sufficient financial resources to meet the demands for care of their eligible populations.

NON-INSTITUTIONAL AND PUBLIC HEALTH SERVICES

As noted in the introduction to this chapter, there are numerous avenues through which ambulatory and community health services are provided. While only the most prevalent types of providers and services are discussed here, each contributes to the availability of the many health care needs of a community. The list is nearly endless and a number of services warrant further discussion.

Home health services are provided by visiting nurse associations, some hospitals, public health departments, and other agencies. These services allow people to remain in their homes yet receive essential health services, thereby reducing costs and increasing the quality of life for many (26). These services, however, often require that the patient have special facilities or equipment and family support at home. For example, home dialysis for chronic renal failure, discussed in Chapter 8, is substantially less expensive than institutional services but requires a specially trained family member.

Rural health care has required unique and innovative solutions in many communities, especially in the absence of physicians and extensive facilities. In rural Alaska, many towns are served by physicians and other professionals who regularly fly-in to treat patients. Satellites have also been used experimentally to facilitate communications with specialists in urban medical centers since even ordinary communications in remote areas may be difficult. In rural Kentucky, nurses in the Frontier Nursing Service provide much of the care to the rural mountain people. These hardy nurses have progressed from horseback to jeep in recent years but continue to provide primary health care, often by traveling from house to house through rugged and remote territory. Rural health care in many areas remains a challenging test of the ingenuity and resourcefulness of the health services system and of community residents.

In urban areas, some creative and innovative efforts to provide health care to people with limited access to services have been attempted. Among the most interesting of these has been the development of "free" clinics in many cities (27). These clinics provide primary medical care and referrals for specialty care and emphasize counseling and patient education. Clients of the free clinics are often working poor who are unable to qualify for publicly assisted care but do not have the financial resources necessary to obtain services from the private sector. The clinics are usually developed by coalitions of community groups or collectives of individuals dedicated to providing care in a non-bureaucratic atmosphere through an egalitarian organizational structure. Although they employ physicians, there is often an effort to demystify the role of the physician and to rely heavily on other types of health providers such as nurse practitioners. Free clinics have had to struggle to survive since they are funded through donations from patients, community groups, and sometimes local health departments. They have also faced opposition from traditional health care providers in some communities and have had difficulties in arranging backup support for hospitalization, specialty referrals, and other services.

Other community health services not discussed in detail here include school health services, prison health services, dental care provided by solo, group, and institutionally-based practitioners, foot care from podiatrists, and drug dispensing from pharmacists who often also extensively advise and educate consumers. Finally, many indigenous health practitioners offer their services in this country and abroad. These practitioners include chiropractors, medicine men, naturopaths, and others. The supportive and sometimes curative role of these individuals is often underestimated.

PUBLIC HEALTH SERVICES

Among the most important contributions to reductions in mortality and morbidity in the twentieth century have been public health measures such as the improvement of sanitation, assurance of potable water supplies, and upgraded housing. In recent years there has also been an increased awareness of the need to control air and water pollution, to reduce exposures to carcinogens, and to improve and assure the quality of the environment. The contributions of these efforts to health far exceeds, dollar for dollar, efforts to treat illness once it occurs. Although a comprehensive discussion of these services is beyond the scope of this book and is available elsewhere (28), these services are essential to a comprehensive consideration of health care.

Public health activities have a long history. Their origins in the United States involved attempts to reduce diseases resulting from poor sanitation and to quarantine against infectious diseases, especially from immigrants. Public health activities developed at both the local and national level. The first state public health departments were organized in Louisiana and in Massachusetts in the mid-nineteenth century. Public health departments at the local level now perform a wide range of functions from health education to the direct provision of services. At the national level, the federal government is involved in the surveillance of disease and numerous other public health activities.

Public health services have addressed serious national problems related to health and illness. Increasing numbers of unwanted births and a lack of family planning services for example, has lead many public health departments to operate family planning clinics offering contraceptive services and advice. Identification of, treatment for, and education about venereal disease has long been a major activity of public health agencies. Typical activities of state and local public health agencies are summarized in Table 4–8.

Many health departments operate specific federally funded categorical programs. These programs range from detection of serious diseases in infants, such as phenylketonuria, to immunizations. The Women, Infants, and Children Program, for example, is a federal effort to improve the nutritional status of low income pregnant women and young children. Screening programs have been developed to detect sickle cell anemia, cervical cancer, and hypertension. Major efforts have been expended to avoid and react to accidental poisoning, especially in children.

Health education is an important activity of many health departments. The avoidance of some illnesses is possible through a better informed public. For example, use of seat belts combined with defensive driving could substantially reduce the number of deaths and injuries from automobile accidents. Avoidance of tobacco products, reduced exposures to radiation and carcinogens, and better nutrition are all examples of health education objectives which have societal benefits through reduced mortality and morbidity. Although few health education program efforts have been extensively evaluated, there is evidence that they have had only mixed success and that people will continue to kill or injure themselves relying on medical services to undo the damage where possible.

Other efforts, by occupational medicine specialists in industry and government, have been directed toward reducing accidents and exposure to disease causing agents, including chemicals, dangerous working conditions, and even noise, in the workplace. Over the years these efforts, which have been controversial and often unpopular among special interest groups, have substantially improved employment conditions in the nation. However, far more remains to be done in this area, particularly in the identification and removal of potential sources of illness such as excessive radiation, chemical contamination, and unsafe facilities and equipment.

Finally, there is an increasing awareness that ambulatory and community health services are only part of the answer to the advancement of health. Self reliance is essential if health is truly the nation's goal. Each individual has to live responsibly by avoiding unnecessary risks of injury and illness, eating adequate diets, exercising, and avoiding excessive stress. There is an increasingly popular movement toward self-reliance for prevention and treatment of disease. Protocols and instructional books have been published to assist people in evaluating their health and needs for care. This movement is a response to the reality that medicine is limited in its ability to prevent and treat disease (29).

TABLE 4–8. Typical Services Provided by Public Health Departments

State Departments:	Licensing boards
	Hospital licensing
	Nursing home licensing
	Vital statistics
	Health planning (statewide agencies)
	Health data systems
	Chronic disease surveillance
	Communicable disease surveillance
	Sanitation control and monitoring
	State laboratory services
	Development of immunization programs
	Tuberculosis control
	Veterinary public health
	Administration and categorical programs
	Emergency medical services
	development
	Support of direct health programs
Local Health Departments:	
	Vital statistics
	Sanitation inspections
	Health education
	Cancer, hypertension, diabetes screening
	Maintenance of disease registries
	Epidemiology
	Supervision of water and sewage
	systems
	Insect control
	Environmental health
	Dairy product supervision
	Information services to physicians
	Public health nursing services
	Tuberculosis screening
	Immunization/vaccination
	Operation of health centers
	Mental health centers
	Family planning clinics
	Venereal disease clinics

ORGANIZATION OF AMBULATORY CARE SYSTEMS

The preceding sections of this chapter have outlined the scope and nature of ambulatory and community health care services. The remainder of the chapter discusses the organization of ambulatory care services. Within this framework, the design criteria that are desirable in ambulatory care systems are presented.

Although no single unified structure currently exists in the United States for providing health services, and ambulatory care services, especially, are often poorly organized, experience and research has led to an ever expanding understanding of the factors that are associated with the optimal design of ambulatory care systems. These are summarized in Table 4–9 and some are discussed in detail in the following section.

TABLE 4–9. Design Criteria for Ambulatory Care Systems

Criteria Topic	Criteria Requirements
Community Criteria	
Availability and Distribution of Resources	Adequate number of facilities and practitioners
	Geographic dispersion
	Adequate transportation
Utilization of Resources	Integration of community resources
	Effective referral network
	Appropriate mix of services
	Constrained excess capacity (few underutilized services)
Consumer Criteria	
Convenience and Satisfaction	Physical access assured
	Availability (hours of operation, after hours coverage) assured
	Efficient scheduling (appointments, follow-ups, waiting times)
	Financial access (insurance coverage, reasonable prices)
	Caring providers
Quality Services	Continuity and coordination of care (medical records, follow-ups, etc.)
	Comprehensive services
	Technical quality of care assured
	Multilingual staff and other special needs assured
	Health education and instruction provided
Provider Criteria	
Work Environment	Pleasant and humane
	Appropriate roles for all providers
	Adequate income
	Productivity encouraged
	Personnel duties match skills and training
Patient Care Services	Efficient use of resources (personnel, capital, and technology)
	Use of most appropriate personnel
	Adequate support services available
System Concerns	Technological progress readily adopted

SYSTEM DESIGN CRITERIA: THE CONSUMER

Perhaps the most important criterion that has been identified for the system from the consumer's perspective has been access to care. As discussed in Chapter 3, there are many complex factors that affect the utilization of health care services and the structure of the system itself, especially in ambulatory care systems, can be a critical factor in facilitating access to care.

Ambulatory care services are affected by several access factors. The number and distribution of providers throughout a community determine, in part, the physical access of individuals to the health care system. Decisions such as the hours of operation and the scope of services provided are important to assure that services can actually be utilized. Facilities should be located so that the target patient population will be able to have access to the facilities. The hours of operation must be consistent with employment patterns, traffic flows, and other factors. Assurance of physical access and availability of services is further complicated by such considerations as public transportation, parking, accessibility for the handicapped, and changing population characteristics. Access to care is a highly complex topic for which researchers have attempted to construct equally complex theories and models (30). All health care professionals should assign high priority to assuring access to care.

Comprehensive services should be available to all consumers which fulfill legitimate health care needs. Who should decide what are legitimate needs, however, is a major issue. For example, a consumer may seek care for a cold believing that this is a high priority need due to discomfort while providers may believe that little relief can be offered and services should be directed toward those who are more ill. And, who should assure that all services are available? For example, should providers be required to offer services such as preventive care and health education or is this a responsibility of government, insurers, or the consumer?

The scope of services is also related to controversies over who is most skilled for providing care. Numerous examples of "turf" struggles are developing in ambulatory care. For example, both general internists and family practitioners seek the central role in providing primary care services. Nurse practitioners and MEDEX are seeking an increasing role in providing services independent of physicians. Optometrists and opthalmologists seek increasing shares of the eye care market. Pharmacists seek to expand their functions beyond dispensing drugs. Deciding who provides which service most appropriately will be among the most complex and politically charged issues to be tackled in the future.

The availability of services and access to care are often affected by special needs of consumers. For example, individuals without an adequate knowledge of the English language have difficulty in utilizing health services unless multilingual staff or translators are able to assist them. Health education in areas such as the correct use of drugs, dietary habits and practices, and infant care are essential when the population served lacks such information. Provision of drugs may be essential when clients are unable to afford needed supplies. The health administrator, planner, or provider must consider the total environment within which services are provided and not assume that the physical presence of a facility or service alone will assure needed care.

The organization of services requires consideration of how units of service are related to each other. Rationalization of ambulatory care requires that services not be duplicated. The absence of duplication assures that individuals are not subjected to unnecessary and repetitive services which can be harmful, such as in the case of excess radiation, and costly. However, in some instances, such as second opinions for surgery, there may be some justification for duplication.

Reductions in redundant services can be achieved through improved coordination and continuity in ambulatory care. Ambulatory services have a central role in the achievement of coordination for all health care services. Coordination and continuity imply that there is some centralization of responsibility for care on the part of both the patient and the provider. A primary care provider who directs the care of the patient with respect to specialized services can promote coordination. Common medical records in group practices also promote coordination. Returning to a previous provider for subsequent care when indicated can promote continuity. Both the patient and the provider have responsibility for assuring the maximum degree of coordination and continuity.

In reality, of course, there are limits to the actual degree of coordination and continuity that can be achieved. Patients become dissatisfied with providers and seek care elsewhere, communications break down, referral patterns change, access to the same provider is not always possible, and numerous other problems can develop. But there is some evidence that coordination and continuity are associated with higher levels of patient compliance (31) which may in turn lead to better health outcomes. It is also likely that greater continuity and coordination will result in an overall higher degree of access and thus patient satisfaction (32), may increase the overall rationalization of the system, and finally may reduce health care costs through less duplication of services.

The consumer also expects high quality services. As discussed in Chapter 12, quality of care is difficult to define and measure. However, reasonable efforts should be taken to assure that unnecessary procedures are not performed and that individuals are treated by practitioners using an acceptable degree of skill, judgment, and current knowledge. Operationalizing these concepts is difficult, especially in ambulatory care where many episodes of treatment are brief and for poorly defined problems.

The quality of care provided should reflect not only adequate technical skills but also the performance of a caring function on the part of the provider. Consumers are capable of detecting some aspects of the technical quality of care (33), but are even more perceptive of the extent to which the provider and the system care about the patient. Since there are limitations to medical practice and much health care is supportive rather than curative, consumer feelings about the treatment process are especially important and may contribute to higher levels of well-being and contentment.

SYSTEM DESIGN CRITERIA: THE PROVIDER

The provider, as well as the consumer, must be satisfied with the structure of the system. Provider satisfaction requires acceptance of individual and organizational roles in the provision of services. From the perspective of the individual worker, whether nurse, physician, technician, or aide, the rewards and structure of the work environment must stimulate productivity and a high quality of performance.

SYSTEM DESIGN CRITERIA: THE COMMUNITY

To many, all of the arguments for designing the system to match the needs of consumers or providers center on the system's role in serving the community. Should the ambulatory care system primarily serve the consumer or the provider, or is there a happy middle ground in which both can be satisfied?

For the community, ambulatory care first and foremost should provide primary and specialty services in response to the needs of the community or population. Although these needs are not always easy to determine, there is at least a minimum scope of services that are critical to any community. Second, the provision of ambulatory care services should be relatively efficient, however defined, so that community resources are not wasted, and should be distributed so that all members of the community have access to care. And third, the organization of ambulatory care systems should perform an integrating function by relating together providers of service and, in a sense, should orchestrate care for clients. This extends far beyond the provision of primary medical and dental services, however, and must also include public health services, voluntary agency efforts, community health education, and all other activities that contribute to the health and well-being of a community.

Whether it is possible or even desirable to establish any single managerial entity to coordinate all of these activities has yet to be determined. But such a function is now performed in a fragmented way by many individuals and organizations from public health departments to the private practitioner. In some countries, such as England and Sweden, such activities are much more centrally organized. In the United States the health planning agencies discussed in Chapter 11 are an early effort to move toward a somewhat more structured system for health care. The extent to which the nation moves further in this direction will be determined in a highly charged political arena.

There are many other forces affecting the design of community systems for ambulatory care. The changing technology of health care directly affects the types of services provided on an ambulatory basis. For example, the rapid expansion of testing and monitoring of the body, discussed in Chapter 8, which can be performed relatively easily on an outpatient basis has resulted in more ambulatory care services. New screening techniques have resulted in community programs to detect diseases such as hypertension, cancer, and diabetes with services offered in such unlikely places as shopping centers.

Third party insurers and governmental programs such as Medicaid and Medicare impact on ambulatory care through their policies on coverage, benefits, and reimbursement levels. By increasingly paying for care provided on an ambulatory basis, they have encouraged a shift from inpatient to outpatient care for many services. Continuation of these trends is likely with the resultant further expansion of outpatient services.

TOWARD AN INTEGRATED SYSTEM

This chapter has discussed the current providers of ambulatory and community health services and the characteristics that are likely to be advantageous to strengthened ambulatory care systems. The variety of services, professionals, and organizations involved in ambulatory care is immense and no single unified structure can encompass them all. The interrelationships between providers and political realities further complicate the system. All of the chapters of this book discuss issues which impinge on ambulatory care and the relationship between ambulatory and other health services has as yet to be fully elucidated. However, progress has been achieved by researchers and practitioners alike in developing an understanding of ambulatory care and in determining the role these services should assume in the overall health services system. The fragmented system that exists now is unlikely to continue in its present form and many new innovations and initiatives should result in a structure that is more efficient and responsive to the needs of both consumers and providers.

REFERENCES

1. Burton L, Smith H: *Public Health and Community Medicine.* 2nd ed. Baltimore, Williams and Wilkins Company, 1975.
2. Noble J (ed): *Primary Care and the Practice of Medicine.* Boston, Little, Brown, 1976.
3. Roemer M: From poor beginnings, the growth of primary care. *Hospitals* 49(5):38–43, 1975.
4. Wolfe S, Badgley RF: *The Family Doctor.* New York, Milbank Memorial Fund, 1972.
5. Peterson OL, Andrews LP, Spain RS, et al: An analytical study of North Carolina general practice 1953–1954. *Journal of Medical Education* 31(12, part 2):1–165, 1956.
6. Petersdorf R: Internal medicine and family practice, controversies, conflict and compromise. *New England Journal Medicine* 293:326–332, 1975.
7. Mechanic D: *The Growth of Bureaucratic Medicine.* New York, John Wiley and Sons, Inc., 1976.
8. Becker M, Maiman L: Sociobehavioral determinants of compliance with health and medical care recommendations. *Medical Care* 13:10–24, 1975.
9. U.S. Department of Health, Education, and Welfare, National Center for Health Statistics: *National Ambulatory Medical Care Survey: Background and Methodology.* Publication Number (HRA) 76-1335. Washington, Government Printing Office, 1976.
10. U.S. Department of Health, Education, and Welfare: *1976 Summary: National Ambulatory Medical Care Survey.* Advance Data, Number 48, National Center for Health Statistics, April 13, 1979.
11. Medical Group Management Association: *The Organization and Development of a Medical Group Practice.* Cambridge, Ballinger Publishing Company, 1976.
12. Rorem R: *Private Group Clinics.* Chicago, University of Chicago Press, 1931.
13. Goodman L, Bennett E, Odem R: Current status of group medical practice in the United States. *Public Health Reports* 92:430–443, 1977.
14. Graham F: Group versus solo practice, arguments and evidence. *Inquiry* 9(2):49–60, 1972.
15. Kimball L, Lorant J: Physician productivity and returns to scale. *Health Services Research* 12:367–379, 1977.

16. Yankauer A, Connelly J, Feldman J: Physician productivity in the delivery of ambulatory care, some findings from a survey of pediatricians. *Medical Care* 8:35–46, 1970.

17. Evashwick C: The role of group practice in the distribution of physicians in nonmetropolitan areas. *Medical Care* 14:808–823, 1976.

18. Egdahl R: Foundations for medical care. *New England Journal of Medicine* 288:491–498, 1973.

19. Bauman P: The formulation and evolution of the Health Maintenance Organization policy, 1970–1973. *Social Science and Medicine* 10:129–142, 1976.

20. Roemer M, Shonick W: HMO performance: the recent evidence. *Milbank Memorial Fund Quarterly* 51:271–317, 1973.

21. Strumpf G, Garramone M: Why some HMOs develop slowly. *Public Health Reports* 91:496–503, 1976.

22. Berraducci A, Delbanco T, Rabkin M: The teaching hospital and primary care, closing down the clinic. *N Eng J Med* 292:615–620, 1975.

23. Williams S, Shortell S, Dowling W, Urban N: Hospital sponsored primary care group practice: a developing modality of care. *Health and Medical Care Services Review* 1(5/6):1–13, 1978.

24. Torrens P: Administrative problems of neighborhood health centers. *Medical Care* 9:487–497, 1971.

25. Morehead M, Donaldson R, Seravalli M: Comparisons between OEO neighborhood health centers and other health care providers of ratings of the quality of health care. *American Journal of Public Health* 61:1294–1306, 1971.

26. Van Dyke F, Brown V: Organized home care: an alternative to institutions. *Inquiry* 9(2):3–16, 1972.

27. Schacter L, Elliston E: Medical care in a free community clinic. *Journal of the American Medical Association* 237:1848–1851, 1977.

28. For example, see Anderson C, Morton R, Green L: *Community Health*. St. Louis, C. V. Mosby, 1978.

29. McKinlay J, McKinlay S: The questionable contribution of medical measures to the decline of mortality in the United States in the twentieth century. *Milbank Memorial Fund Quarterly* 55:405–428, 1977.

30. Aday L, Andersen R: A framework for the study of access to medical care. *Health Services Research* 9:208–220, 1974.

31. Starfield B, Simborg D, Horn S, et al: Continuity and coordination in primary care: their achievement and utility. *Medical Care* 14:625–632, 1976.

32. Williams S, Shortell S, LoGerfo J, et al: A causal model of health services for diabetic patients. *Medical Care* 16:313–326, 1978.

33. Lebow, J: Consumer assessments of the quality medical care. *Medical Care* 12:328–337, 1974.

CHAPTER 5

The Hospital

William L. Dowling

Patricia A. Armstrong

The modern hospital is the key resource and organizational hub of the American health care system, central to the delivery of patient care, to the training of health personnel, and to the conduct and dissemination of health related research. The hospital represents the community's collective investment in health care resources, presumably available for the benefit of all, and it is often the first place people think of when they need medical care. Since the turn of the century, the indispensable workshops of the physician, hospitals have become even more the economic and professional heart of medical practice as the accelerating pace of advances in medical knowledge and technology has brought medical care more and more into the institutional setting. As highly advanced, scientific institutions, hospitals manifest the complexity and detached efficiency of a clinical laboratory. As human service organizations, they are charged with the emotions of life and death situations and of triumphs and tragedies.

Hospitals are also big business. Collectively, they are the second or third largest "industry" in the United States in terms of the number of people they employ. By far the largest part of the health care system, hospitals employ about three-fourths of all health personnel and consume over 40% of the nation's health expenditures. About 60% of all federal expenditures for health services and about 50% of all state and local government health expenditures are spent on hospital care (1).

Ironically, the magnitude of the hospital sector and the central role hospitals play in the delivery of health services, both reflecting the accomplishments of hospitals in making available the benefits of medical progress, now put hospitals at the root of many of the health care system's most pressing problems—cost inflation, duplication of services, bed surplus, overemphasis on inpatient specialized services versus ambulatory primary care services, and "depersonalization" of care, among others (2, 3). Further, as "community" or "quasi-public" institutions heavily dependent on public dollars, hospitals are "open systems," subject to influence from outside, and therefore susceptible to the efforts of community groups and external agencies to use them as instruments of social change and health system reorganization (4, 5). Little wonder hospitals always seem to be "in the middle of things."

The hospital "system" is a mix of public and private for-profit and not-for-profit institutions. Hospitals range from small institutions in less-populated communities and isolated rural areas providing basic medical care to large regional referral centers providing a comprehensive scope of sophisticated, highly-specialized services. Some hospitals provide only inpatient care, while others have expanded their role to include ambulatory care provided through emergency rooms and outpatient clinics. A number provide home care and other outreach services as well.

The purpose of this chapter is to characterize the hospital system in the United States, emphasizing major issues and trends. Because the character of the modern hospital reflects its past, the chapter begins with a discussion of the historical development of hospitals. The second section describes the hospital system as it exists today. The third section describes the internal organization of hospitals. And the last section discusses a number of major issues confronting hospitals at the present time. It should be noted that the discussion of hospitals in this chapter focuses primarily on their inpatient role. Hospitals do play, however, a substantial role in the provision of outpatient care (6, 7). The number of emergency room visits and the number of outpatient referrals for diagnostic and therapeutic services in community hospitals has been increasing four times faster than the number of admissions, and the ratio of outpatient visits to inpatient admissions in community hospitals is now almost six to one. Over a quarter of the nation's community hospitals have organized outpatient departments and 90% have emergency departments (8). Chapter 4 discusses ambulatory care in the hospital setting.

HISTORICAL DEVELOPMENT OF HOSPITALS

The history of hospitals in this country (Fig. 5–1) can be traced back to the almhouses and pesthouses which existed in some form in almost all cities of moderate size by the mid-1700s (9, 10). Almshouses, also called poorhouses or workhouses, were established by city governments to provide food and shelter for the homeless poor, including many aged, chronically ill, disabled, mentally ill, and orphaned people. Medical care was a secondary function of the poorhouse, but in some facilities those who became ill were isolated in infirmaries where care, such as it was before the advent of modern medicine, was provided, typically by other residents. Not until the late 1800s did the infirmaries or hospital departments of city poorhouses break away to become medical care institutions on their own—the first public hospitals.

Pesthouses were operated by local governments as isolation or quarantine stations in seaports where it was necessary to isolate people who contracted contagious diseases aboard ship. During epidemics, these institutions were used to

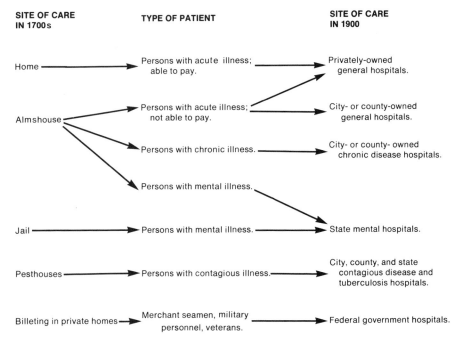

Figure 5–1. Evolution of institutional care sites.

isolate victims of cholera, smallpox, typhus, and yellow fever. Their primary purpose was to control the spread of infectious diseases by removing infected individuals from the community. As with almshouses, medical care was a secondary function; in this case secondary to protecting the community from outbreaks of contagious diseases. Pesthouses were often established during epidemics and discontinued or closed down when the threat of disease subsided. These institutions were the predecessors of the contagious disease and tuberculous hospitals that later emerged.

Almshouses and pesthouses were maintained for the poor and the homeless— and they were avoided by everyone else. These institutions were dismal places: they were crowded, unsanitary, and poorly heated and ventilated. Nutrition was often inadequate, nursing care incompetent, and separation of different types of residents minimal. Contagious persons, the disabled, the dying, and the insane were often crowded together. Cross infection was rampant, and mortality rates high. Persons who were able were cared for at home or in the homes of neighbors.

The first community-owned or voluntary hospitals in this country were established in the late 1700s and early 1800s, often at the urging of influential physicians trained in Europe who needed facilities to practice obstetrics and surgery in the manner in which they had been taught, and also to provide preceptor-type instruction for medical students. These early hospitals depended upon philanthropy, and contributions were solicited from both private citizens and local government. Voluntary hospitals generally preceded both religious and public hospitals in the United States, representing a departure from patterns in England and Europe.

Voluntary hospitals admitted both indigent and paying patients. For example, in its first year of operation (1751), the Pennsylvania Hospital admitted 24 paying patients and 40 poor patients. These hospitals were supported by community contributions and philanthropy, rather than by a church or the state. Except in the largest cities where the concentration of poor was too great, the early voluntary hospitals cared for people in their communities who were unable to pay on a charitable basis, drawing on philanthropy and donations of time by members of the medical staff (9, 11).

The first hospitals of this type were the Pennsylvania Hospital, Philadelphia, 1751; New York Hospital, New York City, 1773; Massachusetts General Hospital, Boston, 1816; and New Haven Hospital, New Haven, 1826. Additional voluntary hospitals were established in Savannah, Georgia, in 1830, Lowell, Massachusetts in 1836, and Raleigh, North Carolina, in 1839. Voluntary hospitals cared for patients with acute illnesses and injuries, but did not admit persons with contagious diseases or mental illnesses. Isolation of these unfortunates from the rest of the community was seen as a governmental responsibility. Therefore, during the same period, a number of city, county, and state mental hospitals were established. These included hospitals in Williamsburg, Virginia, 1773; Lexington, Kentucky, 1817; Columbia, South Carolina, 1829; Worchester, Massachusetts, 1832; Augusta, Maine, 1834; Brooklyn, New York, 1838; and Boston, Massachusetts, 1839.

Although voluntary hospitals provided better accommodations and care for the sick than the poorhouses that preceded them, the efficacy of care improved little, and it was not until the late 1800s that hospitals became accepted by persons of all economic strata as the best setting for the care of serious illness and injury. Prior to that time, most people who became ill were cared for at home. In 1873, there were only 178 hospitals, with 35,604 beds in the United States. By 1909, the number of hospitals had increased to 4,359, with 421,065 beds; and by 1929, to 6,665 hospitals with 907,133 beds. This rapid growth in the number of hospitals can be attributed to advances in medical science that rapidly transformed the hospital's role from a custodial institution in which to isolate and shelter the poor to a curative institution in which communities concentrated their health care resources in support of the practicing physician for the benefit of all (11, 12).

FORCES AFFECTING THE DEVELOPMENT OF HOSPITALS

Four major developments in health care were particularly significant in transforming hospitals into the institutions of today: advances in medical science increased the efficacy and safety of hospitals; the development of technological sophistication and specialization necessitated the institutionalization of much of medical care; the development of professional nursing brought about more humane treatment of patients; and advances in medical education added teaching and research to the hospital's role (9, 11, 13, 14).

Advances in Medical Science. Most notable in terms of their impact on hospitals were the discovery of anesthesia and the rapid advances in surgery that followed, and the development of the germ theory of disease and the subsequent discovery of antiseptic and sterilization techniques. By the early 1800s, enough was known about anatomy and physiology so that surgeons were able to perform a variety of fairly complex surgical procedures. However, the inability to deaden pain meant that surgery had to be carried out with extreme speed. In addition, infections from surgery were common. Ether was first used as an anesthetic in surgery by Long in 1842, and then by Morton in 1846, and its use spread rapidly after that. Great advances in the efficacy of surgery followed.

Prior to the germ theory of disease, a few scientists, most notably Holmes in the United States and Semmelweis in Vienna, had observed and reported that fever, infection, and mortality could be reduced through cleanliness. Both concluded that "childbed" fever, which was the cause of high maternal mortality rates, was an infection transmitted by doctors, midwives, and medical students to women in labor. In 1861, Pasteur proved that bacteria were living, reproducing, micro-organisms which could be carried by air or on clothes and hands. It became clear that germs were the cause rather than the result of infection, and could be destroyed by chemicals and heat. Lister built on Pasteur's work, and in 1867 introduced carbolic acid spray in operating rooms as an antiseptic to keep air and incisions clean. In 1886, steam sterilization was introduced, providing a means of freeing medical equipment from micro-organisms. Surgical infection rates fell. Advances in surgery led to the need for skilled pre-operative and post-operative care and operating room facilities, which could only be provided in hospitals. By 1900, 40% of all hospitalizations were for surgery.

Development of Specialized Technology.   By the late 1800s, medical technology began to proliferate. The first hospital laboratory opened in 1889, and x-rays were first used for medical diagnosis in 1896. These developments greatly increased the diagnostic effectiveness of hospitals. The discovery of blood types in 1901 made blood transfusions safe; the electrocardiogram (EKG) was first used in 1903; and the electroencephalogram (EEG) in 1929. In addition to increasing the efficiency of medical care, these advances in technology affected the site and the organization of care. Since the tools of the new technology could no longer be carried around in the doctor's black bag, hospitals became the central resource where the equipment, facilities, and personnel required by modern medicine were housed. In addition, since one person could no longer be competent in all areas of medical practice, specialization began to occur within medicine, and new professional and technical occupations began to emerge. Again, the hospital became a convenient place for physicians and support personnel to come together to provide patient care.

Development of Professional Nursing.   Humane treatment of patients awaited the development of professional nursing. Prior to the late 1800s, the only humane nursing care was provided by Catholic sisters and Protestant deaconnesses who were dedicated to caring for patients, and who were fairly well trained. Some religious orders established their own hospitals, and occasionally they were called upon by city officials to provide nursing services in public institutions. Almshouses used untrained female residents to provide nursing care and most hospitals relied on poorly paid unskilled labor.

The transformation of nursing into a profession is credited to Florence

Nightingale, who completed four months of nurses' training in a deaconness school in Germany. In 1854, Florence Nightingale and 38 nurses were sent by the British government to Crimea to take charge of nursing care for wounded soldiers. The nurses found conditions for caring for the soldiers deplorable, and instituted cleanliness and sanitation, dietary reforms, simple but humane care, discipline, and organization. As a result, the mortality rate dropped dramatically. Upon her return to England, Florence Nightingale wrote of her experiences in Crimea and on the contributions of sanitation to the recovery of wounded and ill patients. In 1860, she founded the Nightingale School for Nursing in England.

In the United States, President Lincoln called upon the Catholic sisterhoods to provide nursing care for the wounded during the Civil War, but more nurses were needed. Dorthea Dix was appointed Superintendent of Nursing for the Union Army. She began a recruitment program and encouraged a one-month hospital training program for new nurses. By the end of the War, there were 2,000 lay nurses in the country. The first permanent schools of nursing were established at Bellevue Hospital, New Haven Hospital, and Massachusetts General Hospital in 1873. Although there was some initial reluctance on the part of hospital administrators and trustees to establish nursing schools, the benefits of good nursing soon became apparent. In addition, student nurses provided better care, and were less expensive than the untrained women employed to do this work previously. By 1883, there were 22 nursing schools and 600 graduates; by 1898, this had grown to 400 schools with 10,000 graduates.

Advances in nursing contributed to the growth of hospitals in two ways. The first was increased efficacy of treatment: cleanliness, nutritional diets, and formal treatment routines all contributed to patients' recovery. Second, considerate skilled patient care made hospitals acceptable to all people, not just the poor. The public's fear of hospitals began to give way to an attitude of confidence and respect.

Advances in Medical Education.   Changes in medical education brought about by the Flexner Report in 1910 had a major impact on the development of hospitals. Prior to 1900, there was great variation in the nature and quality of medical education. There were no standards of academic training for physicians. Most medical schools were proprietary and were not connected with universities. Schools were dominated by influential practitioners, and most instruction was through didactic (often unscientific) lectures. Apprenticeship practices varied greatly. There was little clinical or laboratory instruction, and little research.

The Flexner Report, sponsored by the Carnegie Foundation, led to changes in the content and methods of instruction to emphasize the scientific basis of medicine. The standards of education established by the Flexner Report were widely accepted by both the profession and the public and, as a result, schools that did not meet the standards were forced to close. State laws were established requiring graduation from a medical school accredited by the American Medical Association as the basis for a license to practice medicine. A four-year course of study at a medical school based in a university became standard, as did clinical training in the wards of a hospital.

These changes expanded the role of the hospital to include education and research as well as patient care. The hospital's role in education became even more prominent as specialization in medicine led to a proliferation of internships and residencies in the 1920s and 1930s. The requirements of medical education necessitated the expansion of hospital facilities and services and the addition of equipment and personnel. Hospitals were called upon to assume a greater responsibility for coordinating and organizing these resources. Quality of care improved through advances in medical education, especially for patients with complex and serious illnesses. On the other hand, specialization led to a fragmentation of care among different physician specialists and ancillary personnel and a lack of interest in chronic, routine, and other "uninteresting" medical conditions.

Thus, the growth of hospitals in the United States was a direct result of advances in medical science that made hospitals effective and safe. These advances, but particularly the discovery of sulfa drugs in the mid-1930s and antibiotics in the mid-1940s, changed the prevalent causes of death from acute, infectious diseases to the diseases of old age, particularly heart disease, cancer, and stroke. Hospitals have not been quick to respond to the health care problems of an aging population. Their resources continue to be concentrated on curable, short-term illnesses which respond quickly to medical treatment, rather than on chronic, long-term illnesses which must be managed over long periods of time. Hospitals are just now beginning to expand their role to include extended or skilled nursing care units, inpatient or outpatient rehabilitation programs, day care, home care, and other "nontraditional" services (15, 16, 17).

Growth of Health Insurance.   Another factor which has significantly affected the development of hospitals is the growth of health insurance. Private insurance for hospital care grew rapidly, especially between 1940 and 1960, increasing both the proportion of the population with insurance and the adequacy and scope of coverage. Today, the out-of-pocket cost of hospital care at time of use is relatively modest for most people, because most of the bill is covered by some third-party purchaser—either government or private health insurance.

A variety of factors led to the growth of hospital insurance. From the consumer's perspective, of course, a hospital stay is expensive enough to warrant the purchase of insurance protection. The hospital industry's interest in insurance began with the Depression of the 1930s when the number of patients who couldn't pay their bill increased markedly, and hospital use declined. The financial solvency of many hospitals was threatened, and the number of hospitals dropped from 6,852 in 1928 to 6,189 in 1937. Further, a study of non-profit hospitals in 1935 showed that total income was 3% less than total expenses. As a result, acting through the American Hospital Association, hospitals took the initiative in actively encouraging the development of hospital insurance plans, primarily Blue Cross (13, 18). These developments are discussed in detail in Chapter 10.

The growth of health insurance has had a substantial impact on hospitals. First, assuring the financial stability of hospitals, insurance subsequently provided the flow of funds that made possible the great expansion of facilities and services and the prompt implementation of new medical technology that have characterized the hospital industry since the end of World War II. Insurance also contributed to the increased demand for health services. Since hospital services are generally better covered by insurance than services provided outside the hospital, patients are reluctant to substitute less expensive out-of-hospital services. This has resulted in a bias toward hospital use versus the use of ambulatory care programs, home care programs, or nursing care facilities as sources of care, and a general overuse of expensive hospital services (19, 20).

Another problem in the hospital industry can be traced at least partially to cost-based reimbursement, the method of payment used by Medicare, Medicaid, and most Blue Cross plans. Cost reimbursement does not provide hospitals with an incentive to contain costs. The result has been inefficiency, duplication of services, and overbuilding (21, 22, 23). On the other hand, cost reimbursement has enabled hospitals to keep up with advances in medical technology and demands from their communities and physicians for access to a broad range of services. A key issue yet unresolved is how to balance the accessability and costliness of hospital services.

Role of Government.   Government's role in the hospital industry has changed substantially over time in both form and level. During colonial times, government involvement was mainly at the local level through ownership of almshouses and pesthouses, and grants to help construct and support voluntary hospitals. State government limited its role to running contagious disease and mental hospitals, and the federal government to running hospitals for merchant seamen, military personnel, and veterans. Gradually, the forms of involvement have multiplied and the balance has shifted to the federal level.

The "initial thrust" of federal involvement began in 1935 with federal categorical grants-in-aid to state and local governments to assist in the establishment of traditional public health programs: public health departments, communicable disease programs, maternal and child health programs, and public assistance for specific groups such as crippled children, the aged, blind, and disabled, and poor families with dependent children. These programs were part of the general social reform movement which came about during the Depression with the recognition that state and local government and voluntary efforts were not sufficient to meet social needs.

Direct federal involvement in the hospital industry began in 1946 with the Hill-Burton (Hospital Survey and Construction) Act. Few hospitals had been constructed during the Depression and World War II, and by the end of the War, it was generally felt that a severe shortage of hospitals existed. The Hill-Burton program was enacted to help states and communities plan for and construct hospitals and other health facilities by providing federal grants on a matching basis to supplement funds raised at the community level. The Act required states to define hospital service areas, inventory existing facilities, and identify areas of greatest need. The program then provided funds for construction in priority areas. Although the initial emphasis of the program was to provide funds for the construction of new hospitals, priorities changed over time from construction to modernization and from inpatient to outpatient facilities. Funds were available through the program for the construction of nursing homes as well.

The Hill-Burton program assisted in the construction of nearly 40% of the beds in the nation's short-term general hospitals and was the major single factor in the increase in the nation's bed supply from 3.5 short-term beds per 1,000 population in 1946 to 4.5 beds per 1,000 today. Another positive impact of the program is that hospital facilities are more evenly distributed across rural and urban areas and high and low income states than they would have been without the program. However, the program also contributed to the over-building of hospitals, and to the preponderance of small rural hospitals existing today.

The survey requirements in the Act introduced the concepts of planning and regionalization for the first time, and in 1964, the Act was amended to provide federal support for the establishment and operation of comprehensive health planning agencies. In 1974, Hill-Burton was replaced by the National Health Planning and Resources Development Act, as discussed in Chapter 11. However, the idea of a functionally differentiated, integrated, regionalized hospital system first envisioned in Hill-Burton has yet to be realized; indeed, one of the lessons of Hill-Burton is that "bricks and mortar" alone are not enough to change the behavior of physicians and hospitals. Another provision of the Hill-Burton Act, that facilities aided by the program provide "community service" in the form of "a reasonable volume of care to persons unable to pay," has only recently begun to be strictly enforced (24).

From assisting with the financing of hospital construction, the federal government's involvement in the hospital industry has expanded to financing the provision of care and regulating the construction, operation, and utilization of hospitals. Fifty-five percent of all hospital bills are now covered by government programs, primarily Medicare and Medicaid (25) and this puts the federal government in a position to exercise a great amount of control over how hospitals operate. The regulation of hospitals is discussed later in this chapter and in Chapter 11.

CHARACTERISTICS OF THE HOSPITAL SYSTEM

The hospital industry is complex and diverse, and therefore difficult to describe simply. However, hospitals can be classified generally in one of three ways: according to length-of-stay, according to the predominant type of service provided, and according to ownership (26). In terms of length-of-stay, the most common type of hospital is the short-stay or short-term hospital where most patients are suffering from acute conditions requiring hospital stays of less than 30 days. The average length-of-stay in short-term hospitals is about eight days. In long-term hospitals, most of which are chronic disease, psychiatric, or tuberculosis hospitals, the average length-of-stay ranges from three to six months (8).

The second method of classification is by type of service. Predominant is the general hospital offering a wide range of medical, surgical, obstetric, and pediatric services. Specialty hospitals, on the other hand, provide care for a specific disease or population group. Examples of specialty hospitals are children's hospitals, maternity hospitals, chronic disease hospitals, psychiatric hospitals, and tuberculosis hospitals. During the first part of the twentieth century, the number of specialty hospitals grew quite substantially in areas of emerging medical specialization, like eye, ear, nose and throat, obstetrics, orthopedics, and rehabilitation. These were largely the result of philanthropists responding to the initiative of prestigious physician specialists who wanted to develop their own hospitals. Due to financial difficulties and advances in medical science which make general hospitals more appropriate and efficient, specialty hospitals are less common today. Most have either closed or converted to general hospitals (9, 11).

The third method of classifying hospitals is according to form of ownership: government or public ownership, private for-profit (proprietary) ownership, and private not-for-profit (religious or voluntary) ownership.

PUBLIC HOSPITALS

Public hospitals are owned by agencies of federal, state, or local government. Federally-owned hospitals are maintained primarily for special groups of federal beneficiaries: American Indians, merchant seamen, military personnel, and veterans. State governments have generally limited themselves to the operation of mental and tuberculosis hospitals, reflecting government's early role of protecting the healthy by isolating the "insane" and persons with contagious diseases from the rest of society. Most local government hospitals are short-term general hospitals, and these institutions comprise 31% of the nation's short-term hospitals and accommodate 21% of all admissions and 28% of all outpatient visits to short-term hospitals (Table 5–1). Local government hospitals can be divided into two types: 1) city, county, or hospital district institutions; mostly small or moderate in bed size, with medical staffs comprised of private physicians and serving both indigent and paying patients. These hospitals tend to be located in small cities and towns. Their costs are met primarily through third-party reimbursement, and they receive little tax support. For all practical purposes, they function the same as community-owned hospitals. And 2) large city or county hospitals in major urban areas. These hospitals serve mostly the poor and near-poor and minorities. They are generally staffed by salaried physicians, mostly residents. Most are affiliated with medical schools. Their costs usually exceed their patient revenues, and so their deficits must be made up through tax refunds (27).

The large urban public hospitals play an important role in the health care system. They are the place of last resort for the poor, both because they care for all patients regardless of ability to pay, and because they provide services that private hospitals cannot finance or do not wish to offer: alcohol and drug abuse treatment, psychiatric services, care for persons with chronic and communicable diseases, abortion and family planning services, and so forth. They are located in areas where health resources, especially private physicians, are in short supply, and their outpatient departments are the only accessible source of ambulatory care for many inner-city residents. Large urban public hospitals average 10.2 outpatient visits per inpatient admission, compared to 5.7 outpatient visits per admission in privately owned hospitals. In addition, these hospitals play a major role in medical education: 70% are affiliated with a medical school and 75% offer residency training programs (8, 28). Over half of all practicing physicians received at least some of their training in public hospitals.

It was thought that enactment of the Medicare and Medicaid programs would greatly reduce the demand on public hospitals by giving the aged and the poor the means to purchase care from other sources. The expected exodus did not occur, however, probably because the "gatekeepers" of the community hospitals, private

TABLE 5–1. Hospitals, Beds, Admissions, and Outpatient Visits by Ownership and Type of Service, 1977

	Hospitals		Beds		Admissions		Outpatient Visits	
	Number	Percent	Number	Percent	Number	Percent	Number	Percent
Total—All Hospitals	7,099		1,407,097		37,059,782		263,775,060	
Federal	377	5	123,590	9	2,017,517	5	53,142,462	20
Nonfederal								
Psychiatric	541	8	261,207	19	587,222	2	5,018,148	2
Tuberculosis	19	1	3,315	1	12,473	1	34,925	1
Long-term	189	3	45,119	3	89,354	1	1,341,707	1
Short-term:	5,973	84	973,866	69	34,353,216	93	204,237,818	77
		(Percent of Short-term)		(Percent of Short-term)		(Percent of Short-term)		(Percent of Short-term)
Nongovernmental Not-for-profit	3,371	56	679,501	70	24,284,417	71	139,044,760	68
Investor-owned for-profit	751	13	80,322	8	2,848,799	8	8,355,428	4
State and local government	1,851	31	241,043	22	7,220,000	21	56,837,630	28

Source: American Hospital Association: *Hospital Statistics*. Chicago, The Association, 1978.

practitioners, are in short supply in inner-city areas. In addition, some of those who are located close enough to be accessible limited the number of "welfare" patients they would accept. Cultural and social barriers also discouraged the poor from approaching community hospitals. As a result, inpatient and outpatient utilization of public hospitals dipped only slightly in 1967, the first full year of operation of both Medicare and Medicaid, and then continued a steady upward climb which continues to this day (29, 30).

Despite the increasing demand that large urban public hospitals are called upon to meet, their problems are great. Characteristically, these hospitals are old and outmoded. They tend to be underequipped, underfinanced, and understaffed. They have difficulty attracting physicians and rely heavily on interns, residents, and foreign-trained physicians. Their administration is constrained by the bureaucratic red tape and rigidity of city or county government. Public hospitals have responded to these difficulties in a variety of ways. Most are affiliated with medical schools to attract faculty as supervisory physicians and to facilitate the recruitment of interns and residents. In some areas, a special agency or commission has been created to run the public hospital in order to buffer it from government bureaucracy. In some cases, the agency is completely separate from city or county government but is empowered by enabling legislation to borrow, issue bonds, and tax, much like a school district. A number of public hospitals are attempting to improve their position by becoming the source of highly specialized tertiary services, like burn care, neonatal intensive care, or kidney dialysis, for the entire community. Other aspects of this strategy include opening the medical staff to private physicians, adding amenities, and improving facilities to encourage the physicians to bring their patients to the public hospital, at least for the more specialized services (31, 32).

FOR-PROFIT HOSPITALS

For-profit, investor-owned, or proprietary hospitals are operated for the financial benefit of the individual, partnership, or corporation that owns the institution. Around the turn of the century, more than one-half of the nation's hospitals were proprietary. Most of these hospitals had been established by one or a small group of physicians to have a place to hospitalize their own patients, and most were quite small. Gradually, these institutions were closed or sold to community organizations, and until 1972, the number of proprietary hospitals declined steadily, although the decline in beds reversed itself around 1960 as the better-situated proprietary hospitals expanded to meet population increases, and as new proprietary hospitals, typically larger than those that were closing, were built (Table 5–2). As of 1977, proprietary hospitals comprised 13% of the nation's short-term hospitals, with 8% of the beds and 4% of the outpatient visits (Table 5–1) (33, 34).

The trend most significant over the past few years has not been in the number of proprietary hospitals *per se,* but rather the building or buying-up of a substantial number of hospitals by large, investor-owned corporations to form multi-unit, for-

TABLE 5–2. Characteristics of Proprietary Short-term Hospitals, United States, Selected Years

Year	Number of Hospitals	Number of Beds	Admissions
1950	1,218	42,000	1,661,000
1960	856	37,000	1,550,000
1970	769	53,000	2,031,000
1971	750	54,000	2,088,000
1972	738	57,000	2,161,000
1973	757	63,000	2,334,000
1974	775	70,000	2,553,000
1975	775	73,000	2,646,000
1976	752	76,000	2,734,000
1977	751	80,000	2,849,000

Source: American Hospital Association: *Hospital Statistics.* Chicago, The Association, 1978.

profit, hospital systems. At present, the ten largest investor-owned corporations own or lease about 340 hospitals, totaling 52,000 beds. These corporations manage another 220 hospitals, totaling 25,000 beds—most of which are non-profit hospitals—and the growth of management contracts is now more rapid than is the number of owned hospitals. It appears that both trends will continue, at least for the foreseeable future (35, 36).

Investor-owned hospital corporations claim that they are able to earn a profit by operating their hospitals more efficiently than non-profit hospitals. They point to the availability of management specialists, the application of modern management techniques, cost savings in construction and maintenance, economies of scale, and group purchasing as the key factors enabling them to keep costs down enough to make a profit and pay taxes, without cutting quality. For-profit hospitals have also been able to respond promptly to population shifts because of their ability to raise capital quickly (37). Critics of for-profit hospitals claim that their profits are attributable to the practice of "cream skimming": admitting only patients with less serious medical conditions and patients who are able to pay the full costs of their hospitalization. By not admitting poorly-insured patients, for-profit hospitals can avoid bad debts, which may run as high as 10% of total patient charges in non-profit and public hospitals in certain locations. By not admitting seriously ill patients, for-profit hospitals can avoid providing expensive or unprofitable services, and few offer educational programs. The quality of care in for-profit hospitals has also been criticized: the 13% lower employee-to-bed ratio in for-profit hospitals, for example, is pointed to as an indicator of lower quality and less sophisticated services rather than more efficient management. Another criticism is that, even if for-profit hospitals are more efficient, their cost savings are not passed on to patients. Rather, it is claimed that their charges are set at the same level as other hospitals in the community, whatever their costs. Also questioned is the extent to which for-profit hospitals are willing to push the physicians on their medical staffs to be aggressive and stringent about quality and utilization controls when they depend on these physicians for patients. However, this argument also applies to non-profit hospitals (38).

There is little firm evidence to support these criticisms, however, or even to accurately compare for-profit and non-profit hospitals. What "cream-skimming" does occur is likely to be due more to where for-profit hospitals are located (e.g., in rapidly growing suburban areas) than to the actual turning away of patients who cannot pay. Not admitting patients with complex conditions requiring sophisticated services and not providing high-cost, low-use specialized services are cited by for-profit hospitals as examples of how they avoid duplication by referring out patients requiring costly services—long a goal of those who would reform the health care system. Although the poor reputation of the small, physician-owned, proprietary hospitals of the past was often well deserved, the new investor-owned hospital corporations are most concerned about how the community views the institutions they run. A slightly higher proportion of for-profit hospitals are accredited by the Joint Commission on Accreditation of Hospitals than comparable-sized non-profit hospitals. It seems appropriate to conclude that the "jury is still out" on the implications of the recent growth of investor-owned hospitals. Perhaps the greatest challenge is to determine how for-profit and non-profit hospitals can effectively and successfully co-exist in a pluralistic system (39, 40, 41).

NON-PROFIT HOSPITALS

Fifty-six percent of the nation's short-term hospitals are non-profit or voluntary institutions, owned and operated by community associations or religious organizations. These hospitals accommodate over two-thirds of all short-term hospital admissions and outpatient visits (Table 5–1).

COMMUNITY HOSPITALS

Taken together, non-federal short-term hospitals, whether for-profit, non-profit, or public, are commonly referred to as "community" hospitals because they are typically available to the entire community and meet the bulk of the public's need for hospital services. Community hospitals represent over 80% of the nation's hospitals, and they provide care for over 90% of all patients admitted to hospitals each year and accommodate 77% of all outpatient visits. In 1977, there were 5,973 community hospitals with about 974,000 beds (Table 5–1). The average length-of-stay in these hospitals is 7.6 days, down from the jump to 8.4 days that occurred in 1967 and 1968 after Medicare and Medicaid went into effect. The steady decline in length-of-stay since then is presumably due in part to the emphasis placed on utilization review in hospitals.

The major role of community hospitals is to provide short-term inpatient care for patients with acute illnesses and injuries. However, their outpatient role has been growing in importance as discussed in Chapter 4. In 1977, they recorded 73,000,000 emergency room visits, 55,000,000 clinic or outpatient department visits, and 76,000,000 visits by patients referred to departments such as laboratory, x-ray, or physical therapy for diagnostic or therapeutic procedures. Taken together, these three types of outpatient visits totaled 204,000,000, or six outpatient visits for every inpatient admission (8).

Community hospitals are feeling pressures to expand their roles even more to become true "community health centers" (3, 15, 16) . The fundamental rationale is that these hospitals represent their community's collective investment in health resources, assembled in one institution and financially supported by all. Hence, access to these resources should not be limited to patients who happen to need inpatient hospitalization. Community hospitals might also play a more central and substantial role in planning and coordinating the entire range of community health services, even those provided by other agencies and organizations (42). For a variety of reasons, including a lack of physician interest, health insurance coverage biases, poor reimbursement, the small size of the average community hospital, and resistance by nursing homes and other community health agencies to hospital encroachment, hospitals have been slow to expand their roles. However, many hospitals, especially the larger institutions, have added services in areas such as ambulatory care, long-term and rehabilitation care, mental health care, and home care, which indicate a movement in the direction of a broadening role (Table 5–3). It appears that the persistent rise in the public's utilization of community hospitals has finally peaked, and this has motivated many hospitals to search for new services they might offer. Perhaps this development, more than the underlying rationale, will finally give impetus to the several-decades-old concept of the hospital as a community health center (43, 44).

Almost one-half of all community hospitals have less than 100 beds, the average size being 165 beds in 1977 (8). Small hospitals tend to care for less seriously ill patients than larger hospitals. Their average length-of-stay is shorter and their care less intensive and less specialized. Small hospitals cannot support as broad a scope of services as larger hospitals and find it difficult to keep up with developments in medical technology. They also cannot support the range of management specialists found in larger hospitals (45).

PATTERNS OF FINANCING AND OWNERSHIP

Patterns of hospital financing and ownership differ from country to country. Most countries recognize health care as an essential service in which government should have a major role. In Great Britain, and many other industrialized nations, government owns and operates most of the hospitals and employs the physicians who work in them. In other countries, the government limits its role to financing

TABLE 5–3. Trends in Selected Hospital Facilities and Services (Community Hospitals), United States, 1960–1977

Facility or Service	Percent of Hospitals with Facility or Providing Service		
	1960	1977 All Hospitals	1977 300–400 Bed Hospitals
Ambulatory Care			
Emergency Service	91	89	97
Outpatient Department	54	28	52
Outpatient hemodialysis	NA*	11	24
Outpatient psychiatry	NA	14	34
Outpatient rehabilitation	NA	13	31
Outpatient Volume	(70,700,000 visits) (1962)	(204,200,000 visits)	
	(2.9 visits/admission)	(6.0 visits/admission)	
Inpatient Care			
Intensive Care Unit	10	74	99
Skilled nursing care unit	NA	13	12
Self-care unit	3	2	6
Home care program	3	7	16
Long-term Care and Rehabilitation			
Physical therapy	41	81	99
Occupational therapy	9	22	54
Skilled nursing care unit	NA	13	12
Inpatient rehabilitation unit	7(1962)	6	18
Outpatient rehabilitation unit	NA	13	31

Mental Health Care

Inpatient unit	11	19	49
Outpatient unit	NA	14	34
Partial hospitalization program	NA	9	20
Emergency services	NA	21	48
Foster and/or home care	NA	1	2
Consultation and education	NA	13	33
Clinical psychologist	NA	17	38

Other

Dental	27	36	57
Social work	15	57	93
Family planning	2(1962)	6	15
Abortion service	NA	20	38
Alcohol/drug dependency	NA	7	15
Speech therapist	NA	26	60

*NA—not available, not applicable, or none.

Source: American Hospital Association: *Hospital Statistics.* Chicago, The Association, 1978.

care provided by private hospitals and private practitioners, but in countries like Canada, where some form of comprehensive national health insurance is in effect, hospitals operate primarily on public funds and hence are essentially controlled by government. In the United States, government's role has essentially been limited to financing care for needy groups like the aged and the poor. This role has grown, however, to the point where hospitals now receive 55% of their income from government sources (primarily Medicare and Medicaid). The rest comes from private health insurance (27%), direct payments by patients (6%), and philanthropy (2%) (25). In short, the United States has a pluralistic public-private financing system with largely privately-owned hospitals. However, as the portion of hospital income financed by government has increased (from about 25% in 1960 to 55% today), so has the amount of regulation, as discussed in Chapter 11.

Government's limited role in the ownership of hospitals in the United States has been shaped by four major forces. First, the government was still relatively weak in the 1800s when the short-term hospital as it exists today was evolving as a result of advances in medical science. Innovations and progress generally came from the private sector. At that time, poverty was not so severe (or was not perceived as so severe) that the needy could not be taken care of through charity and philanthropy in private hospitals. It was generally felt that the private sector could handle the provision of care for the poor as well as for those who could pay. The exception was in major cities with large concentrations of poor. There public hospitals were established to care for the needy.

Second, government responsibility for the public's health was viewed narrowly prior to the Depression of the 1930s and was limited mainly to public safety (i.e., protecting healthy citizens from persons with communicable diseases and mental illnesses), to providing care for special groups such as merchant seamen, military, and veterans, and to assisting the needy. State governments operated communicable disease and mental hospitals; the federal government operated hospitals for its beneficiary groups; and city and county governments in large urban areas operated hospitals for the poor.

Third, our strong tradition of reliance on the private sector means that government becomes involved only when the private sector clearly fails to provide a critical service. For example, chronic disease, mental, and tuberculosis hospital care would have been difficult to finance privately. The long stays that used to prevail would have been expensive and not readily insurable. Hospitalization generally meant loss of one's job and income, especially since the incidence of hospitalization for these conditions was greatest among the poor. As a result, these areas of care have traditionally fallen to the public sector. The private sector proved better able to finance short-term hospital care through direct payments and private health insurance, and so the government's role has been supplementary. For example, the government helped to finance the construction of hospitals through the Hill-Burton program beginning in 1946, and helped to finance care for the groups that could not afford to pay, primarily the aged and the poor.

And fourth, government involvement has been resisted by the medical profession. Physicians represent a particularly powerful group in the United States, and they have long been concerned that government involvement in the health care system would compromise their economic and professional interests.

INTERNAL ORGANIZATION OF COMMUNITY HOSPITALS

From the outside, a community hospital appears as one organization with a clear goal of providing high quality patient care toward which the efforts of the professional and technical groups working in the institution are devoted. However, from the inside, it is apparent that there are at least two different organizations with two distinct sets of goals: the administrative organization which is responsible for the efficient management and operation of the institution as a whole; and the medical staff organization, responsible for the patient care provided by individual physicians. Further, there are three loci of authority within a hospital: the governing board, the medical staff, and the administration, and much balancing goes on between them (46, 47). Each authority group has a distinct responsibility. The board is ultimately responsible for everything that goes on in the hospital, both administrative and professional. It oversees the operation of the hospital and carries out its responsibility in three ways. First, it adopts policies and plans to guide the hospital's operation. Second, it chooses and delegates responsibility for the day-to-day management of the hospital to the hospital administrator and supervises his or her performance. Third, it appoints physicians to the medical staff, approves the medical staff's organization for governing itself and for supervising the professional activities of its members, and delegates responsibility to the medical staff for the provision of high quality patient care (48, 49).

In practice, the three areas of authority are neither so clear nor distinct. For example, it might seem that there is a clear distinction between governance matters and the medical staff's responsibility for patient care. Court decisions have made it clear, however, that the hospital as an institution has a corporate responsibility or legal liability for assuring that patients receive high quality patient care, and so the governing board must make sure that only qualified physicians practice in the hospital and that quality review mechanisms are established and working (50). But, only the medical staff has the expertise to actually carry out the assessment of the qualifications and care provided by physicians. Although the medical staff is clearly subordinate to the governing board in terms of authority for the affairs of the institution, physicians are independent of strict control by the board because the board does not share their expert knowledge and special skill.

Employees of the hospital working in clinical areas often find themselves in the middle when physicians' actions conflict with hospital policy. Legally, they should follow hospital policy; however, professionally they are expected to follow the physicians' orders regarding patient care, and their day-to-day working relationships are with the medical staff (51). The independence of physicians from the hospital is exacerbated because most are in private practice and not employed by the institution. On the other hand, physicians must have access to a hospital to practice modern medicine, and only the governing board has the power to grant physicians the privilege of practicing in the hospital. This unique relationship between physicians and hospitals is not without its stresses and strains, and it makes the governance and management of hospitals a challenging responsibility (52, 53).

The distinction between adopting policies to guide hospital operations, and managing operations on a day-to-day basis is not always clear either. Problems arise when the governing board becomes involved in administrative matters, like acting directly on employee grievances that come to their attention rather than referring them to the administration. On the other hand, the administration may make decisions that go beyond board policies. Thus, the community hospital is not a united front, but rather is an organization with at least two separate lines of authority, administrative and medical, and with some ambiguity between what is governance and what is management. Power at the top is shared, both because the board depends on the expertise of the medical staff and because of the independent contractor status of physicians. Administrators are also becoming more and more influential because of their expertise in dealing with the increasingly complex operational and regulatory issues confronting hospitals (54). Since the internal powers do not always agree among themselves on priorities and programs, hospitals often experience internal tensions and find it difficult to respond in a systematic way to environmental conditions and changing community needs.

THE GOVERNING BOARD

The governing board of the community hospital has evolved in function and structure as the hospital itself has developed new roles. During the late 1800s and early 1900s when advances in medical science were transforming hospitals from custodial institutions for the sick poor to sources of effective and safe care for the entire community, board members were mostly wealthy benefactors who had made substantial donations to establish and equip the hospital and to meet its deficits. The primary function of the board at that time was trusteeship, that is, preserving the assets they and others like them donated. The trustees' job was seen as providing the facilities and equipment the medical staff needed to care for their patients. There was little trustee involvement in medical matters. The administrator was essentially a clerk, and administrative duties were divided among the board members (9).

After World War I, the complexity and size of hospitals grew to the point that board members could no longer administer and financially support the hospital. Business managers were hired to handle administrative and financial matters; the business manager, along with the superintendent of nurses, reported to the board, and the board coordinated work between the two. As the complexity of the hospital and the competence of managers increased, the business manager gradually assumed responsibility for overseeing nursing and all other departments as well, so that only one person reported directly to the board. The manager's title became Superintendent. The board of trustees moved into an oversight role, relinquishing day-to-day management matters to the Superintendent (55).

The governing board's role changed further as hospitals continued to grow, as management decisions took on greater complexity and significance, and as philanthropy yielded to patient revenue as the primary source of financial support. The board's role became overall policy making and planning, and board membership was used to augment and supplement the skills of the administrative staff. Boards began to be composed of fewer philanthropists and more individuals with specific management skills such as business executives, attorneys, bankers, architects, contractors, and so forth (55, 56). Even so, community hospital boards remained relatively closed to external scrutiny, with their membership essentially comprised of self-perpetuating groups of community influentials (57, 58, 59). Board decisions were mostly in the areas of finance, personnel, and physical plant, the areas of board expertise, and boards typically deferred to the medical staff on medical and patient care matters, delegating fully the responsibility for the qualifications and quality of care provided by the medical staff.

During the 1960s four major forces caused further change in the governing board's role: 1) continuing advances in medical science, the proliferation of medical technology, and the rapid growth in the size and sophistication of hospitals gave rise to public concern about the cost of hospital care, while making the hospital even more central in the delivery of health care and valuable to the public; 2) public expectations about the hospital's responsibility to the community changed. Hospitals began to be viewed as community resources with a definite obligation to respond to community needs; 3) regulation of hospital construction, costs, quality, and utilization, and labor relations became more and more stringent, particularly following Medicare and Medicaid; and 4) the Darling legal case established the concept of corporate or institutional responsibility for assuring the quality of patient care (52, 60, 61).

As a result of these forces, the governing board's role broadened and became even more demanding (62, 63). Boards became active in environmental surveil-lance, becoming knowledgeable about community concerns and external trends, and interpreting their significance for the hospital (64, 65). External pressures forced hospitals to re-examine their priorities and programs, and boards found it necessary to provide clearer direction and stronger leadership in long-range planning. Boards have also assumed an active role in seeing that community concerns and interests are brought into hospital decision-making and many ex-panded the community representation within their membership (66, 67). The board finds itself in the role of balancing and mediating between the demands and pressures on the hospital from the community and external agencies on the one hand, and from the medical staff, employees, and other internal groups on the other (68). Finally, boards have been forced to take a more active role in quality assurance rather than abdicating this responsibility to the medical staff. Although the function of quality monitoring is still delegated to the medical staff, the staff is now being held accountable for how well this function is carried out. The board is responsible for assuring that the mechanisms for evaluating the credentials of physicians and evaluating the care they provide are established and working. Courts have held the board and the hospital responsible in malpractice cases where reasonable precautions were not taken to ensure 1) careful selection of the medical staff; 2) establishment of high standards of care; 3) monitoring and supervision of care; and 4) enforcement of policies, rules, and regulations. In practice, board control over medical staff performance remains limited and depends more on the attitudes of the medical staff, the character of hospital-medical relations, and moral suasion than on formal sanctions such as suspending or terminating a physician's privileges, an action that is very rare.

As governing boards became more actively involved in medical and patient care matters, both in determining the hospital's role and relationships with other institutions, and in overseeing quality assurance mechanisms, physicians began to seek more involvement in hospital planning and policy making. At the same time, boards felt a greater need for more direct physician participation in their deliberations (69, 70). As a result, more and more boards have added physicians to their membership, although some argue against this as a conflict of interest (71). At the present time, more than half of all community hospital boards include physicians (72, 73). Less frequent but emerging is the trend toward the administrator serving on the board, generally with a change in title to President or Executive Vice President, in a corporate type of structure (65).

Today, governing boards are being challenged and scrutinized as never before. They are being called upon to demonstrate their effectiveness in assuring that the hospitals they govern meet community needs and provide high quality care while at the same time functioning efficiently within a complex structure of guidelines and regulations, all in an environment of constant change. Not all boards are up to this task. Boards have been criticized as too inward-looking, passive, uninformed, reluctant to get involved in "medical" matters, and reluctant to change the status quo. It appears, however, that the pressures discussed above are causing boards to take active steps to broaden and strengthen their membership, educate themselves more fully, and streamline their structure so that they will be better equipped to provide the strong leadership that will be required in the future (74, 75, 76).

HOSPITAL ADMINISTRATION

Hospital administration has grown in importance and status as hospitals have grown in size and sophistication (55, 77, 78). The job of implementing board policy and responsibility for the day-to-day management and supervision of the hospital is delegated by the board to the hospital administrator. The administrator has responsibility for managing the hospital's finances, acquiring and maintaining equipment and facilities, hiring and supervising hospital personnel, and coordinating hospital activities. The breadth of the administrator's responsibility is illustrated by a typical community hospital organization chart, Figure 5–2. A key aspect of the administrator's job is to coordinate and serve as the channel of communication between the governing board, medical staff, and hospital departments. Another is planning for the future development of the hospital's services. Large hospitals have several assistant administrators, responsible for nursing (Director of Nursing), professional services, support services, and hospital finances (Comptroller).

In addition to financial, personnel, and physical plant matters, administration plays an important role in patient care as well. For example, administration is responsible for coordinating the patient care departments with each other and with the support departments, assuring that they are adequately equipped and staffed and technically up-to-date, and assuring that they function smoothly. Administration must assure that physician orders for the treatment of patients are carried out correctly and promptly by hospital personnel, but also that orders do not conflict with governing board policies or hospital rules. The administrator is also actively involved in planning for new patient care services and in assuring that the hospital

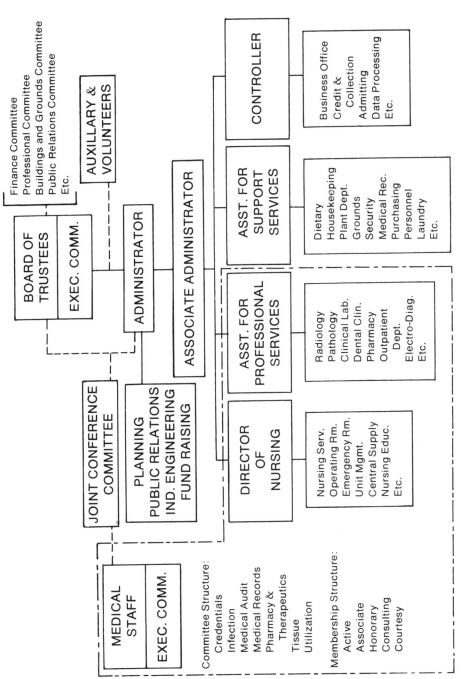

Figure 5-2. Prototype hospital organization chart. (*Source:* Reprinted with permission from Chamber of Commerce of the United States, *A Primer for Hospital Trustees*, Washington, D.C., 1974.)

147

meets accreditation, licensure, and other standards. Because the medical staff is not employed by the hospital, establishing a cooperative working relationship with the medical staff is essential for the administrator to effectively handle the many tasks that involve both administrative and medical questions. Finally, administration acts as the liaison with the community and external agencies, both bringing information from these sources into hospital decision making and planning, and representing the hospital to these outside parties. Because of the growing impact of external and regulatory pressures on hospitals, this "boundary spanning" role has become one of the most important aspects of the administrator's job. Hospital administration has advanced rapidly as a profession. Schulz and Johnson (79) describe the transition as moving from business manager (1920s–1940s), to coordinator (1950s–1960s), and now to corporate chief (with full authority for directing all aspects of the hospital's operation) and management team leader (promoting participative decision making by board, medical staff, nursing staff, and administrative representatives). Administrators are now full participants in the development of policies and plans as well as in their implementation and in the external as well as internal affairs of the hospital (80, 81, 82).

HOSPITAL MEDICAL STAFF

The governing board delegates responsibility for the provision of high quality patient care to the medical staff which is formally organized to carry out this responsibility and is accountable to the board for it (83). Unlike many advanced countries, where hospital medical staffs are composed of salaried physicians, the medical staffs of community hospitals in the United States are composed mostly of private practitioners who are not employees of the hospital. The relationship between the hospital and its medical staff is a mutually dependent and sometimes stressful one. The hospital is dependent upon the medical staff to admit and care for patients and to monitor the quality of patient care. In a sense, the clients of the hospital are the physicians, since it is they who admit patients, decide how long the patients will stay, and order hospital services. On the other hand, physicians are dependent upon hospitals because to practice modern medicine they must have access to the diagnostic and therapeutic services of the hospital on behalf of their patients. This is particularly true of specialties like obstetrics and surgery. Thus, a *quid pro quo* relationship exists; physicians agree to abide by hospital policies and medical staff rules and to devote time to the medical staff's quality monitoring activities (in the past, they also contributed time to care for patients who could not pay), in return for the privilege of using the community's hospital to care for their private patients (84, 85, 86).

Different categories of appointment to the medical staff carry different privileges and responsibilities (87):

Active medical staff members have full hospital privileges and provide most of the medical care in the hospital. They are responsible for the administrative activities of the organized medical staff. They can vote, hold office, and serve on committees;

Associate medical staff members consist of physicians new to the hospital. After a year or two probationary period, during which their work is closely watched, associate staff physicians are considered for advancement to the active medical staff. They may serve on some hospital and medical staff committees, but they cannot hold office;

Courtesy medical staff membership is comprised of physicians who would be eligible for active membership on the staff but who admit patients to the hospital only occasionally (usually because they are on the active staff of another hospital). They are not involved in any administrative functions;

Consulting medical staff are those physicians recognized for their professional expertise and who are willing to act as consultants to the hospital's medical staff, although they practice primarily in other hospitals;

House staff are the interns and residents. They function under the supervision of attending physicians, but are employees of the hospital.

In carrying out its delegated responsibility for assuring the quality of care, the medical staff governs itself, establishes qualifications for appointment to the staff and for clinical privileges, establishes standards of care and rules and regulations to guide the provision of care, and supervises the professional performance of its members. This is accomplished within the medical staff bylaws which set forth the form, functions, and responsibilities of the medical staff. The bylaws must be approved by both the medical staff and the governing board (87, 88, 89).

The administrative head of the medical staff organization is the chief-of-staff. The chief-of-staff is responsible for: 1) acting as a liaison between the governing board, the administrator, and the medical staff; 2) chairing the executive committee of the medical staff and serving as an ex-officio member of all committees and usually of the governing board; 3) establishing medical staff committees and appointing their members; 4) enforcing governing board policies; 5) enforcing medical staff bylaws, rules, and regulations; 6) maintaining standards of medical care in the hospital; and 7) providing for continuing education for the medical staff (87).

Although the chief-of-staff is usually elected by the medical staff for a one or two year term, this position is also in a sense a part of the hospital's administrative structure, directly accountable to the hospital's governing board. As such, the chief-of-staff is looked to by the board for advice on medical matters as well as for assurance that the medical staff's responsibilities are being carried out. Administration of medical staff affairs can be a time consuming job, but in most community hospitals the chief-of-staff fills this role in addition to a busy private medical practice. Larger hospitals often hire a full-time salaried medical director to carry out many of the administrative duties of the chief-of-staff, and this idea is spreading although not without controversy (90, 91, 92).

Most of the organizational responsibilities of the medical staff are carried out by committees (93, 94). The *executive committee* is the key administrative and policy-making body of the medical staff. It governs the activities of the medical staff, and all other committees are advisory to it. It is comprised of the chief-of-staff, the chiefs of the clinical departments, and members at large elected by the active medical staff. The *joint conference committee* is the formal liaison between the governing board and medical staff, and includes members from both groups plus the administrator. This committee is a forum for discussing medico-administrative matters of mutual concern. The *credentials committee* reviews the qualifications of applicants to the medical staff and makes recommendations regarding appointments, annual reappointments, and clinical privileges. Recommendations are transmitted through the executive committee of the hospital's governing board which has final decision-making authority regarding medical staff membership and privileges.

A second type of medical staff committee advises or oversees specific functional areas or departments; examples include emergency room, nursing, pharmacy, special care, and disaster committees. A third type of committee is the evaluative or quality assurance committee responsible for monitoring the patient care provided by individual physicians. These include medical audit, utilization review, and tissue committees. Finally, a continuing education committee plans educational programs for the medical staff. In larger hospitals most of these committee functions are duplicated in each clinical department.

There is a small but growing body of empirical evidence in support of the presumption that the structure of the medical staff affects quality and other aspects of hospital performance (95). Roemer and Friedman (96) studied the extent to which the degree of structuring of the medical staff influences the costliness, quality, and scope of hospital services, and found that a relationship does exist. They concluded that a fairly highly structured medical staff organization functions better than a low or moderate structure. They found that effectiveness is enhanced by a core of full-time salaried physicians within the medical staff, a comprehensive department and committee structure, clearly specified policies, rules, and regulations, and thorough documentation of medical staff activities. This type of organization pattern offers the private physicians who use the hospital the benefits of full-time hospital based physicians who provide administrative support and supervision and take the leadership in developing standards of care and educational programs. An interesting finding is that a core of full-time salaried physicians tends to stimulate the other physicians to take their quality monitoring responsibilities more seriously. The mix of both salaried and private practice physicians tends to provide an environment conducive for change and improvement. It is apparent that hospitals are moving slowly, but surely, and not without conflict, toward more highly structured forms of medical staff organization which can be held more directly accountable for quality. At the same time, medical staff officers are being asked to participate more actively in governing board and management decision making. Clearly, the hospital-physician relationship of the future will be closer than in the past (97, 98, 99).

TRENDS AND ISSUES IN THE HOSPITAL INDUSTRY

The high and persistently climbing cost of hospital care is of such great concern that it is central to much of the public policy in health. The hospital cost inflation rate since the mid-1960s has been almost three times the general economy-wide inflation rate (See Chapter 10). The key question is how to slow the trend. The special problems small and rural hospitals have attracting resources, keeping up with advances in medicine, and maintaining their financial viability raise questions about their future role and about how they should be related to larger institutions offering the specialized services they are not able to provide. A significant trend in the hospital industry is the growth of unions, particularly professional unions, and this raises questions about the impact of collective bargaining on patient care as well as about employee-employer relations. Another trend that has had great influence on hospitals is regulation: external regulatory agencies and third-party insurers are exerting more and more control over hospitals. These trends, their impact on hospitals, and the issues they raise are discussed in this section.

HOSPITAL COST INFLATION

The nation's health expenditures have been increasing dramatically with hospital spending leading the way. On a per capita basis, hospital expenditures increased from $50 per person in 1960 to $300 per person in 1977. This $300 was double the per capita spending for physicians' services, more than five times what was spent for drugs or nursing home care, and more than six times what was spent for dental services. Because the cost of hospital care has been increasing so much faster than the other elements of health care, hospitals are consuming a larger and larger share of the nation's health expenditures. About 40% of our health expenditures now go for hospital care compared to about 33% in 1960 (1).

To explain the causes of the dramatic cost inflation in the hospital sector, total hospital spending can be broken down into its parts (100, 101, 102). In 1965, $9,000,000,000 was spent for care in community hospitals. By 1975, this figure had reached $39,000,000,000, a 328% increase in ten years. About 5% of the $30,000,000,000 increase was due to growth in the population. Another 7% was due to increases in the per capita use of hospitals: the use rate rose from 1,072 days of hospital care per 1,000 population in 1965 to 1,218 days in 1975. About 36% was due to general inflation which affected the prices of all goods and services throughout the economy. The largest component of the cost increase, however, was attributable to changes in the nature of hospital output (i.e., in the intensity, scope, sophistication, and quality of hospital care) which in turn caused hospitals to employ more and better labor inputs (accounting for 24% of the 1965 to 1975 expenditure increase) and more and better non-labor inputs (accounting for the remaining 28%). In short, expenditures for hospital care have increased because more people are using hospitals more; because hospital care is more intensive and sophisticated; and because, like other businesses, hospitals must pay more for the equipment, personnel, and supplies they need (8, 103). Not answered in this breakdown of the cost increase are questions about how efficiently hospitals operate and about how much of the care they provide might be provided in less expensive settings.

A wide range of factors has caused the increase in the amount of hospital care people use (19, 104). First, availability: 566 new community hospitals have been built since 1960, and the bed supply has increased 25% from 3.6 beds per thousand population in 1960 to 4.5 beds per thousand today (8). Second, advances in medical science have brought new diagnostic and therapeutic services to hospitals and increased their effectiveness in dealing with injury and illness. Third, physicians are trained in sophisticated hospitals, and they learn to rely on the hospital's specialized equipment and personnel to back them up in caring for patients. Fourth, the population is aging such that the proportion of the population over age 65 increased from 9% in 1960 to almost 12% today, and the aged use about three and one-half times as much hospital care as the younger population. Another factor is urbanization: hospitals are more accessible to people who reside in urban areas. In addition, because of the high mobility of the population, many people do not have a family physician. Instead, they turn to the hospital emergency room and outpatient department as a substitute.

Perhaps the most important factor affecting hospital use, however, is the increase in the affluence, education, and sophistication of the population, and the resulting increase in people's ability and inclinations to seek health care. Facilitating this is the growth of private health insurance and the enactment of public financing programs for the aged and the poor. Insurance has removed much of the strain of paying for hospital care: now only 5.9% of hospital bills are paid directly out-of-pocket by patients (25). In addition to generally increasing hospital use, insurance has biased patterns of utilization toward the hospital, because the costs of services tend to be covered better by insurance if the services are provided in a hospital rather than in a physician's office or nursing home (20).

Separate and distinct from the fact that people are using hospitals more is the fact that the costs per inpatient day and outpatient visit have been increasing, both because of economy-wide inflation, and because the care provided by hospitals is changing over time (105). Hospital services are continually increasing in intensity, scope, and sophistication as a result of advances in medical science and community and physician preferences to have available in their local hospital the widest possible range of the most up-to-date services. As a result, the cost per inpatient day has increased over six times between 1960 and 1977, from about $30 per day to $200 per day. The average hospital stay now costs almost $1,500 (8).

Regarding intensity, patients today receive more lab, x-ray, and other diagnostic and therapeutic services than patients who were treated for the same conditions a few years ago (19, 102). Several factors have contributed to the increased intensity. Advances in medical science have made more diagnostic and therapeutic procedures available, and both patients and physicians want to take advantage of all that modern medicine has to offer. The nature of physician training in sophisticated hospitals may lead them to order more procedures. Another factor is the fear of malpractice suits which leads to defensive medical practice: physicians are inclined to order the extra lab test or x-ray procedure "just to make sure." The shortening length-of-stay has resulted in patients receiving more services each day than if the same services were spread over a longer period of time. Many people feel that another factor is that physicians are not directly affected financially by the costs of the services they order on behalf of their patients. A most important factor again is hospital insurance which has led patients to want the best of care regardless of costs.

Regarding the broadening scope of services offered by community hospitals, advances in medical science have created new diagnostic and treatment technology not dreamed of a few years ago. Fetal monitoring, diagnostic radioisotope procedures, computerized tomography, open-heart surgery, organ transplants, microscope surgery, radiation therapy, renal dialysis and so forth, require expensive equipment, expensive facilities, and skilled personnel. Communities and physicians alike have come to expect a wide range of services to be available in their local hospitals. As a result, there has been an increase in the scope and sophistication of services being offered by even relatively small community hospitals serving limited populations (106).

The increased investment by hospitals in equipment and facilities is reflected by a substantial increase in assets per bed. In 1960, the capital investment per bed in community hospitals was about $17,000. This figure is now well over $60,000. Expenditures for equipment, facilities, and supplies have been increasing faster than expenditures for personnel. As a result, nonpayroll expenses as a portion of total expenses increased from 38% in 1960 to 50% in 1977. However, the use of personnel has increased as well, from 2.3 employees per patient in 1960 to 3.6 in 1977, an increase of almost 60%. In addition, the skill levels of hospital personnel has increased, and more hospitals are employing physicians. The average hospital salary increased over 200% between 1960 and 1975, from $3,239 to $10,082 (8).

Another cost increasing factor is debt financing of capital projects. In the past, hospital construction projects were financed mostly by community fund raising drives, philanthropy, and government programs like Hill-Burton. As these sources of capital declined in importance, hospitals have been forced to borrow a higher proportion of the funds needed for capital projects, adding interest expense to the cost of these projects (107).

A final, and increasingly significant cost-increasing factor is the administrative costs of complying with regulations. Programs now exist to regulate hospital construction, rates and reimbursement, quality and utilization, plant safety, and labor relations to name a few (as discussed in Chapters 11 and 12). The array of complex and often conflicting requirements these agencies impose on hospitals contributes substantially to increased costs. The current situation is approaching the point where the solution is becoming part of the problem: hospitals must spend money to comply with regulations, and this adds to the costs that regulation was designed to control.

The problem of hospital cost inflation is complex, and complex problems generally call for multi-faceted solutions (21, 22, 105, 108). It would seem that any solution must first encourage the most prudent possible hospital use consistent with good medical practice. There is growing evidence that perhaps as many as one-fourth of all patient days of care provided by hospitals are not medically necessary. This is suggested by the great variation in hospital use rates from area to area and by the substantially lower hospital use rates experienced by Health Maintenance Organizations (HMOs). Less expensive alternatives such as ambulatory, long-term, and home care can be substituted for all or some portion of the hospital stays of many patients.

The public's use of hospitals might be constrained by building higher copayment and deductible provisions into health insurance policies, and limiting benefits, although the arguments against shifting more of the economic burden of health care back to the consumer are many. Other strategies include: 1) attempting to counterbalance the physicians' inclination to use the hospital by changing their financial incentives and developing more HMOs; 2) attempting to strengthen external review of the appropriateness of hospital use through Professional Standards Review Organizations (PSROs); 3) encouraging the planning of more ambulatory care, day care, home care, skilled and intermediate nursing care and other out-of-hospital care programs and improving insurance coverage for them; and 4) constraining the hospital bed supply through planning and certificate-of-need.

The question of how to deal with the increasing complexity and intensity of hospital care is equally difficult. It is physicians, not hospitals, who decide what diagnostic and therapeutic services to order for patients. Hence, changes in physician incentives and training must be part of the solution (109). Again, HMOs would seem to provide an appropriate set of incentives in this regard (109). Another approach would be to control malpractice insurance premiums and pressures which apparently cause physicians to practice defensive medicine. The financial incentives inherent in hospital reimbursement might be modified so as to discourage increases in the intensity of services.

Planning and certificate-of-need, affiliations, mergers, and shared services among hospitals, and a movement toward regionalized hospital systems may help curtail the duplication of specialized services frequently found in multi-hospital communities, achieve economies of scale, and reduce the nation's bed supply (110, 111, 112). There is increasing discussion at the federal level and among third-party purchasers of offering to buy-out unneeded hospitals. Finally, cost-containment incentives must be brought to bear on the individual institutions to encourage improvements in efficiency and productivity through modern management techniques.

A number of Blue Cross plans have experimented with incentive or prospective reimbursement schemes as an alternative to cost reimbursement in an attempt to introduce incentives to cut costs, and more than a dozen states have enacted rate regulation programs to create an environment of financial stringency that will act to slow the rate of cost increases in hospitals. Evidence to date on the effectiveness of the existing prospective reimbursement and rate regulation programs is mixed, and it is unlikely that financial controls or incentives are in and of themselves the panacea to the cost inflation problem. Rather, the answer undoubtedly lies in a coordinated program of controls and incentives to contain the pace of capital investment, discourage unnecessary utilization, reduce existing duplication and overbedding, increase productivity, and shift some economic incentives back to consumers and physicians. The key contribution of prospective reimbursement or rate regulation may be to provide the financial environment to make these other programs work (113, 114, 115, 116).

SMALL AND RURAL HOSPITALS

Considerable attention is being directed toward the special problems of the country's many small and rural hospitals. In part because Hill-Burton priorities in the early years channelled funds to thinly-populated, rural areas, the United States is a nation of many small hospitals: about one-half of all community hospitals are less than 100 beds. These hospitals face a number of problems which threaten their future viability. First, they are losing patients: admissions to community hospitals with less than 100 beds have declined as has their average daily census

(Table 5–4). Between 1967 and 1977, the number of hospitals with less than 100 beds fell from 3,442 to 2,833. Labor requirements are high in small hospitals for the services offered, and small hospitals tend to operate at less efficient levels of occupancy than larger hospitals (Table 5–5). These efficiency limitations, coupled with the limited financial means of some rural populations, have resulted in many small hospitals incurring substantial operating losses. Small hospitals offer a more limited range of services than larger institutions, because they have neither the patient volume nor the physicians or specialized personnel to support much beyond the basic essential services. Small hospitals are often located in areas where they have a difficult time attracting qualified personnel. Together, all of these problems may lead to difficulty in achieving accreditation or meeting hospital certification and licensure standards.

Finally, small hospitals find it especially difficult to keep up with and respond to the increasingly complex and demanding regulatory environment without the range of management specialists common to larger institutions, and as a result, many are contracting with investor-owned corporations or larger hospitals to take over their management (40, 45, 117, 118). It would appear that the future viability of small hospitals will depend on their adapting their mission and the services they offer to fit their resources, establishing relationships with other institutions, and seeking additional resources to support new programs to broaden their role in health care delivery in the communities they serve (119, 120, 121, 122).

Consolidation of Community Health Resources.   Because it is especially difficult for smaller hospitals to assemble the array of equipment and personnel or attain the patient volume needed to support a broad range of services, it is critical to consolidate around the small hospital to the greatest extent possible whatever health resources do exist in the community. Ideally, the hospital building or "campus" might include physicians' offices, facilities for public health nurses and

TABLE 5–4. Change in Average Daily Census by Hospital Size, United States, 1970–1977

Bed Size	Average Daily Census		Percent Change
	1970	1977	
6–24	3,989	2,516	−37
25–49	30,370	21,827	−28
50–99	74,093	65,336	−12
100–199	134,117	136,210	+ 2
200–299	113,793	131,283	+15
300–399	99,404	100,265	+ 1
400–499	69,895	86,022	+23
500 and over	135,810	171,503	+26

Source: American Hospital Association: *Hospital Statistics.* Chicago, The Association, 1978.

TABLE 5–5. Selected Indicators by Hospital Size, United States, 1977

Hospital Bed Size	Full-time Equivalent Personnel per 100 Census	Percent Occupancy
6–24	328	45.6
25–49	298	53.4
50–99	284	62.7
100–199	294	69.3
200–299	307	76.0
300–399	320	77.8
400–499	326	79.6
500 and over	349	80.1

Source: American Hospital Association: *Hospital Statistics*. Chicago, The Association, 1978.

health-related community organizations, a nursing home, and so forth. Consolidation would enable limited health resources to be stretched further and provide opportunities for jointly supporting personnel like a home-care nurse, laboratory technician, or physician assistant. The hospital need not own all of these facilities; just grouping the community's health-related activities together would be an important step. The extreme form of consolidation would be a merger of two small hospitals existing in the same or nearby communities, although there is often considerable resistance among small hospitals and their communities to a merger. A small hospital might also find the means of taking over or providing the location for an area nursing home.

Functional Differentiation.   The difficulties of providing expensive but essential services in smaller hospitals may lead to more formal functional differentiation among hospitals with regard to the levels and types of care provided. Small hospitals may drop some services and give up some types of patients they now treat, adding other services in their place. Criteria or guidelines for referrals may be developed similar to the criteria which now exist for quality and utilization review. Such criteria would specify the conditions or diagnoses that would be treated in the small hospital and those that would be referred to larger hospitals. Such criteria for referral might become a formal part of accreditation and licensure standards. By limiting the types of patients they treat, small hospitals could be exempted from inapplicable equipment, facility, and personnel standards.

Functional differentiation by level of complexity or severity of illnesses would not necessarily mean reducing the role of the smaller hospital. Smaller hospitals might expand their services in the areas of ambulatory care, preventive and health maintenance services, convalescent, extended, and long-term care, home care, and outreach services.

Regionalization.   The key to the future of smaller rural hospitals still seems to lie in the concept of regionalization, the much discussed but little implemented idea of formally relating small hospitals with larger urban hospitals (123, 124).

Regionalization begins with the concept that each level of hospital—small basic service hospitals, moderate size community hospitals, and large regional referral centers—should provide only those services they can offer efficiently and at a high level of quality. Communities would be assured access to a full range of services, not by each hospital attempting to provide every service, but rather by the development of closer relationships among networks of hospitals and their medical staffs to encourage the referral of patients to the institutional setting most appropriate to their needs. Such relationships could range from informal agreements to formal affiliations, jointly provided programs, or mergers of institutions into multi-hospital systems.

The specific objectives of regionalization include: 1) a two-way flow of patients, with patients referred to larger hospitals for specialized services and returned to smaller hospitals for convalescent care, long-term care, follow-up care, and home care; 2) continuing education for physicians, nurses, and other personnel from the small hospitals through participation in the educational programs of the larger hospital; 3) assistance from administrative, nursing, and professional department heads and specialists from the larger hospital representing skills not available in the small hospitals; 4) consolidation (in the larger hospital) and sharing of services the small hospitals cannot provide as efficiently or at the same level of quality as the larger hospital; 5) regularly scheduled visits by physician specialists from the larger hospitals to conduct clinics and serve as consultants in the small hospitals; 6) sharing of personnel; and 7) joint purchasing (125).

The success of regionalization depends on the support of the community, the governing board, and the medical staffs of both the small and larger hospitals (126). There are few examples of effective regional relationships. In part this reflects community and professional pride and a desire for independence. In part, it reflects the difficulty of working out the essential elements of regionalization: 1) the movement of referrals in both directions so that the small hospitals do not lose patients but maintain their census by providing basic, convalescent and follow-up care; 2) granting physicians from the small hospitals privileges in the larger hospital and making them feel welcome to admit and treat their patients there when they need the specialized services of the larger hospital; and 3) broadening the role of the small hospital to include convalescent and follow-up care, long-term care, home care, and so forth. In the long run, regionalization may preserve rather than threaten the independence and viability of smaller hospitals.

UNIONIZATION OF HOSPITAL PERSONNEL

Unionization of hospital employees is growing at an increasing rate. Surveys conducted by the American Hospital Association show that in 1961, 224 hospitals, 3.2% of the nation's community hospitals, were organized and had collective bargaining agreements with one or more unions. By 1967, collective bargaining agreements existed in 555 hospitals (7.7%); by 1970, 1,046 hospitals (14.7%); by 1973, 1,197 hospitals (19.7%); and by 1976, 1,327 hospitals (23.1%) (127, 128). Unionization is most common in large hospitals, particularly federal and public hospitals. California and the industrialized eastern states have the most unionized hospitals, and unionization is most common in metropolitan areas. In addition, there tend to be more unionized hospitals in states which had labor laws prior to 1974.

A variety of factors deterred the growth of unionization in hospitals until recently (129). Most hospitals are fairly small, and small organizations may be better able to settle employee problems informally than formally by collective bargaining. It is also more costly for unions to attempt to organize many small units rather than a few larger firms. A large number of different occupations are found in hospitals (about 125) suggesting that many unions would be necessary to represent all of the interests of hospital workers. The public has tended to be less supportive of union activities in essential service organizations like hospitals, feeling that humanitarian services should not be interrupted by strikes or work stoppages. In addition, many health professionals themselves have been ambivalent about whether unionization is consistent with their professional values. The labor force in hospitals is composed of a high proportion of women and part-time workers. High turnover rates are not unusual. Unions have been reluctant to attempt the difficult task of organizing this type of labor force. Finally, a significant barrier to unionization has been the absence of facilitating labor legislation in the hospital industry, since hospitals were exempted from the Taft-Hartley Act until 1974.

When Congress began to consider bringing hospitals under Taft-Hartley, hospitals pressed for special protection against strikes, priority for National Labor Relations Board action on disputes, and mandatory mediation requirements. Hospitals also wanted to limit the number of bargaining units with one each for professional, technical, clinical, and maintenance and service workers (130, 131).

In 1974, hospitals became subject to Taft-Hartley, but with special provisions. A hospital or union must give 90 days' notice to the other party of a desire to change an existing contract. The Federal Mediation and Conciliation Service (FMCS) must be given 60 days' notice, and 30 days' notice if an impasse occurs in bargaining for an initial contract after the union is first recognized. A cooling-off period of at least ten days is required before a strike can occur, to enable the hospital to plan for the care of patients. The FMCS may appoint a Board of Inquiry to mediate among the parties if it determines that a strike would impair delivery of health care to the community. Neither the hospital nor the union are required to accept the Board's recommendation, although they must provide information and witnesses called for by the Board (132).

With the exemption from Taft-Hartley removed, several factors have made the hospital industry vulnerable to rapid unionization (129, 133). First, many hospitals lag behind industry in personnel practices. A substantial number have no professional personnel director, and policies for resolving grievances, discipline, promotion, seniority, overtime, and night shift work are often poorly spelled out. Professional departments such as nursing often handle their own personnel matters, often ignoring the concerns of their non-professional workers. Wages and fringe benefits in hospitals also appear to have lagged behind other industries.

Second, supervisory training is often insufficient. Department heads and supervisors are commonly promoted because of their professional or technical skills rather than their managerial or supervisory capabilities. In addition, supervisors and professional department heads may have divided loyalties between being part of hospital management on one hand, and members of professional associations which act as unions on the other.

Third, the reluctance of professional workers to unionize has diminished. The change in attitude is attributable in part to their professional associations acting as their unions. Professional associations are more acceptable than national trade unions might have been. In addition, the professional associations point to collective bargaining not only as a means of improving wages but also as a means of negotiating over staffing standards and work perogatives that could affect the quality of patient care. The underlying issue of the balance between administrative and professional control over work and the work setting is especially important in professional organizations like hospitals and adds a unique dimension to unionization in this industry. Also unique is the fear that a strike could cause harm to patients (134, 135, 136, 137).

REGULATION OF HOSPITALS

External regulation of hospitals has grown rapidly since the mid-1960s. There are external controls over: 1) institutional quality standards (licensure, certification, accreditation); 2) construction and expansion of facilities and services (Section 1122 of the 1972 Social Security Amendments, National Health Planning and Resources Development Act, state certificate-of-need); 3) costs or rates (Blue Cross, Section 223 of the Social Security Amendments, state rate regulation); and 4) utilization (Blue Cross, Medicare, Medicaid, PSROs). Hospital regulations come from both public agencies and private organizations. All states license hospitals, and more and more are enacting certificate-of-need and rate regulation programs. Many of the federal controls are tied to the Medicare and Medicaid programs as conditions for participation or payment: certification, cost ceilings, and capital expenditure review, to name a few. The major private sector organizations which exert control over hospitals are Blue Cross plans and the Joint Commission on Accreditation of Hospitals (138, 139). These and related mechanisms are discussed in Chapters 10, 11, and 12; those that most directly affect hospitals are discussed below.

Controls on Quality.   The regulatory structure for controlling quality includes state licensure, federal certification, and voluntary accreditation (140, 141, 142). Licensure is a state function generally carried out by the department of health, whereby minimum standards are established and enforced regarding the equipment, personnel, plant, and safety features an institution must have to operate. Licensing agencies are empowered to set standards, conduct inspections, issue licenses, close facilities that cannot comply with the agency's standards, and provide consultation services. In many states, however, these agencies are underfinanced and understaffed, and so standards are not enforced stringently. In addition, there is a tendency to focus on fire, safety, and physical plant standards rather than standards for medical services.

Hospitals must be certified by the designated state agency in order to participate in Medicare and Medicaid. The purpose of certification is to assure that care for beneficiaries of these programs is only purchased from institutions which can meet acceptable minimum quality requirements. In most states, the Department of Health, Education, and Welfare (HEW) contracts with the health department to carry out the actual inspection process. Virtually all community hospitals are certified, so it can only be concluded that the administration of this program is not very stringent.

Accreditation is a professionally sponsored, voluntary process carried out by the Joint Commission on Accreditation of Hospitals (JCAH), a private organization formed in 1951 as a joint effort of the American College of Physicians, American College of Surgeons, American Hospital Association, and American Medical Association. The JCAH establishes quality standards and surveys hospitals that choose to seek accreditation voluntarily. Standards relate to both the "structure" and "process" aspects of quality, and considerable emphasis is given to the organization of the medical staff. About three-fourths of the nation's community hospitals, and over 95% of those over 200 beds, are accredited. Accreditation is designed to encourage institutions to maintain the highest possible levels of performance rather than just minimum standards. Accredited hospitals are deemed to meet HEW's certification requirement. Although the relevance and rigor of the JCAH's standards and survey procedures are not above challenge, there is little question that from a historical perspective the JCAH has been a major force in elevating institutional standards.

Controls on Facilities and Services.   Areawide hospital planning began with Hill-Burton in 1946 (143). States were required to define hospital service areas, inventory existing facilities, and identify the areas of greatest need as determined by bed to population ratios. Hospitals not eligible for or not in need of Hill-Burton funds were not constrained by the program's plans or priorities. Voluntary areawide planning was promoted by the American Hospital Association and the U.S. Public Health Service beginning in 1959; unfortunately it too had no "teeth" (138). In 1965, the Regional Medical Program was established to encourage regional planning for the dissemination of advances in the treatment of heart disease, cancer, and stroke. Federally-sponsored health planning began in earnest in 1966 with the Comprehensive Health Planning Act. State planning agencies (314 A agencies) and areawide, private, non-profit planning agencies (314 B agencies) were set up with federal aid to coordinate the development of health facilities and services and to discourage overbuilding and duplication. These agencies had little economic or political power, however, and no legal means of stopping capital projects, and it is generally agreed that few were effective (144).

The 1972 Social Security Amendments (Section 1122) added "clout" to facility and services regulation by authorizing denial of Medicare and Medicaid reimbursement for building and depreciation expenses for capital projects over $150,000 not approved by the designated state agency. Proposed projects were reviewed by area Comprehensive Health Planning (CHP) agencies, but approval powers remained with the state. There is some evidence that Section 1122 and state certificate-of-need programs have constrained the growth in beds although not in equipment and other capital investments (145). These issues are discussed further in Chapter 11. The most recent federal planning and regulation program is the National Health Planning and Resources Development Act of 1974 which establishes a network of state and areawide planning agencies. This program links federal funding more closely with state regulation and requires states to establish certificate-of-need programs which require prior approval by the state agency of plans to build or modernize facilities or add new services costing in excess of $100,000 (110, 111, 146, 147).

Cost Controls.   Programs to control hospital costs or regulate hospital rates have been introduced by federal and state agencies and by private third-party purchasers as a result of their concern over the rapid rise in their expenditures for hospital care (116, 148, 149, 150). Most Blue Cross plans reimburse hospitals on the basis of costs, and so they are directly affected by cost increases which they must pass on to subscribers in the form of premium increases. State insurance commissioners become involved because of their authority over Blue Cross premiums. Much of the pioneering work in attempting to incorporate cost containment incentives in reimbursement schemes must be credited to a number of the major Blue Cross plans. However, the impact of these incentives was limited by Blue Cross' close relationship with hospitals, its lack of mandatory sanctions, and because its economic "clout" was limited to only its share of a hospital's patients.

Public involvement in cost controls and rate regulation began in earnest after the rapid post-Medicare inflation in hospital costs in the mid to late 1960s. Medicare had adopted cost-based reimbursement and so was directly affected by cost increases, just like Blue Cross. Section 223 of the 1972 Social Security Amendments authorized Medicare to set upper limits on routine inpatient service costs for reimbursement purposes, and Section 1122 limited Medicare reimbursement for capital expenditures made without approval of the designated state planning agency.

The Economic Stabilization Program (ESP), which President Nixon imposed in 1971 to deal with economy-wide inflation, set caps on the amount that hospitals could raise their rates from year to year. Hospitals were subject to ESP until 1974. It appears that this stringent program did slow rate increases and to a lesser degree cost increases during the 1971–74 period, although costs soared dramatically as soon as the controls were removed. In the late 1970s, the Carter administration is pushing for the reestablishment of federal cost and revenue controls for the hospital industry (151). In addition to federal efforts, about a dozen states concerned about controlling their Medicaid expenditures have empowered state agencies or special public utility-type commissions to regulate hospital rates. In general, these agencies approve prospectively the rates hospitals may charge for their services based on budget review or formula methods for projecting hospital costs or financial need for the coming year. Hospitals are then reimbursed at these rates rather than on the basis of the costs they actually incur. Thus, hospitals are at risk to keep their costs below the prospectively set rates. Evidence regarding the effectiveness of state prospective rate-setting programs in containing costs is sparse but suggests that this strategy may have considerable potential. The critical question may well be whether this cost containment potential can be exploited with enough care and sensitivity that the quality and financial viability of the hospital system is protected (113, 152, 153, 154).

Control of Utilization.   The most recent form of regulation in the hospital industry is the attempt to control utilization (155, 156, 157). Medicare first required that hospitals and extended care facilities establish utilization review programs as a condition for certification as participating providers. Physician committees were to review the medical records of discharged Medicare patients to determine the necessity of the hospital care provided. This requirement was seen as a way to discourage inappropriate admissions and unnecessarily long lengths-of-stays and hence as a means of keeping Medicare and Medicaid expenditures down. However, utilization review raises a number of sensitive issues, because establishing standards and monitoring physician practices with regard to hospitals may be seen as infringing on professional judgment regarding patient care.

Building on the utilization review requirements, the 1972 Social Security Amendments established Professional Standards Review Organizations (PSROs) to strengthen the appropriate monitoring process. PSROs are non-profit associations of physicians that review the care provided Medicare and Medicaid patients in all institutions in their area under contract with HEW. PSROs are to establish objective standards of treatment against which utilization can be judged. They can delegate the actual review function to hospital medical audit and utilization review committees, but must monitor the outcome of hospital-based reviews to assure their effectiveness.

The question of whether or not the hospital industry "should" be regulated is a moot point at this time because a complex regulatory environment already exists. That environment is fragmented because a great number of individual regulatory programs have evolved as specific responses to specific problems. Attempts to coordinate and nationalize the multiplicity of regulatory programs to impact on the entire delivery system in a positive manner are relatively recent (119). Regulation has become expensive for hospitals as well, calling for more careful cost-benefit analysis of regulatory requirements. The main criticisms of current external regulatory practices are "1) excessive reporting and inspection, which often takes the form of duplication and sometimes leads to conflicting requirements; 2) multiple centers of authority and accountability; 3) lack of incentives to institutions and professionals to achieve effective delivery of health care; and 4) subsidization of some groups and services by others through cost shifting" (158, 159). These and related issues of regulation are discussed further in Chapter 11.

REFERENCES

1. Gibson RM, Fisher CR: National health expenditures, fiscal year 1977. *Social Security Bulletin,* 41(7):3–20, 1978.
2. Knowles J: The hospital. *Scientific American* 229:128–137, 1973.
3. Somers AR: *Health Care in Transition: Directions for the Future.* Chicago, Hospital Research and Education Trust, 1971.
4. Schulz R, Johnson AC: *Management of Hospitals.* New York, McGraw-Hill, 1976, p. 33–36.
5. Shortell SM: Organization of hospital resources, In American Hospital Association: *Hospitals in the 1980s.* Chicago, American Hospital Association, 1977.

6. Goldsmith S: *Ambulatory Care.* Aspen Systems Corporation, Germantown, Maryland, 1977.

7. Williams S, Shortell S, Dowling W, et al: Hospital sponsored primary care group practice: a developing modality of care. *Health and Medical Care Services Review* 1(5/6):1–13, 1978.

8. American Hospital Association: *Hospital Statistics.* Chicago, The Association, 1978.

9. MacEachern MT: *Hospital Organization and Management,* 3rd ed. Chicago, Physicians Record Company, 1957.

10. Rosenberg S: The hospital in America: a century's perspective, in *Medicine and Society.* Philadelphia, American Philosophical Society Library, Publication No. 4, 1971.

11. Rosen G: The hospital—historical sociology of a community institution, in Friedson E (ed): *The Hospital in Modern Society.* Glencoe, New York, The Free Press, 1963, p. 1–36.

12. Corwin EH: *The American Hospital.* New York, The Commonwealth Fund, 1946, p. 193–213.

13. Commission on Hospital Care: Expansion of hospitals, 1840–1900, in *Hospital Care in the United States.* Cambridge, The Commonwealth Fund, Harvard University Press, 1947, p. 454–526.

14. Davis K: The hospital's position in American Society, in Owen J (ed): *Modern Concepts in Hospital Administration.* Philadelphia, W.B. Saunders Company, 1962, p. 6–16.

15. Brown RE: The general hospital has a general responsibility. *Hospitals* 39(12):47–54, 1965.

16. McKeown T: Medical education and medical care: an examination of traditional concepts and suggestions for change, in Knowles J (ed): *Doctors, Hospitals, and the Public Interest.* Cambridge: Harvard University Press, 1965, p. 254–270.

17. Somers AR: *Health Care in Transition: Directions for the Future, op. cit.,* p. 27–38.

18. Somers AR: *Health Care in Transition: Directions for the Future, op. cit.,* p. 39–72.

19. Feldstein M: *The Rising Cost of Hospital Care.* Washington, D.C., Information Resources Press, 1971.

20. *Trends Affecting the U.S. Health Care System.* Bureau of Health Planning and Resource Development, Health Planning Information Service, DHEW Publication No. HRA 76-14503, 1976, p. 195–199.

21. Davis K: Rising hospital costs: possible causes and cures. *Bulletin of the New York Academy of Medicine* 48:1354–1371, 1972.

22. McCarthy CM: Supply and demand and hospital cost inflation. *Medical Care Review* 33:923–948, 1976.

23. *Trends Affecting the U.S. Health Care System. op. cit.,* p. 124, 173–75.

24. *Trends Affecting the U.S. Health Care System. op. cit.,* p. 91–95.

25. Gibson RM, Fisher CR: National health expenditures, fiscal year 1977. *op.cit.,* p. 10.

26. Schulz R, Johnson AC: *Management of Hospitals. op. cit.,* p. 30–43.

27. Cooney J: Public hospitals: we must love them or leave them, study says. *Modern Hospital* 118(5):87–92, 1972.

28. Dumbaugh K, Bentkover J, Neuhauser D: Public hospitals: an evolution, in Levin A (ed): *Health Services: The Local Perspective, Proceedings of the Academy of Political Science* 32(3):148–158, New York, The Academy, 1977.

29. Conference Report: Impact of government programs on public hospitals—directions for the future. *Public Health Reports* 83:53–60, 1968

30. Tetelman A: Public hospitals—critical or recovering? *Health Services Reports* 88:295–304, 1973.

31. Levin PJ: Public hospitals must adapt to changes in the delivery system. *Hospitals* 51(8):81–88, 1977.

32. *The Future of the Public General Hospital—An Agenda for Transition.* Report of the Commission on Public General Hospitals (R. Nelson, chairman). Chicago, Hospital Education and Research Trust, 1978.

33. Steinwald B, Neuhauser D: The role of the proprietary hospital. *Law and Contemporary Problems* 35:817–838, 1970.

34. Stewart DA: The history and status of proprietary hospitals. *Blue Cross Reports,* Research Series No. 9, Chicago, Blue Cross Association, 1973.

35. Miller A: An address before the New York Society of security analysts. Bal Cynwyd, Pa, American Medicorp, Inc., 1977.

36. Special report on the nation's leading proprietary and voluntary multiunit hospital systems. *Modern Healthcare* 125:46–59, 1978.

37. Kushman JE, Nuckton CF: Further evidence on the relative performance of proprietary and nonprofit hospitals. *Medical Care* 15:189–204, 1977.

38. *Trends Affecting the U.S. Health Care System. op. cit.,* p. 299–305.

39. Hill DB, Stewart DA: Proprietary hospitals versus non-profit hospitals: a matched sample analysis in California. *Blue Cross Reports,* Research Series 9, Chicago, Blue Cross Association, 1973.

40. Ruchlin H, Pointer D, Cannedy L: A comparison of for-profit investor-owned chain and nonprofit hospitals. *Inquiry* 10(4):13–23, 1973.

41. Schweitzer SO, Rafferty J: Variations in hospital product: a comparative analysis of proprietary and voluntary hospitals. *Inquiry* 13:158–166, 1976.

42. Terris M: The comprehensive health center. *Public Health Reports* 78:861–866, 1963.

43. Somers AR: *Health Care in Transition: Directions for the Future. op. cit.,* p. 99–126.

44. Somers AR: Towards a rational community health care system: the Hunterdon model. *Hospital Progress* 54(4):46–54, 1973.

45. Spitzer WD: The small general hospital: problems and solutions. *Milbank Memorial Fund Quarterly* 48:413–477, 1970.

46. Coe R: *Sociology and Medicine.* New York, McGraw-Hill, 1970, p. 264–288.

47. Georgopoulos BA (ed.) *Organizational research in Hospitals.* Ann Arbor, University of Michigan Press, 1973.

48. Broehl WD: Policy formulation and implementation: the governing board in Moss AB, Broehl WG, Guest RH (eds): *Hospital Policy Decisions: Process and Action.* New York, G.P. Putnam & Sons, 1966, p. 23–79.

49. Melkonian D, Raichel T: Organization of a hospital. *Provider Review Manual.* Chicago, Blue Cross Association, 1974, p. 18–50.

50. Southwick A: The hospital as an institution—expanding responsibilities change its relationship with the staff physician. *California Western Law Review* 9:429–467, 1973.

51. Smith HL: Two lines of authority are one too many: the hospital dilemma. *Modern Hospital* 84:59–64, March 1955.

52. Perkins R: The physician's view of the hospital: a love-hate relationship. Parts 1 and 2, *Hospital Medical Staff* 4(4):1–7, 1975; 4(5):10–14, 1975.

53. Scott WR: The medical staff and the hospital: an organizational perspective. *Hospital Medical Staff* 1:33–38, 1973.

54. Perrow C: Goals and power structure: a historical care study, in Friedson E (ed): *The Hospital in Modern Society.* Glencoe, New York, The Free Press, 1963.

55. Johnson EL: Changing role of the hospital's chief executive officer. *Hospital Administration* 15:21–34, 1970.

56. Gilmore K, Wheeler J: A national profile of governing boards. *Hospitals* 46:105–108, 1972.

57. Blankenship LV, Elling RH: Organizational support and community power structure: the hospital. *Journal of Health and Human Behavior* 3:257–369, 1962.

58. Burling T, Lentz EM, Wilson RN: The board of trustees, in *The Give and Take in Hospitals*. New York, G. P. Putnam & Sons, 1956, 39–50.

59. *Trends Affecting the U.S. Health Care System. op. cit.,* p. 339–341.

60. Perloff E: Health care issues for the 70s: for the trustee, deepening responsibilities. *Hospitals* 44(1):84–89, 1970.

61. Springer E: The Darling case: ten years later. *Hospital Medical Staff* 4(6):1–7, 1975.

62. Schulz R, Johnson AC: *Management of Hospitals. op. cit.,* p. 47–67.

63. Willits RD: What boards of trustees do. *Trustee* 27(5):1–8, 1974.

64. Marmor T: Public accountability and consumerism, in American Hospital Association *Hospitals in the 1980s*. Chicago, The Association, p. 189–202.

65. Pfeffer J: Size, composition and function of hospital boards of directors: a study of organization-environment linkage. *Administrative Science Quarterly* 18:349–364, 1973.

66. Bellin L: Changing composition of voluntary hospital boards—an inevitable prospect for the 1970s. *HSMHA Health Reports* 86:674–681, 1971.

67. Cathcart HR: Including the community in hospital governance. *Hospital Progress* 51(10):72–76, 1970.

68. Kovner A: Hospital board members as policy-makers. *Medical Care* 12:971–982, 1974.

69. Jorgenson CJ: Should doctors be on your board? *Hospital Administration* 15(4):6–13, 1970.

70. Guest R: The role of the doctor in institutional management, Georgeopoulos B (ed): in *Organizational Research in Health Institutions*. Ann Arbor, University of Michigan Press, 1972.

71. Hahn JA, Bornemeier W: AHA, AMA leaders present views on physician board membership. *Hospital Topics* 48(7):24–25, 1970.

72. Schulz R: Does staff representation equal active participation? *Hospitals* 46(24):31–35, 1972.

73. A profile of the hospital trustee. *Trustee* 28(1):21–23 and 26, 1975.

74. Kovner A: Improving community hospital board performance. *Medical Care* 16:79–89, 1978.

75. Prybil LD, Starkweather DB: Current perspectives on hospital governance. *Hospital and Health Services Administration* 21:67–75, 1976.

76. Study points way to better governance. *Hospitals* 48(19):35–38, 1974.

77. Schulz R, Johnson AC: *Management of Hospitals. op. cit.,* p. 129–164.

78. Thompson J, Filerman G: Trends and developments in education for hospital administration. *Hospital Administration* 12:13–32, 1967.

79. Schulz R, Johnson AC: *Management of Hospitals. op. cit.,* p. 147–164.

80. Kovner A: The hospital administrator and organizational effectiveness, in Georgeopoulos B (ed): *Organization Research on Health Institutions. op. cit.,* p. 355–376.

81. Kuhl IK: *The Executive Role in Health Services Delivery Organization*. Washington, D.C., Association of University Program in Health Administration, 1977.

82. White R: The hospital administrator's emerging professional role, in Arnold MF, Blankenship LV, Hess JM (eds): *Administering Health Systems*. Chicago, Aldine-Atherton, 1971.

83. Williams KJ: Basic principles of medical staff organization. *Hospital Progress* 51(3):50–55, 1970.

84. Perkins R: The physician's view of the hospital: a love-hate relationship. *op. cit.,* part 2, p. 12.

85. Schulz R, Johnson AC: *Management of Hospitals. op. cit.,* p. 68–69.

86. Williams KJ: Medical staff issues—past and present. *Hospital Medical Staff* 1(1):2–13, 1972.

87. Joint Commission on Accreditation of Hospitals: *Accreditation Manual for Hospitals.* Chicago, The Commission, p. 78–89, 1978.
88. Blaes SM: Why and how should medical staff laws be revised? *Hospitals* 47(23):100–106, 1973.
89. Mills DH: Staff bylaws: an internal code of conduct. *Hospital Medical Staff* 5(8):7–9, 1976.
90. Fischer DC: Catholic Hospital Guidelines—Physician-directors: logical next step. *Hospital Progress* 56(3):28–33, 1975.
91. Harvey JD: The hospital medical director: an administrator's view. *Hospital Progress* 51(11):80–84, 1970.
92. Williams KJ: Does your hospital need a medical director? *Medical Economics* 15(22):228–236, 1973.
93. Jack WW: Medical staff functions and leadership. *Hospital Progress* 51(11):76–79, 1970.
94. Roemer M, Friedman E: *Doctors in Hospitals.* Baltimore, John Hopkins University Press, 1971, p. 29–48.
95. Shortell SM: Hospital medical staff organization: structure, process, and outcome. *Hospital Administration* 19:96–107, 1974.
96. Roemer M, Friedman E: *Doctors in Hospitals. op. cit.*
97. Johnson EA: An emerging medical staff organization. *Hospital Administration* 17:26–38, 1972.
98. Paxton HT: No more autonomy for hospital medical staffs. *Medical Economics* 48(Nov22):35–44, 1971.
99. *Trends Affecting the U.S. Health Care System. op. cit.,* p. 333–338.
100. Altman SH, Eichenholz J: Inflation in the health industry: causes and cures, in Zubkoff M (ed): *Health: A Victim or Cause of Inflation?* New York, Milbank Memorial Fund, 1976. p. 7–30.
101. McMahon JA, Drake DF: Inflation and the hospital, in Zubkoff M (ed): *Health: A Victim or Cause of Inflation?* New York, Milbank Memorial Fund, 1976. p. 130–148.
102. Raske K: Components of inflation: an analysis of the causes of increases in hospital cost. *Hospitals* 48(13):67–70, 1974.
103. Drake DF, Raske KE: The changing hospital economy, *Hospitals.* 48(22):34–40, 1974.
104. *Trends Affecting the U.S. Health Care System. op. cit.,* p. 162–176.
105. Schulz R, Johnson AC: *Management of Hospitals. op. cit.,* p. 202–222.
106. *Trends Affecting the U.S. Health Care System. op. cit.,* p. 321–328.
107. *Trends Affecting the U.S. Health Care System. op. cit.,* p. 179–181.
108. McMahon JA, Drake DF: Inflation and the Hospital. *op. cit.*
109. Redisch MA: Physician involvement in hospital decision making, in Zubkoff M, Raskin E, Hauft RS (eds): *Hospital Cost Containment—Selected Notes for Future Policy.* New York, Milbank Memorial Fund, 1978, p. 217–243.
110. Institute of Medicine: *A Policy Statement—Controlling the Supply of Hospital Beds.* Washington, D.C., National Academy of Sciences, 1976.
111. McClure W: *Reducing Excess Hospital Capacity.* Minneapolis, Interstudy, 1976.
112. *Trends Affecting the U.S. Health Care System. op. cit.,* p. 99–108.
113. Dowling WL: Prospective rate setting—concept and practice. *Topics in Health Care Financing* 2:1–37, 1976.
114. Griffith JR, Hancock W, Munson FC: Practical ways to contain hospital costs. *Harvard Business Review* 51(6):131–139, 1973.
115. Thueson J: Hospitals' programs and progress in cost containment reported. *Hospitals* 51(18):131–138, 1977.
116. *Trends Affecting the U.S. Health Care System. op. cit.,* p. 137–140, 200–210.
117. Kernaghan SG: Legislation: the painful shot in the arm. *Hospitals* 48:65–75, 1974.

118. Cooper JK, Heald K, Samuel SM, et al: Rural or urban practice: factors influencing the location decision of primary care physicians. *Inquiry* 12:18–25, 1975.

119. American Hospital Association: *Delivery of Health Care in Rural America.* Chicago, The Association, 1977, pp. 38–61.

120. American Medical Association: *Health Care Delivery in Rural Areas.* Chicago, The Association, 1976.

121. Madison DL: Recruiting physicians for rural practice. *Health Services Reports* 88:758–762, 1973.

122. United States Public Health Service: *Building a Rural Health System.* DHEW Pub. No. (HSA) 76-15028. Rockville, Md., Bureau of Community Health Services, 1976.

123. Phillips D: Reaching out to rural communities: hospital's expanding role as a social agency parts 1 and 2. *Hospitals* 46(11):33–38, 46(12):53–57, 1972.

124. Rannels HW, Ross DE, Waxman CR: The community hospital and regional health care responsibilities—how to do it! *Medical Care* 13:885–896, 1975.

125. McNerney WJ, Riedel D: *Regionalization and Rural Health Care.* Research Series No. 2. Ann Arbor, Bureau of Hospital Administration, University of Michigan, 1962.

126. Strowbridge RH: How to cope with the big problems of a small or rural hospital. *Trustee* 26(8):3–7, 1973.

127. Frenzen PD: Survey updates unionization activities. *Hospitals* 52(15):93–98, 1978.

128. Juris, H Rosmann, Maxey C, et al: Nationwide survey shows growth in union contracts. *Hospitals* 51(6):122–130, 1977.

129. Schulz R, Johnson AC: *Management of Hospitals, op. cit.,* p. 237–255.

130. American Hospital Association. *Taft Hartley Amendments: Implications for the Health Care Field, Report of a Symposium.* Chicago, The Association, 1976.

131. Rosmann J: One year under Taft-Hartley. *Hospitals* 49(24):64–68, 1975.

132. Pointer D, Metzger N: *The National Labor Relations Act: A Guidebook for Health Care Facility Administrators.* New York, Spectrum Publications, 1975, pp. 41–60.

133. Rakich, JS: Hospital unionization: causes and effects. *Hospital Administration* 18(1):7–18, 1973.

134. Davis LJ, Foner M: Organization and unionization of health workers in the United States—the trade union perspective. *Internatl J of Health Services* 5:19–36, 1975.

135. Phillips DF: New demands of nurses: San Francisco area nurses' strike, parts 1 and 2. *Hospitals* Vol. 48, No. 16, Aug. 16, 1974; 48(18):41–44, Sept. 16, 1974.

136. Bloom BS: Collective action by professionals poses problems for administrators. *Hospitals* 51(6):167–174, 1977.

137. Wilmot IG: Management's viewpoint, in AMA, *Taft-Hartley Amendments: Implications for the Health Care Field.* Chicago, The Association, p. 78–94, 1976.

138. Somers AR: *Hospital Regulation: The Dilemma of Public Policy.* Princeton, N.J., Princeton University, Industrial Relations Section, 1969.

139. Schulz R, Johnson AC: *Management of Hospitals. op. cit.,* p. 256–271.

140. Somers AR: *Health Care in Transition: Directions for the Future. op. cit.,* p. 101–131.

141. Schulz R, Johnson AC: *Management of Hospitals. op. cit.,* p. 185–201.

142. Schlicke CP: American surgery's noblest experiment: the story of hospital accreditation. *Archives of Surgery* 106:379–385, 1973.

143. Somers, AR: *Health Care in Transition: Directions for the Future. op. cit.,* p. 132–161.

144. *Trends Affecting the U.S. Health Care System. op. cit.,* p. 91–109.

145. Salkever DS, Bice TW: Certificate-of-need legislation and hospital costs, in Zubkoff M, Raskin E, Hauft RS (eds): *Hospital Cost Containment: Selected Notes for Future Policy. op. cit.,* pp. 429–460.

146. Chassin MR: The containment of hospital costs: a strategic assessment. *Medical Care* (suppl) 16:21–26, 1978.

147. *Trends Affecting the U.S. Health Care System.* op. cit., p. 91–109.

148. *Controlling the Cost of Health Care.* NCHSR Policy Research Services, DHEW Publication No. (HRA) 77-3182, 1977.
149. Zubkoff M, Rankin IE, Hanft RS (eds.): *Hospital Cost Containment—Selected Notes for Future Policy.* New York, Milbank Memorial Fund, 1978.
150. Somers AR: *Hospital Regulation: The Dilemma of Public Policy. op. cit.,* p. 162–191.
151. Dunn W, Lefkowitz B: The hospital cost containment act of 1977: an analysis of the administration's proposal, in Zubkoff M, Raskin E, Hauft RS (eds): *Hospital Cost Containment—Selected Notes for Future Policy. op. cit.,* p. 166–214.
152. Bauer K: Hospital rate setting—this way to salvation? in Zubkoff M, Raskin E, Hauft RS (eds): *Hospital Cost Containment—Selected Notes for Future Policy. op. cit.,* N.Y. Milbank Memorial Fund, 1978, p. 324–369.
153. Chassin MR: The containment of hospital costs: a strategic assessment, *op. cit.,* p. 36–45.
154. Hellinger FJ: An empirical analysis of several prospective reimbursement systems, in Zubkoff M, Raskin E, Hauft RS (eds): *Hospital Cost Containment—Selected Notes for Future Policy. op. cit.,* pp. 370–400.
155. Chassin MR: The containment of hospital costs: a strategic assessment, *op. cit.,* p. 27–35.
156. Goran MJ, Roberts JS, Kellogg M, et al: The PSRO hospital review system. *Medical Care* 13(suppl):1–33, 1975.
157. *Trends Affecting the U.S. Health Care System. op. cit.,* p. 131–136.
158. American Hospital Association; *Hospital Regulation.* Report of the Special Committee on the Regulatory Process. Chicago, The Association, 1977, pp. 17–26.
159. O'Donoghue P: *Evidence About the Effects of Health Care Regulation: An Evaluation and Synthesis of Policy Relevant Research.* Denver, Spectrum Research, Inc., 1974.

CHAPTER 6

The Nursing Home:
Neither Home
Nor Hospital

Robert L. Kane

Rosalie Kane

This chapter discusses the long-term care needs of society with a particular emphasis on the role of the nursing home. The discussion also serves to emphasize the broader social and environmental concerns that must be considered in any examination of health services. The nursing home vividly illustrates past failures to maintain this broader perspective.

The nursing home has assumed a residual role in our health and social systems. In a sense, it is the station of last resort for a variety of different groups. Although most identified with the aged and elderly clientele, it also serves the chronically and seriously ill of all ages. In recent times it has become the successor to the state mental hospital, housing both elderly and not-so-elderly former state hospital patients who were transferred to so-called community treatment. Nursing home patients have been termed "the copeless." However, it is our social system which seemingly cannot cope with the problems created by prolonged adult dependency. The makeshift solution—the nursing home which is largely insulated from public scrutiny and involvement—cares for the severely disabled, the terminally ill, the deranged, the senile, the frail, and the homeless once the fragile layer of family or other resources has been exhausted by the chronicity of the problem. Our society has built more varied supports for dependent children than for dependent adults.

From a broader social perspective, the nursing home reflects our growing tendency to substitute institutions for services that used to be performed by natural, or at least commonly available, social groups such as the extended family and community charities. Historically, the nursing home can trace its origins to the almshouse as well as to the hospital. This mixed parentage has produced a confusion that plagues those who seek to improve the situation. Even today it is not clear whether nursing home care and related alternatives should be considered a social or a medical service. This unresolved conflict produces a variety of problems to be addressed in this chapter.

HISTORICAL DEVELOPMENT

The historical vacillation between "indoor" and "outdoor" relief (institutional care versus support payments) that began with Elizabethan Poor Laws can still be seen today in discussions of alternatives to nursing home care, most specifically home care. Given the fluctuating pattern of enthusiasm for either alternative, a definitive and permanent decision one way or the other seems unlikely.

The proprietary nursing home of today had its origins in the third decade of this century with the passage of the original federal Social Security legislation; the development of nursing home policy in one state is described elsewhere (1). Pensions provided the first financial base for small homes to care for elderly persons no longer able to care for themselves. In many instances, the homes grew out of a family's efforts to care for an aged parent or spouse or from a boarding house situation.

For the next several decades, nursing homes remained literally a cottage industry. The exceptions were the large, usually local, governmental institutions for the indigent elderly, facilities operated by voluntary agencies, and state mental institutions containing substantial numbers of elderly persons classified as senile.

The 1950 amendments to the Social Security Act provided for aid to the permanently and totally disabled, including those in long-term medical institutions. This offered a major source of federal support for nursing home care and an inducement to move patients out of hospitals.

With the passage of titles XVIII and XIX of the Social Security Act in 1965, substantial resources became available to support the care of elderly. The nursing home industry was directly affected. Not only was there a stimulus to growth, there was also a series of regulations designed to assure at least a minimum standard of care. In another sense, the passage of Medicare and Medicaid is important as a social value landmark; nursing home care was placed under medical jurisdiction and the nursing home has continued ever since to be monitored as a cousin of the hospital.

Figure 6–1 traces the growth in the number of nursing homes, and nursing home beds, over a ten year span that includes the introduction of Medicare and Medicaid. Not only is there a marked increase in the numbers, but there is also a growing predominance of nursing care services over simple domiciliary care. The growth in nursing home resources was paralleled by a growing cost for this care. By 1975, nursing home expenditures had reached $9,000,000,000, representing 8.7% of total personal health care expenditures for that year. This was a dramatic increase over 1950 when nursing home care had been only 1.7% of personal health care expenditures.

The source of payment has also changed. As shown in Figure 6–2 during the early 1970s and thereafter public funds for nursing home care exceeded private funds. In 1975, just over 53% of nursing home expenditures were supported by

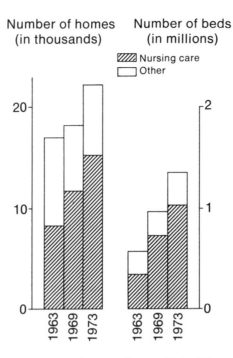

Figure 6–1. Growth of the nursing home industry, United States, 1963–1973. (*Source:* United States National Center for Health Statistics: *Health Resources Statistics,* Washington, D.C., U.S. Government Printing Office, 1975.)

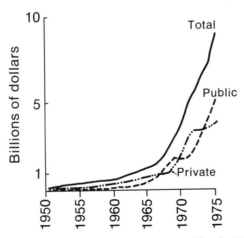

Figure 6–2. Nursing home expenditures by source of funds, United States, 1950–1975. (*Source:* United States National Center for Health Statistics: *Health Resources Statistics,* Washington, D.C., U.S. Government Printing Office, 1975.)

Medicaid, only 3% by Medicare, 2% by Veterans' programs and about 42% came from patients and their families. The relatively low expenditures under Medicare might seem surprising at first until one remembers that Medicare covers only short stays (up to 60 days) for skilled care.

DESCRIPTIVE DATA ON NURSING HOMES

At this point, it is useful to examine descriptions of nursing homes and the people who live and work in them. A few facts are important to clarify the marked differences between nursing homes and hospitals. Pertinent data are summarized in Table 6–1; unless otherwise indicated, all data is based on the 1973–74 and 1977 National Nursing Home Surveys (2–7). The 1973–74 data indicate that: 1) nursing homes are generally small scale operations; the average size is about 75 beds; 2) nursing homes are primarily operated under proprietary auspices; about 75% of the homes and 70% of the beds are operated for profit; 3) nursing homes are not heavily staffed. In all, there is about two-thirds of a full-time equivalent person per bed. About two-thirds of the staff are nursing personnel; 4) nursing homes are generally full; over 70% have waiting lists; and 5) in 1974, the average monthly charge for nursing home care was around $500; about one percent of residents did not pay anything and about three percent paid over $1,000 a month.

These data are based on a national sample. There is considerable variation from place to place. For example, the breakdown of total nursing home beds per 1,000 people aged 65 and above ranges from a high of 105 in Minnesota and Wisconsin to a low of under 30 in West Virginia and Florida. Instructively, the occupancy rate is uniformly high whatever the availability of beds.

THE NURSING HOME SCENE

Nursing homes in the United States imply some form of supervised care for medical and medically related problems. The term embraces those facilities which offer skilled nursing care, those which are personal care homes, and those with intermediate levels of care. The level of care is usually defined by the level of nursing effort required. A large proportion of people in nursing homes in the United States would, in other countries, be served in old age homes under social service auspices. Under those circumstances, the term "nursing home" is reserved to connote a more chronic hospital situation funded under health auspices.

The nursing home, in turn, is categorized as a "long-term care" facility. Technically, long-term care alludes to any care for a chronic problem on either an ambulatory or institutional basis. In practice, the term is used to refer to a prolonged service in a chronic care institution or its equivalent. A major point of contention currently is the definition of an "equivalent" to chronic institutional care. Suggestions include combinations of home health care, geriatric day centers, and day hospitals. Much work is still needed to determine whether such equivalents are truly substitutive for the nursing home or whether they are added requirements applicable to specific segments of a comprehensive health program for the elderly.

The picture of the nursing home is quite different from the profile of the general hospital. The latter tends to be larger (on the order of 160 beds) with more personnel (about 250 per 100 beds); only about 15% of general hospitals are proprietary. Length-of-stay is expressed in terms of days rather than months or years. The spectrum of problems treated is shifted toward the more acute illnesses. The costs of a single hospital day approach the average monthly nursing home charge. Even this brief list of differences suffices to predict the difficulties that can be anticipated in imposing a set of hospital-derived values onto the nursing home.

The residents of nursing homes are most easily categorized by their age (Fig. 6–3); three-quarters of the residents are over age 75. About 70% of the residents are women and 80% of these are 75 years and over. From the perspective of the general population, about 5 people per 1,000 live in nursing homes, but the proportion rises sharply over age 65. The data in Table 6–2 demonstrate, however, that nursing home residents do not reflect the general United States population over age 65. Nursing home residents are more likely to be women, over age 75, white, and widowed or never married.

The predominate reason for admission to a nursing home is illness and need

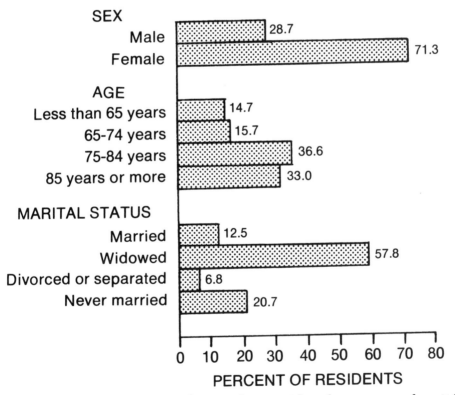

Figure 6–3. Percent distribution of nursing home residents by sex, age, and marital status, United States, 1977. (*Source:* United States National Center for Health Statistics: *Advance Data, No. 29,* Hyattsville, Maryland, May, 1978.)

TABLE 6-1. Selected Data on Nursing Homes by Medicare and Medicaid Certification Status, Mid-1970s

			Certification Status		
				Medicaid Only	
	Total	Both Medicaid and Medicare*	SNHs†	ICFs‡	Not Certified
All homes (percent)	100.	26.5	22.4	28.1	23.1
Average bed size	75.	105.0	92.0	57.0	45.0
Percent proprietary	76.	78.0	72.0	79.0	73.0
Average total full-time equivalent employees per 100 beds	66.3	72.3	68.7	57.5	58.5
Nursing staff	41.4	46.1	42.9	35.8	33.6
Registered nurse	4.9	6.5	5.2	2.4	3.7
Licensed practical nurse	5.8	6.4	6.5	4.9	4.2
Aide	30.7	33.2	31.2	28.5	25.7
Average occupancy rate (percent)	88.2	85.6	89.2	89.2	89.0

Average total monthly charge (dollars)	479.0	592.0	484.0	376.0	329.0
Median length-of-stay (years)	1.5	1.1	1.7	1.9	2.1

*Extended care facilities. This term was used to define facilities "for patients who require skilled nursing and rehabilitation services on a daily basis to help them achieve their optimal level of functioning." Of these homes, 8% were certified by Medicare only.

†Skilled nursing homes (SNH). This was the Medicaid equivalent of the extended care facility (ECF). SNH and ECF were subsequently merged into a single category, skilled nursing facility, when Medicare and Medicaid regulations were combined. Of these homes, 35% were certified as both SNFs and ICFs.

‡Intermediate care facilities (ICF). These were defined as facilities which provide health-related care and services to those who do not need SNF care, an admittedly imprecise definition.

Sources: United States National Center for Health Statistics: Selected operating and financial characteristics of nursing homes, United States: 1973–74 national nursing home survey. *Vital and Health Statistics*: Series 13, Data from the National Health Survey; No. 22—DHEW Publication No. (HRA) 76-1773. Government Printing Office, Washington, D.C., 1975.

United States National Center for Health Statistics: Utilization of nursing homes, United States: National nursing home survey, August, 1973–April, 1974. *Vital and Health Statistics*: Series 13, Data from the National Health Survey; No. 28—DHEW Publication No. (HRA) 77-1779. Government Printing Office, Washington, D.C., 1977.

United States National Center for Health Statistics: Charges for care and sources of payment for residents in nursing homes, United States: National nursing home survey, August 1973–April, 1974. *Vital and Health Statistics*: Series 13, Data from the National Health Survey; No. 32—DHEW Publication No. (PHS) 78-1783. Government Printing Office, Washington, D.C., 1977.

TABLE 6–2. Number and Percent of Nursing Home Residents 65 Years and Over, August, 1973–April 1974, and the Noninstitutionalized Population of the United States 65 Years and Over in March, 1974, by Selected Characteristics

Characteristic	Nursing home residents 65 years and over	Noninstitutionalized U.S. population 65 years and over
	Number	
Total 65 years and over	961,500	20,602,000
	Percent	
Total	100.0	100.0
Sex		
Male	27.6	41.4
Female	72.4	58.6
Race/ethnicity		
White	94.8	91.0
All other races	5.2	9.0
Marital status		
Married	12.2	54.3
Widowed	69.4	36.7
Divorced or separated	3.4	3.5
Never married	15.0	5.6
Age		
65–74 years old	17.0	63.5
76 years and over	83.0	36.5

Source: United States National Center for Health Statistics: Characteristics, social contracts and activities of nursing home residents, United States: 1973–74 national nursing home survey. *Vital and Health Statistics:* Series 13, Data from the National Health Survey; No. 27—DHEW Publication No. (HRA) 77-1778. Government Printing Office, Washington, D.C., 1977.

for treatment. This category accounts for over 80% of total admissions and for an even larger proportion of admissions for residents over age 75. Social reasons (e.g., no family support) account for only about six percent and economic reasons (e.g., no money or resources) for only one percent of admissions. Disruptive behavior or mental deterioration accounts for 12% overall, but for a third of admissions for those under age 65.

About 40% of patients enter the nursing home directly from their residences. Another 35% are transferred from general hospitals. The rest come primarily from other institutions such as mental hospitals or long-term care specialty hospitals (8%), other nursing homes (14%), or boarding homes (2%).

The nursing home is the repository of the chronically ill. Patients frequently suffer from more than one problem. Table 6–3 presents the prevalence of chronic conditions. It is noteworthy that mental illness remains the most prevalent problem. Among the elderly it is called senility, a term perhaps overladen with diagnostic impressions, and among the young, mental illness and mental retardation. The other major problems affecting one out of every three residents are those associated

TABLE 6–3. Chronic Conditions and Impairments of Nursing Home Residents, Based on Reporting by a Sample of Nursing Homes, United States, August, 1973–April, 1974

Chronic Condition or Impairment	Prevalence per 1,000 Residents
Senility	583.0
Arthritis or rheumatism	342.5
Heart trouble	335.1
Mental illness	186.3
Amputation of extremities or limbs, or permanent stiffness or any deformity of foot, leg, fingers, arm, or back	139.4
Diabetes	132.6
Paralysis or palsy due to stroke	113.5
Glaucoma or cataracts	103.1
Any chronic trouble with back or spine	98.6
Mental retardation	67.8
Paralysis or palsy not related to stroke, arthritis, or rheumatism	61.6
None of the above	53.6

Source: United States National Center for Health Statistics: Health, United States, 1976–1977. DHEW Publication No. (HRA) 77-1232. Government Printing Office, Washington, D.C., 1977.

with advanced age—heart disease and arthritis. The prevalence of chronic impairments is accompanied by functional limitations; 32% could not hear a telephone conversation; 46% could not read ordinary newsprint; 28% had lost bowel and bladder control; 51% had problems with mobility; and 31% were either chairbound or bedridden (7). More than one of these functional limitations may, of course, occur in any person, just as multiple diagnoses are frequent. Figure 6–4 displays the patterns of disability from a national sample of nursing home patients in 1977.

Nursing homes do not tend to offer a rich therapeutic milieu. Data from utilization review records suggest that psychoactive drugs are widely used. A recent survey showed that patients without psychiatric diagnoses were more likely to receive such drugs than were those labeled as mentally ill (8). This ubiquitous use suggests that sedation is used as a major means of control, quite possibly to minimize the need for active nursing and medical staff.

PAYING FOR NURSING HOME CARE

The costs of nursing home care reflect to a fair degree the services provided, but it is not at all clear which is the chicken and which the egg. The recent scandals involving Medicaid abuse and fraud leave an impression that, even when the

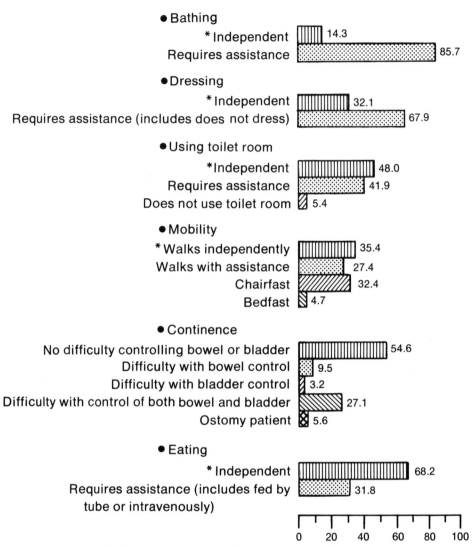

LEVEL OF DEPENDENCY

● Bathing
  * Independent — 14.3
  Requires assistance — 85.7

● Dressing
  * Independent — 32.1
  Requires assistance (includes does not dress) — 67.9

● Using toilet room
  * Independent — 48.0
  Requires assistance — 41.9
  Does not use toilet room — 5.4

● Mobility
  * Walks independently — 35.4
  Walks with assistance — 27.4
  Chairfast — 32.4
  Bedfast — 4.7

● Continence
  No difficulty controlling bowel or bladder — 54.6
  Difficulty with bowel control — 9.5
  Difficulty with bladder control — 3.2
  Difficulty with control of both bowel and bladder — 27.1
  Ostomy patient — 5.6

● Eating
  * Independent — 68.2
  Requires assistance (includes fed by tube or intravenously) — 31.8

0   20   40   60   80   100

* Includes small percentage for whom category was unknown.

Figure 6–4. Percent distribution of nursing home residents by level of dependency in performing selected activities of daily living, United States, 1977. (*Source:* United States National Center for Health Statistics: *Advance Data, No. 29,* Hyattsville, Maryland, May, 1978.)

payments are low, they are misused by some. Table 6–4 summarizes the changes in charges across the years before and after the introduction of Medicare and Medicaid. Interest here is primarily on Medicaid due to the focus on nursing homes. Costs are related to the amount of nursing care given and have increased more than the rate of medical price inflation. Using constant 1964 dollars, costs rose almost 40% between 1964 and 1969 and another 15% in the subsequent five

TABLE 6–4. Average Monthly Charge and Percent Distribution by Level of Nursing Care, United States, 1964, 1969, and 1973–74

Level of Nursing Care Received	1964		1969		1973–74	
	Average Total Monthly Charge	Percent of Residents	Average Total Monthly Charge	Percent of Residents	Average Total Monthly Charge	Percent of Residents
All residents	$185	100	$335 (257)*	100	$479 (296)	100
Intensive nursing care	221	33.0	374 (286)	33.7	510 (315)	40.6
Other nursing care	197	30.3	335 (256)	43.0	469 (289)	42.1
Personal care	162	25.6	293 (224)	18.0	435 (268)	16.4
No nursing or personal care	97	11.1	230 (176)	5.3	315 (194)	0.9

*Cost in 1964 dollars adjusted by medical care price index.

Source: United States National Center for Health Statistics: Charges for care and sources of payment for residents in nursing homes, United States: National nursing home survey, August, 1973–April, 1974. *Vital and Health Statistics*, Series 13, Data from the National Health Survey; No. 32—DHEW Publication No. (PHS) 78–1783. Government Printing Office, Washington, D.C., 1977.

year period. In 1977 the average monthly charge for a nursing patient was $669 ($852 for a skilled nursing facility and $409 in non-certified facilities) (6).

The source of payment has also shifted over this time as shown in Figure 6–5. Public funds became pre-eminent and public assistance and welfare gave way to Medicaid. By 1973–74, Medicaid was the primary source of payment for almost half the nursing home residents in the United States, while Medicare covered just over 1%.

Although the individual monthly costs of nursing home care may seem modest, the long lengths-of-stay and the large numbers of residents make this form of care an important component in the overall costs of care. Not only are the dollars involved substantial, the care they purchase is questionable. The investigations into the financing and management of nursing homes spurred by accusations of fraud and abuse revealed a distressing situation in New York State. The investigating commission concluded that "the costs of many elements of nursing home care are unknown in any usable form and, further, that there was no statistical connection between the costs of care and either patient needs or services provided" (9).

Payment for nursing home care under Medicaid was originally calculated as a fixed *per diem* cost that varied according to the level and intensity of nursing care; a patient classified as needing skilled nursing care was paid for at a higher rate than one deemed in need of only intermediate level care. However, such a system was viewed as lacking incentives for better quality of care and a more variable approach was inaugurated. As in other areas of nursing home care, the hospital model was adopted. The 1972 amendments to the Social Security Act required that states reimburse nursing homes on the basis of reasonable costs by July of 1976. Although this date has long since passed, there is still no clear statement of what is a "cost" and what is "reasonable." These definitions partially determine the degree to which nursing homes are permitted to make a profit and affect what constitutes a reasonable return on investment. Because the nursing home industry is primarily proprietary, incentives for investment and services are an important prerequisite for improving the level of care. The question becomes one of calculating the proper base for profits; should this include both capital equity as well as current costs? This issue is still shrouded in controversy (10).

Costs can be divided into several major components for different purposes. Some costs are fixed and others vary with intensity of service and occupancy. At the simplest level, these include the general costs of room, board and maintenance, nursing care, other therapies and medical care. Each may be expected to yield a different rate of return for investors.

A few innovative reimbursement proposals have been suggested to create climates conducive to nursing care. One proposal is for a prospective incentive reimbursement scheme in which facilities would be grouped into homogeneous peer categories and paid a mean *per diem* rate based on four factors: dollar ceiling for the peer group, occupancy rate, health status of patients, and facility evaluation (11). Reimbursement above a fixed range of the group mean would require documentation that these additional funds contribute toward quality-related services. Operating surpluses for fully compliant homes would be partially distributed to the owners and employees and partially used to purchase capital expansion rights.

Another proposal for achieving quality care at the appropriate level is to hold nursing homes responsible for the provision of a minimum custodial care only, and

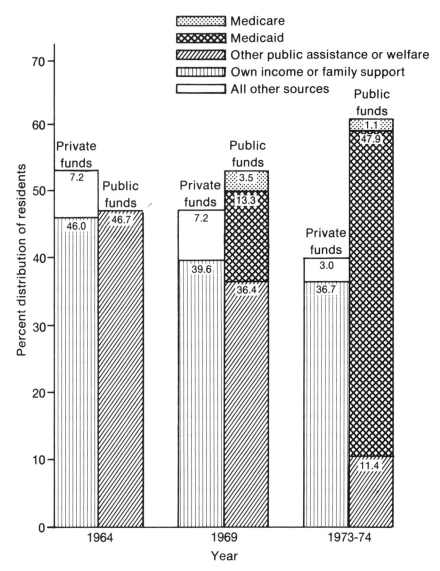

Figure 6–5. Percent distribution of residents by primary source of payment, United States, selected years. (*Source:* United States National Center for Health Statistics: *Charges for Care and Sources of Payment for Residents in Nursing Homes, United States: National Nursing Home Survey, August, 1973–April, 1974.* Series 13, Data from the National Health Survey, No. 32—DHEW Publication no. (PHS) 78–1783. Government Printing Office, Washington, D.C., 1977.)

to permit residents to purchase all other services on the open market (12). Such a system would, according to its advocates, end placement at an inappropriate level and have the added psychological benefit of permitting the resident to control his or her medical care and make personal decisions. The nursing home would become a more home-like environment under these conditions. This is attractive as a theoretical model but there are many potential problems that would need to be addressed in pilot tests of the plan. How is custodial care to be defined? If it includes necessary bedside nursing, would a level of care system again become necessary, or would the patient also purchase intensive nursing services on the open market? Will the services be available on the open market? And, perhaps most crucial, what safeguards will be developed to protect those residents who do not have the capacity to exercise their purchasing power and who do not have family as guardians? A rather complex administrative system with guardianship mechanisms would surely be necessary.

Kane (13) has proposed a model whereby nursing homes would be paid in proportion to the degree that their patients achieved good outcomes. Each patient's outcome would be compared against an individualized prognosis generated from data collected by independent reviewers. Payment would be based on average costs for that class of patient multiplied by a prognostic adjustment factor (PAF). Where a patient did better than expected, the PAF would be greater than one; where the outcome was worse than expected, the PAF would be less than one. Such a system is compatible with both prospective and retrospective reimbursement procedures. Its major virtue is the focus on the results of care, thereby minimizing the need for rules and regulations.

MEDICAL CARE IN NURSING HOMES

Nursing homes are not the favorite haunts of physicians. In one study, only 14% of the active physicians in a metropolitan area participated in nursing home care (14). Closer scrutiny of the care that is provided offers little solace (15). A review of the medical records of nursing home patients in a metropolitan area revealed a substantial number of charts with no evidence of a new observation or physical examination for six months or more (16).

Physician indifference to nursing home care is hardly surprising. Few medical schools offer training in geriatrics (17), and the medical model of seeking definitive treatment is unlikely to find satisfactory application among the pool of patients with multiple chronic problems.

Other disciplines may be more appropriate as primary care givers to nursing home patients. The growth of the nurse practitioner movement offers an attractive alternative to sole reliance on physicians. The philosophy of nursing places more emphasis on care rather than on curing and its traditions encourage nurses to work more comfortably with nursing home staffs to upgrade their skills. Geriatric nurse practitioners would thus appear to be an ideal solution to the problem of how to improve the care provided to nursing home patients (18). One demonstration project using a team of geriatric nurse practitioners and social workers provides cause for enthusiasm. The care rendered by the team, supported by physician and clinical pharmacist consultants, was not only better than the alternatives, but was also cost-effective. The savings in other care costs were greater than the entire costs of fielding the team (19).

QUALITY OF NURSING HOME CARE

There is a disappointing dearth of useful data on the quality of nursing home care. What little light is shed tends to be diffuse; a number of problems remain unresolved. Despite a plethora of instruments to measure various aspects of patient functioning, few are well standardized with known measures of validity and reliability. Some exceptions are presented by Sherwood and associates (20) who reviewed a number of social and mental status measures; and the federal government has sponsored the development of a patient classification and assessment tool based on the medical model (21). Few instruments have been applied across large cross-sections of nursing homes. There is little agreement about what constitutes good care. Advocates of the medical and social models continually debate the respective merits of these approaches. Without consensus about goals, evaluation is impossible. Not surprisingly, those studies of quality that are available are not always consistent in their findings, especially when different measures are used. Table 6–5 offers examples of several approaches that have been attempted. Related issues concerning the quality of medical care are presented in Chapter 12.

One can discern a certain hierarchy in these studies. Several reports deal with the question of whether nursing home patients really need the level of care they are receiving. This question is generally couched in terms of those needing less, or at least less expensive, care, but occasionally patients are found to need more care. The judgment about need is most often implicit, based on clinical expertise, but there have also been attempts to develop explicit criteria based on patient needs for nursing care (22).

Most researchers have addressed the assessment of quality by examining the structure of care provided by nursing homes. Using essentially unvalidated measures based on assumptions of what constituted good care, these investigators have ranked nursing homes based on such factors as amount of care or nurse/patient ratios, types and variety of programs, and impressions about the physical facilities.

Mandated programs to assess the need for care and appropriate length-of-stay of Medicaid and Medicare patients have been conducted by state agencies. The model for such assessments is the hospital utilization review (UR) procedure, which may not be directly transferable to the nursing home. These reviews correspond to process measures in the more common parlance of quality of care assessment as presented in Chapter 12. Several investigators have attempted to take advantage of this set of data to describe nursing home care. As the UR function is increasingly assumed by Professional Services Review Organizations, beginning with Medicare patients, the hospital model is likely to be even more in evidence (23, 24).

A few studies have pursued process of care assessment by identifying measures of patient need (at least implicit measures) and determining the degree to which patients receive appropriate services. One study which reviewed the drug regimens among a small set of nursing home patients uncovered a number of notable deficiencies (25).

Miller (26) has pointed to the reciprocal side of nursing home care. His analysis of the information that accompanied a group of newly admitted patients suggests that often the nursing home staff is presented with incomplete and erroneous data.

TABLE 6–5. Summary of Illustrative Quality of Care Studies in Long Term Care

Type of Study and Reference	Variables Examined	Population Studied	Major Findings
1. Appropriateness of Placement/ Utilization Review			
Williams, et al (55)	clinical assessment medical record review	332 patients seen by evaluation and placement unit in Rochester, New York	52% of nursing home patients appropriately placed; 35% of patients referred for nursing home placement actually required it
Levey, et al (56)	weighted score of structural and process variables	129 nursing homes in Massachusetts	quality improved 1965 to 1969; quality related to cost but not to ownership
Zimmer (57)	physical, mental and functional status care requirements; appropriateness of placement	738 admissions to 40 skilled nursing facilities in Rochester, New York	13% required care; 51% required minimal care; 36% require continuing care; 1.3% could have lower level of care
Congressional Budget Office (58)	review of 14 reports	Intermediate Care Facilities, Skilled Nursing Facilities	14–74% of ICF patients and 8–76% of SNF patients inappropriately placed
2. Structural Analysis			

Kosberg and Tobin (59)	36 organizational characteristics, 3 factors; total resources score	214 Chicago nursing homes	resources related to source of funds, location, race of residents, not to ownership, size
Linn (60)	equally weighted score of medical records, meals, available services, patient appearance, administrative policies, accreditation, personnel records, physical facilities, safety equipment and overall impression	56 Florida nursing homes	range of scores 6–73; patients' appearance and attitudes of nursing home operators most important
Anderson, et al (45)	patients/room, staff hours/patients, staff variety, patient participation, therapeutic orientation	118 nursing home owners or administrators in Minnesota	quality associated with fewer welfare patients; cost/day, rural, size, hospital attachment

3. Receipt of Appropriate Services

TABLE 6–5. (*continued*)

Type of Study and Reference	Variables Examined	Population Studied	Major Findings
DHEW Office of Nursing Home Affairs (61)	health needs, nutritional needs, medical services, other services, pharmaceutical services, rehabilitation, administration, physical environment	U.S. sample of 288 SNFs	descriptive data, some problems in each area
Miller, et al (62)	diagnosis, nursing care requirements, dependency physician	8917 Medicaid patients in 288 SNFs in Minnesota	use PSRO approach for special medical care evaluation studies
4. Outcome Measures			
Gottesman and Bourestom (63)	patient behavior, Activities of Daily Living, mental status	40 nursing homes, 1144 patients, 200 aides in Detroit	quality related to patients having possessions, aides with experience, majority of private patients, percent of patients white, and more visitors
Kane, et al (64)	activities, medications	3092 utilization review records of Utah nursing home patients	little change over time; high use of psychoactive drugs
Linn, et al (65)	structural variables above plus physician program; ratings of patients by physician and nurses on placement and 6 months later	1000 male VA patients; 40 nursing homes in Florida	functional status related to RN hours/patient, cost/month, policies, patient appearance and ratings

In only rare instances have researchers examined changes in patients over time to observe the outcomes of nursing home care; several authors have suggested this type of research (27–29). Outcome assessments are critical in an area like nursing home care, where the relationships between what is done and what happens to patients is so poorly delineated. The continued trend toward increasingly rigorous regulations with no demonstrated efficacy is likely to accomplish increases in tension and cost, but may not necessarily lead to improved care. The posture of the regulators comes increasingly to resemble that of the edentulous lion who roars for attention but soon frightens only the uninitiated.

QUALITY OF LIFE

In an ideal situation, quality of care and quality of life should be highly overlapping concepts—the facility achieving a high level of "quality of care" should, by definition, insure residents a good quality of life. As noted above and in Chapter 12, quality of care is difficult to achieve and to measure. But quality of life is an even more elusive commodity, dependent on individual preferences and limited by individual health, regardless of residence in a nursing home. To the extent that particular nursing home settings have been related to the quality of the life of the residents, positive ratings of quality may also be independent of highly competent technical care. In some ways, medical technology may produce a well-ordered, hospital-style environment which is most unattractive for a long-term resident.

A fairly safe generalization is that few persons perceive nursing home admission as a positive event. Dread and despair are the reactions most associated with nursing homes among the prospective client population. It is difficult to assess the facility's role in providing a high quality of life for residents in the face of all the negative connotations that the home carries in the minds of its clientele.

More is known about what is wrong with life in a nursing home than how a program may go about remedying the situation. Books by nursing home residents (30) or by participant observers in long-term care institutions (31) cite the loss of personal freedoms inherent in the role and the extreme difficulty residents may encounter in completing simple actions, such as making a telephone call. The former identity of the nursing home residents tends to become subsumed under the classification "patient." In a demonstration project which attempted to meet social needs of the patients, Jorgensen and Kane (32) noted that the interests and skills of the residents (such as piano-playing) were unknown to nursing home staff prior to the beginning of the project.

Brody (33) catalogued what she called the "iatrogenic diseases of institutional life" as follows:

> dependency; depersonalization; low self-esteem; lack of occupation or fruitful use of time; geographic and social distance from family and friends and cultural milieu; inflexibility of routines and menus; loneliness; lack of privacy, identity, own clothing, possessions and furniture; lack of freedom;

desexualization and infantalization; crowded conditions; and negative, disrespectful or belittling staff attitudes.

It is with such criteria that quality of life can be measured. Some of the items, such as inflexibility of routines and menus, lack of privacy, and negative staff attitudes may be directly attributable to institutional life while others, such as loneliness and geographic distance from family and friends, may also characterize the lives of many elderly persons outside nursing homes; nor are there before-after studies to show how the quality of particular patients' lives deteriorates upon admission to a nursing home.

The nursing home has sometimes been called a decision-free environment for its residents. This quality has taken on an extremely ominous note because of our current understanding of the phenomenon which has been called "learned helplessness" (34). According to the theory, when a person perceives that his or her actions no longer elicit responses, a syndrome develops characterized by depression, cessation of efforts to influence events, and inability to distinguish when one's actions have actually elicited a response. Learned helplessness has been documented in nursing home residents and a number of field studies have demonstrated that startling changes may occur in both affective state and levels of activity when small changes are made that increase actual or perceived control among nursing home residents. In one of these studies regular visits from volunteers, coupled with the residents' power to decide the timing of the visits, produced beneficial effects (35). Two other studies demonstrated that the ability to make small decisions, such as the timing of visits or selection of and caring for a plant, led to lessened depression and an improved level of activity compared to a control group which received similar attention, but in a paternalistic way which offered no decision opportunities (36, 37).

Ferrari (38) studied the effect of perceived control among those on a waiting list for admission to a nursing home. After controlling for level of health, she found that those patients who perceived that it was their own decision to enter the facility prior to admission were significantly more likely to survive after admission than those who perceived they had no choice. This study suggests, first, that the repercussions of perceived helplessness are actually life-threatening and, second, that quality of life within a nursing home may be partially related to procedures of selection, referral, and decision-making prior to admission.

Because individual control is an important dimension affecting the quality of a nursing home resident's life, information is necessary about preferences of particular groups of elderly persons and about which patients fare best under what kinds of conditions. Little data of this nature is available, in part because controlled clinical trials of nursing home conditions raise ethical questions and in part because, in many areas, beds are limited and few choices of placement are possible. Unlike free-market industries, it is impossible to study nursing home preferences by observing movement of patients from facilities with which they are dissatisfied to other facilities. There is some evidence to suggest, however, that the widely known negative effects of relocation of nursing home patients do not occur when the patient requests the transfer and is prepared for the move (39).

Fragmentary findings exist to suggest conditions which may be desirable in nursing homes from a quality of life standpoint. Jorgensen and Kane (32) found that patients were mostly willing to accept nursing home placement if some continuation of their previous lifestyle were possible. In another study (40), a change to heterosexual living spaces improved adjustment to nursing home and social behavior in male residents. The factors most associated with negative adjustment to nursing homes in a group of 20 women were lack of privacy, lack of independence, and distance from families and friends (41). A comparison of institutionalized and non-institutionalized elderly found an association between future commitments (measured by number of planned appointments in the week ahead) and successful aging; those in nursing homes tended to have fewer future commitments (42). Jones (43) hypothesized that crowded conditions caused interpersonal conflict and that friendships tend to be formed, not with people in the same room, but people several doors away. Some of these findings are consistent with the impressions from a study of nursing homes abroad (44) that homogeneous populations, based on ethnicity and culture, single rooms, separation of the mentally alert from the disorganized, and opportunity to pursue former interests, are associated with a higher quality nursing home environment. Studies such as those cited above, however, are not very useful for forming guidelines to assess quality of life since they are isolated pieces of work that have not generally been repeated and do not form a coherent knowledge base.

MEDICAL VERSUS SOCIAL MODELS

How, then, can measures of quality of care and of life be combined? Inevitably one is led back to the distinction between the social and medical models for long-term care.

If the nursing home is not the natural heir to the social responsibility for the elderly, it has at least become the *de facto* answer to fill a void formerly handled by family members in a less complex and less mobile era; a void partially filled by government social services and personal health services in European countries. Like many products of mixed marriages, the nursing home faces a severe identity crisis. It is far from clear whether its dominant lineage is medical or social. While most of the regulations for nursing homes seem to cast the facilities as miniature hospitals, most of the problems are more social than medical.

The question of eminent domain has not been resolved. The issue of predominance between the medical and social models for long-term care is not merely a battle for bureaucratic supremacy between two factions of government. It is a fundamental clash of beliefs in the style of life to be pursued and the appropriate manner of its pursuit. This conflict of credos involves questions of both ends and means—the goals and expectations generated by different perspectives and the paths deemed most approachable to reach them. Under the growing pressure of enforced fiscal austerity, a choice is increasingly necessary. No longer can providers and consumers tolerate the ambiguity resulting from assigning equal weight to both approaches.

The social model is attractive because it emphasizes that health care, albeit crucial, is just one of many services needed to raise the quality of life of the aged. Especially with an elderly population, the often dwindling benefits of heroic medical measures must be balanced against the heavy social and psychological costs. Morbidity and disability are conditions of life for the majority of aged people. A medical model allows the conditions to define a range of life circumstances. The very permanence and intractability of these problems argue for societal provisions to protect the elderly from a permanent patient role for decades before their death.

MEETING HEALTH NEEDS

Although long-term institutional care should be perceived and organized as a social program, medical nihilism cannot be advocated. Clearly medical services are needed for nursing home patients, and perceptive, responsive, skilled practitioners are needed to fill those roles. Earlier, physician disinterest in very elderly patients in general and nursing home practice in particular was discussed. There are two quite distinct approaches to redressing this situation: 1) to elevate medical practice with the elderly through education, credentialling, and research money into a prestigious specialty; and 2) to train and utilize non-physician primary care personnel to serve the institutionalized aged. The effectiveness of the nurse practitioner as a deliverer of care in nursing homes was described above. These two extremes represent a continuum; a mid-point approach would be sensitization of family practitioners and internists to the particular needs of the elderly. Another solution would be a simultaneous emphasis on the development of geriatric medical specialists for differential diagnosis while other personnel are utilized for ongoing care. This approach has been utilized in a number of European countries, particularly Great Britain (44).

What are the advantages and disadvantages of various models for medical care in nursing homes? The geriatrician emphasis carries with it the likelihood of increasingly sophisticated differential diagnosis (45) but has the pitfalls of accentuating the hospital model of nursing home life. On the other hand, it is important that nursing personnel who work on a daily basis with residents and physicians in nursing homes be alert to physical problems and be able to differentiate the disorientation accompanying an acute illness from the disorientation of old age. Whether a cadre of geriatricians is needed to spearhead training and research for such awareness is not yet certain.

More safely, one can assert that a team approach is required for providing health services to the elderly. Many of the interventions that are most effective in terms of increasing comfort and reducing functional disability are provided by physical therapists, dentists, optometrists, podiatrists, and hearing aid specialists. A pharmacist, too, is invaluable for monitoring the drug usage of patients. Although there is often overdependence on the magic of teamwork, health care to long-term institutional residents has the ingredients necessary to justify a team approach— there are clearly differentiated functional tasks for the different team members and, since the mobility of the patient group is limited, the importance of assembling a comprehensive service in a convenient manner is increased. Indeed, in most instances many health personnel are not available to residents of nursing homes, nor is there any mechanism for reimbursing for many needed services. Unpublished data from the National Center for Health Statistics 1973–74 Nursing Home Survey indicates that only 9.9% of nursing home patients receive physical therapy, 15.2% recreational therapy, 5.7% occupational therapy, 0.5% speech therapy, and only 8% any form of professional counselling (46).

If, in the face of finite resources, a choice is required between geriatric specialists or geriatric nurse practitioners mobilizing a team of providers as needed, the latter would seem to offer the greatest positive benefit. Perhaps, if the nursing home is really a "home" as the designation implies, it would not be too far-fetched to consider that home health services should be developed to serve nursing home residents as well as those in their own dwellings.

Regardless of the medical resources adopted, there is great value in maintaining some balance of forces separate from the nursing home itself. The providers of medical services should have an entity distinct from the nursing home if they are to offer a set of standards independent of the institutions. The resultant dynamic tension is not intended to be a source of conflict, but to provide an outside influence that will promote improved quality. This approach represents a segment of the hospital model very worthy of adoption.

MEETING SOCIAL NEEDS

According to a recent summarization (47) there have been three general approaches to improving the quality of life in a nursing home through psychosocial interventions. The first is the use of a variety of therapeutic approaches with explicit goals to change or improve the patient. The second is structural changes in organization, staffing patterns, and relationships in the nursing home community, designed to facilitate individualized care while developing a sense of community. And the third is changes in the relationship between the nursing home and the community designed to break down communication barriers, increase the visibility of nursing homes, and develop more flexible programs to serve the community.

The first approach, the therapeutic one, has been a partial response to the lack of mental health services for the elderly, particularly those in institutions. Reactive depressions are endemic among elderly nursing home residents and paranoid responses are also prevalent. Sometimes these psychiatric disturbances have been lumped together into the catch-all concept of "senility." Senile disorientation is itself often considered hopeless and often no treatment is offered. Among more popular treatments are various talking therapies, ranging from reminiscence groups to current event clubs, more traditional drug therapy and convulsive therapy for depression, and reality orientation therapy to combat and stem off disorientation. The last of these consists of short daily group sessions directed to reinforcing awareness as to time, place, and names with reinforcement on a twenty-four hour basis from staff. Controlled studies of these various, and sometimes conflicting (compare reality orientation to reminiscing), interventions are rare, and it is difficult to separate out the Hawthorne effect (changes in behavior due to the experiment) for a population which has notoriously been neglected. Another therapeutic approach is general behavior modification, sometimes complete with token economies to reinforce desired behaviors.

The shortcoming of all the therapeutic approaches is that they do not compensate for a deficient environment. What good is reality orientation if reality itself is bleak? What use is reminiscing if the elderly perceive it as an exercise in humoring them rather than a genuine interest in and social use for their experiences? What use is counseling to alleviate depression if, as noted earlier, depression is a by-product of the helplessness and perceived lack of control inculcated by the nursing home itself? Austin and Kosberg (48) interviewed the administrators and head nurses of 27 Florida nursing homes and found that the opportunities for patient autonomy and decision-making were minimal. For example, in half the homes, patients were not allowed to visit patients of the opposite sex with their doors closed, in one-third of the homes bedtimes could not be determined by the patients, in no instance could patients determine waking hours, and there was almost never a choice of roommate. Contrast this with the assertion that the most desirable environment for long-term care is a naturalistic environment, designed by the clientele (49).

The second general approach involves the creation of a sense of community through various adjustments of resident-staff mix, and development of community councils for decision-making, creation of an active recreational program, and elevation of staff competency by training as well as by adding professionals. It is certain that there are some nursing homes in the country which are especially attractive environments and this can readily be perceived by visitors. Former United States Senator Frank Moss, previously chairperson of a Senate Long-Term Care Subcommittee, documented some of the ingredients of a good nursing home based on staffing, facilities, and programs and encouraged family members to approach nursing home selection with a checklist of requirements (50).

The third approach, bridging the gap between nursing home and community, is quite promising. In this general category are included a variety of emphases: encouraging volunteers from the community to enter the nursing home; encouraging volunteers from nursing home residents to offer service in the community; integrating day centers with nursing homes; encouraging brief admissions to relieve families; and combining programs for children with those of long-term care facilities. Innovations which increase the visibility of the nursing home in the community not only create opportunities for residents to fulfill community roles, but also reduce potential abuses through the protection of public scrutiny.

Although there is much evidence that the aged are not readily abandoned by family members (51, 52), but rather are placed in nursing homes when the family has exhausted its own resources (53), there is nevertheless a withdrawal of many family members after admission to a home. As Gottesman (54) indicates, the relative of the patient will not hold the nursing home accountable if most contact ceases after the initial referral, especially if "the implicit contract between the nursing home and relatives is one of non-interference by the other from whom the home takes over a difficult burden." Additionally, of course, those who have no remaining families are over-represented among nursing home residents. Therefore, the public attention on nursing homes created by a variety of community-based strategies may be essential to create a public which holds the nursing home responsible.

CONCLUSIONS

Investment in alternatives to nursing home care cannot be adequate to meet the total needs of those now served in nursing homes. For the cost-conscious, it will be discouraging to recognize that community-based programs such as home-health, day-centers, and even protected housing may not provide the level of care needed or chosen by many elderly persons. A continuum of services would, of course, provide more choices and also facilitate transition from one level of care to another, perhaps in the same geographic setting. It is still necessary, however, to develop knowledge and then implement a program which will permit older persons to live in institutions with a minimum of disruption of their previous life-style and preferences and with the opportunity to manage their lives as independently as their condition permits. Money will be necessary, but not sufficient, to achieve such standards.

This chapter has advocated that institutions for the elderly, whether called nursing homes or old age homes, be developed as dwelling places for those who may have health problems for the rest of their lives, rather than as hospitals requiring added social services because the average length-of-stay is long. The distinction may call for reconsideration of the organization of services, the structure of authority, and the funding auspices of long-term care. Sherwood (29) adopted the awkward terminology "long-term-care person," presumably to avoid the designation "patient" or "resident." It is suggested here that the long-term-care person is more in need of a hospitable than a hospital environment.

REFERENCES

1. Thomas, WC Jr: *Nursing Homes and Public Policy.* Ithaca, Cornell University Press, 1969.
2. United States National Center for Health Statistics: *Selected Operating and Financial Characteristics of Nursing Homes, United States: 1973–74 National Nursing Home Survey.* Vital and Health Statistics: Series 13, Data from the National Health Survey; No. 22—DHEW Publication no. (HRA) 76-1773. Government Printing Office, Washington, D.C., 1975.
3. United States National Center for Health Statistics: *Characteristics, Social Contracts and Activities of Nursing Home Residents, United States: 1973–74 National Nursing Home Survey.* Vital and Health Statistics: Series 13, Data from the National Health Survey; No. 27—DHEW Publication no. (HRA) 77-1778. Government Printing Office, Washington, D.C., 1977.
4. United States National Center for Health Statistics: *Utilization of Nursing Homes, United States: National Nursing Home Survey, August, 1973–April 1974.* Vital and Health Statistics: Series 13, Data from the National Health Survey; No. 28—DHEW Publication no. (HRA) 77-1779. Government Printing Office, Washington, D.C., 1977.
5. United States National Center for Health Statistics: *Charges for Care and Sources of Payment for Residents in Nursing Homes, United States: National Nursing Home Survey, August, 1973–April, 1974.* Vital and Health Statistics: Series 13, Data from the

National Health Survey, No. 32—DHEW Publication no. (PHS) 78-1783. Government Printing Office, Washington, D.C., 1977.

6. United States National Center for Health Statistics. *Advance Data, number 35.* Hyattsville, Maryland, September 1978.

7. United States National Center for Health Statistics: *Health, United States, 1976–1977.* DHEW Publication no. (HRA) 77-1232. Government Printing Office, Washington, D.C., 1977.

8. Schmidt L, Reinhardt A, Kane R, et al: The mentally ill in nursing homes: new back wards in the community. *Archives of General Psychiatry* 34:687–691, 1977.

9. Joe T, Meltzer J: *Policies and Strategies for Long-term Care.* Health Policy Program, University of California at San Francisco, San Francisco, 1976 (mimeo).

10. McCaffree K: *Returns to Equity Capital in Nursing Homes.* Center for Health Services Research, University of Washington, Seattle, 1977 (mimeo).

11. Ruchlin HS, Levey S, Muller C: The long-term care marketplace: an analysis of deficiencies and potential reform by means of incentive reimbursement. *Medical Care* 13:979–991, 1975.

12. Ruchlin H, Levey S: An Economic Perspective of Long-term Care, in S Sherwood (ed): *Long-term Care: A Handbook for Researchers, Planners, and Providers.* New York, Spectrum Publications, Inc., 1975.

13. Kane RL: Paying nursing homes for better care. *Journal of Community Health* 2:1–4, Fall, 1976.

14. Solon JA, Greenawalt LF: Physicians' participation in nursing homes. *Medical Care* 12:486–495, 1974.

15. United States Senate: Subcommittee on Long-term Care of the Special Committee on Aging. *Nursing Home Care in the United States: Failure in Public Policy.* Government Printing Office, Washington, D.C., 1975.

16. Kane RL, Hammer D, Byrnes N: Getting care to nursing-home patients: a problem and a proposal. *Medical Care* 15:174–180, 1977.

17. Akpom CA, Mayer S: A survey of geriatric education in U.S. medical schools. *Journal of Medical Education* 53:66–68, 1978.

18. Pepper GA, Kane RL, Teteberg B: Geriatric nurse practitioner in nursing homes. *American Journal of Nursing* 76(1):62–64, January, 1976.

19. Kane RL, Jorgensen L, Teteberg B, et al: Is good nursing home care feasible? *Journal of the American Medical Association* 235:516–519, 1976.

20. Sherwood S, Morris J, Mor V, Gutkin C: *Compendium of Measures for Describing and Assessing Long-Term Care Populations.* Hebrew Rehabilitation Center for the Aged, Boston, January 19, 1977 (mimeo).

21. Jones EW: *Patient Classification for Long-term Care: User's Manual.* DHEW Publication No. (HRA) 75-3107. Government Printing Office, Washington, D.C., 1974.

22. Cavaiola LJ: *A Unified Approach to Patient Classification and Nurse Staffing for Long-Term Care Facilities.* Baltimore, The Johns Hopkins University, 1975.

23. Jessee WF, Ford L, Pebbutt J: Implications of PSROs for long-term care. *Hospitals* 50(15):140–Passim, 1976.

24. Goran MJ, Crystal R, Ford L: PSRO review of long-term care utilization and quality. *Medical Care* 14(Suppl):94–98, 1976.

25. Howard JB, Strong SR. K, Strong Jr. K: Medication procedures in a nursing home: abuse of PRN orders. *Journal of the American Geriatrics Society* 25:83–84, 1977.

26. Miller M, Elliott D: Errors and omissions in diagnostic records on admission of patients to a nursing home. *Journal of the American Geriatrics Society* 24:108–116, 1976.

27. Ruchlin HS: A new strategy for regulating long-term care facilities. *Journal of Health Politics, Policy and Law* 2:190–211, 1977.

28. Kosberg JI: Making institutions accountable: research and policy issues. *The Gerontologist* 14:510–516, December 1974.

29. Sherwood S (ed): *Long-term Care: A Handbook for Researchers, Planners and Providers.* New York, Spectrum Publications, 1975.

30. Tulloch J: *A Home is Not a Home.* New York, Seabury Press, 1975.

31. Gubrium JF: *Living and Dying at Murray Manor.* St. Martin's Press, New York, 1975.

32. Jorgensen LA, Kane R: Social work in the nursing home: a need and opportunity. *Social Work in Health Care* 1:471–482, 1976.

33. Brody E: A million Procrustean beds. *Gerontologist* 13:430–435, 1973.

34. Seligman M: *Helplessness: On Depression, Development and Death.* San Francisco, W. H. Freeman & Company, 1975.

35. Schulz R: Effects of control and predictability on the physical and psychological well-being of the institutionalized aged. *Journal of Personality and Social Psychology* 33:563–573, 1976.

36. Langer E, Rodin J: Effects of choice and enhanced personal responsibility for the aged: a field experiment in an institutional setting. *Journal of Personality and Social Psychology* 34:191–198, 1976.

37. Mercer, S: *Helplessness and Hopelessness in the Institutionalized Aged: A Field Experiment in the Impact of Increased Control and Choice.* Doctoral thesis, University of Utah School of Social Work, Salt Lake City, 1978.

38. Ferrari N: *Institutionalization and Attitude Change in an Aged Population: A Field Study in Dissonance Theory.* Doctoral Dissertation, Western Reserve University, Cleveland, 1962 (mimeo).

39. Ogren E, Linn M: Male nursing home patients: relocation and mortality. *Journal of the American Geriatrics Society* 19:229–239, 1971.

40. Silverstone B, Wynter L: The effects of introducing a heterosexual living space. *Gerontologist* 15:83–87, 1975.

41. Abdo E, Dills J, Schectman H, et al: Elderly women in institutions versus those in public housing: comparison of personal and social adjustments. *Journal of the American Geriatrics Society* 21:81–87, 1973.

42. Schonfield, D, Hooper A: Future commitments and successful aging: I. Random Sample. II. Special groups. *Journal of Gerontology* 28:189–196, 197–201, 1973.

43. Jones DC: Spatial proximity, interpersonal conflict and friendship formation in the intermediate care facility. *Gerontologist* 15:150–154, 1975.

44. Kane RL, Kane RA: *Long-term Care in Six Countries: Implications for the United States.* Government Printing Office, Washington, D.C., 1976.

45. Anderson N, Hopkins RH, Schneider R, et al: *Policy Issues Regarding Nursing Homes: Findings from a Minnesota Survey.* Minneapolis, Institute for Interdisciplinary Studies, June 1969.

46. Knee R: The long-term care facility, in Dobroff R (ed): *Social Work Consultation in Long-term Care Facilities.* United States Department of Commerce, Division of Long-term Care Resources Administration, Publication no. (HRP) 002385. Government Printing Office, Washington, D.C., 1978.

47. Gottesman L, Brody E: Psycho-social Intervention Programs Within the Institutional Setting, in Sherwood S (ed): *Long-term Care: A Handbook for Researchers, Planners and Providers.* New York, Spectrum Publications, Inc., 1975.

48. Austin M, Kosberg J: Nursing home decisionmakers and the social service needs of residents. *Social Work in Health Care* 1:447–456, 1976.

49. Gottesman L, Quarterman C, Cohn G: Psycho-social Treatment of the Aged, in Eisdorfer C (ed): *The Psychology of Adult Development and Aging.* Washington, D.C., American Psychological Association, 1973.

50. Moss FE, Halamandaris VJ: *Too Old, Too Sick, Too Bad.* Aspen Systems Corporation, Germantown, Maryland, 1977.
51. Shanas E: Family responsibility and the health of older people. *Journal of Gerontology* 15:408–411, 1960.
52. Brody E: *A Social Work Guide for Long-Term Care Facilities.* Government Printing Office, Washington, D.C., 1974.
53. Eggert G, Granger C, Morris R et al: *Community-based Care for the Long-term Patient.* Levinson Policy Institute, Brandeis University, Waltham, Massachusetts, 1975.
54. Gottesman L: Organizing Rehabilitation Services for the Elderly. *Gerontologist* 10:287–293, 1970.
55. Williams TF, Hill JG, Fairbank ME et al: Appropriate placement of the chronically ill and aged: a successful approach by evaluation. *Journal of the American Medical Association* 226:1332–1335, 1973.
56. Levey S, Ruchlin HS, Stotsky BA et al: An appraisal of nursing home care. *Journal of Gerontology* 28:222–228, 1973.
57. Zimmer JG: Characteristics of patients and care provided in health-related and Skilled Nursing Facilities. *Medical Care* 13:992–1010, 1975.
58. United States Congressional Budget Office. *Long-term Care for the Elderly and Disabled.* Government Printing Office, Washington, D.C., 1977.
59. Kosberg JI, Tobin SS: Variability among nursing homes. *The Gerontologist* 12:214–219, Autumn, 1972.
60. Lin MW: A nursing home rating scale. *Geriatrics* 21(10):188–192, 1966.
61. United States Department of Health, Education, and Welfare, Office of Nursing Home Affairs. *Long-Term Care Facility Improvement Study: Introducing Report.* Government Printing Office, Washington, D.C., 1975.
62. Miller WR, Hurley SJ, Wharton E: External peer review of skilled nursing care in Minnesota. *American Journal of Public Health* 66:278–283, 1976.
63. Gottesman LE, Bourestom NC: Why nursing homes do what they do. *Gerontologist* 14:501–506, 1974.
64. Kane RL, Olsen D, Thetford C et al: The use of utilization review records as a source of data on nursing home care. *American Journal of Public Health* 66:778–782, 1976.
65. Linn MW, Gurel L, Linn BS: Patient outcome as a measure of quality of nursing home care. *American Journal of Public Health* 67:337–344, 1977.

CHAPTER 7

Mental Health Services: Growth and Development of a System

Mary Richardson

Mental health services have experienced considerable growth and change over the last several decades. Who is treated, and the problems they are treated for, have changed with changing definitions of mental illness, changing viewpoints about the appropriate response to mental health problems, and increasing social recognition and acceptance of mental health services as a treatment, rather than custodial, function. This chapter describes the development of mental health services in this country, the users and reasons for use, the organization and financing of services, recent trends, and the problems of providing care.

DEFINITIONS OF MENTAL ILLNESS

Definitions of mental illness are extremely difficult to formulate and they change over time. The labels applied to psychiatric or emotional disability are usually defined within biological, sociological, and cultural frameworks. There are relatively few disorders which are clearly physiological in origin and which exhibit precise symptomatology. Describing the more subtle maladaptations of human beings to society involves social and cultural values; as value systems change so do conceptions of deviant behavior. Societal tolerance of deviant behavior partially determines what constitutes mental illness. Changing definitions of mental illness increasingly incorporate behaviors previously defined as "normal behavior," or which were even ignored in the past, thus expanding what society tolerates as sick behavior.

MEDICAL AND CLINICAL DEFINITIONS

Historically, mental health was defined along medical-clinical lines with the assumption that mental illness resulted from various internal causes which presumably were treatable by a corresponding therapy. In the late 1800s, Kraepelin, a German physician, outlined a concise system of classification establishing mental illness as a separate and distinct disease entity subject to the rules that applied to physical or somatic diseases. His work legitimized psychiatry as a branch of medicine. Kraepelin described in detail the symptoms, course of the disease, and prognosis of dementia praecox and manic-depressive psychoses. Sigmund Freud, the father of psychoanalysis, described neuroses in a deterministic fashion by proposing that all events could be traced to a specific origin. He described mental illness as related to disturbances and distortions from unconscious developmental difficulties in psychic growth and maturation, and traumatic experiences and conflicts over sexual and self-destructive instincts. Although psychotherapy came to be regarded as a medical and psychiatric specialty, Freud established the psychological viewpoint.

Continuing biomedical research in the twentieth century produced evidence which supported the concept of organic causations for mental illness. The discovery of the spirochete which causes syphilis and general paresis, and discoveries of chromosomal aberrations in mental retardation were cited as such evidence. Studies of schizophrenia, defined as a diagnosis by Bleuler in the early 1900s (replacing dementia praecox), and manic depressive syndromes have suggested possible familial tendencies. For example, 10% of siblings and children of schizophrenic patients also are diagnosed as schizophrenic, possibly indicating a biological basis for this illness. Transcultural studies of mental illness have demonstrated remarkably uniform prevalence rates for schizophrenia in different countries and cultures. However, modern techniques for the study of chromosomal aberrations do not isolate genetic differences, and even with clinical evidence suggesting a biological component, critics would argue that a diagnosis of schizophrenia is highly subjective and that the perception of behavior as being schizophrenic is relative to the environmental context. Studies of other illnesses such as the neurotic syndromes or drug abuse syndromes have so far been unable to identify biogenetic factors.

SOCIAL PSYCHIATRIC AND BEHAVIORAL DEFINITIONS

During the twentieth century there has been increasing acceptance of pluralistic determinants of mental illness including biological, sociological, and social factors. Harry Sullivan was the first American psychiatrist to develop a theory stressing the importance of interpersonal relations in disease etiology. Concurrent with the development of social psychiatric definitions were new psychological and behavioral concepts of mental illness. Carl Jung broke away from the Freudian approach and formed the field of analytic psychology. Erich Fromm, a psychoanalyst never trained in medicine, and others applied anthropological and sociological concepts to Freud's theories. Later John B. Watson discarded Freudian theory and developed behaviorism which recognized only observable behavior as critical to the diagnosis of mental illness. He believed that all behavior was predictable based on environmental stimuli. Psychologists introduced classical conditioning and learning theory to psychiatrists and other psychopathologists.

Social psychiatric and behavioral definitions of mental health reduced reliance on the disease concept of mental illness as internally manifested by the client; rather, social and cultural relativity and personality development were emphasized as significant factors in mental health. The development of humanistic psychology also had origins in the behavioral movements. The Freudian approach was considered too pessimistic and the behavioral approaches too mechanistic. Carl Rogers developed the technique of client centered therapy which recognized the client's role in affecting his or her own rehabilitation. Using this approach, client behavior is compared to expected behavior for the culture or environment of the patient. Differences between adaptive and maladaptive functioning will vary from culture to culture and will be more or less acceptable according to one's economic or social status. The validity of these broader environmentally based approaches are supported by transcultural psychiatric research which documents mental illness in all cultures and suggests that outward manifestations of these illnesses are shaped by the childrearing practices, indoctrinations, sanctions, encouragements and discouragements of each culture.

Definitions of deviant behavior can be predicated on the social and cultural values of the group therapist or provider. As a result, definitions may be based on the values of the care-giver rather than the care-recipient and may change as values change in a society. Consequently, behavior may be tolerated, accepted, or even encouraged within one cultural group but viewed as deviant by another population group. For example, an epidemiologic study of psychiatric disorders in a Pacific Northwest coastal Indian village found differing symptom patterns in men and women (1). Women, suffering more from psychoneuroses, were viewed as ill within this society while males, generally suffering from alcoholism, not only did not seek treatment but were not even considered ill by their community. Thus, social and behavioral definitions of, and treatments for, mental illness can differ within cultural groups, between cultures and societies, and over time in any society. Finally, defining the overlap between social problems and mental illness is difficult. Are deviations such as delinquency or criminal behavior a mental health problem? What about poverty, discrimination, and unemployment? Mental health professionals must determine the extent of their roles as care-givers and as social change agents.

EXTENT OF MENTAL DISORDERS

The American Psychiatric Association classifies mental illness within three general categories: impairment of brain tissue, mental deficiency, and disorders without clearly defined clinical cause. Most disorders treated by mental health professionals fall in the third category but diagnosis of these problems is subjective in actual clinical practice. The American Psychiatric Association published a book containing this classification system, the "Diagnostic and Statistical Manual" (DSM) (2), which is used extensively in diagnosing mental illness. These classifications are generally used in measuring incidence and prevalence of mental illness as well as the utilization of services.

INCIDENCE AND PREVALENCE OF MENTAL ILLNESS

Schizophrenia continues to be a major mental health problem in this country. The affective disorders, which include psychotic depression, mania, and manic depression, constitute another primary component of mental illness in our society. Drug abuse and alcohol-related problems form a third major category. Many people suffer from anxiety, moderate depression, and other emotional disorders. There is some evidence that only about one-fourth of those suffering from a clinically significant disorder have been in treatment (3). Table 7–1 presents the estimated distribution of people with mental disorders by treatment facility. Note that 54.1% of those seeking treatment do so in a primary care medical setting. Figure 7–1 shows the distribution of people seeking care by mental health settings; the majority of contacts occur in outpatient facilities.

There have been a number of attempts to measure the prevalence of mental illness in American society. An estimated 10,000,000 Americans experience one or more episodes of serious mental illness before reaching old age (3). The President's Commission on Mental Health estimated that 20,000,000 to 32,000,-000 Americans are in "need" of mental health services (3). Most reporting of mental illness is from public agencies as a requirement of funding and little information is available from private practitioners and non-public facilities. As a result, even the most valiant attempts to estimate the incidence and prevalence of mental illness are at best approximations. Many studies use such vague terms as "psychiatric impairment" rather than a more definitive diagnosis. Even diagnoses recorded on insurance claims forms are subject to considerable bias since reimbursement is dependent on diagnosis. Perhaps the most current estimates are those presented in the President's Commission on Mental Health, which are based on an analysis of available epidemiological studies (3). Reported prevalence rates for

TABLE 7–1. Estimated Percentage Distribution of Persons with Mental Disorders, by Treatment Setting, United States, 1975

Treatment Setting	Percent of People
Primary care/ outpatient medical sector	54.1
Not in treatment/ other human services sector*	21.5
Specialty mental health sector	15.0

Both specialty mental health
  sector and primary care/outpatient
  medical sector (overlap)
	6.0

General hospital inpatient/ nursing home sector*	3.4

*Excludes overlap of an unknown percent of persons also seen in other sectors.

Source: President's Commission on Mental Health: *Final Report, Volume II, Task Panel Reports.* Washington, D.C., Government Printing Office, 1978.

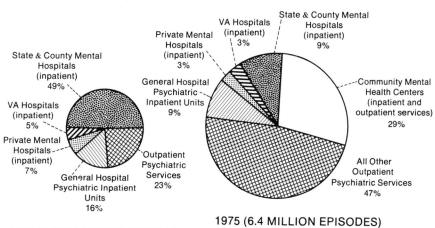

1955 (1.7 MILLION EPISODES)

1975 (6.4 MILLION EPISODES)

Figure 7–1. The percent distribution of inpatient and outpatient care episodes in mental health facilities, by type of facility, United States, 1955 and 1975. (*Source:* President's Commission on Mental Health: *Final Report, Volume II, Task Panel Reports.* Washington, D.C., Government Printing Office, 1978, p. 54.)

201

functional psychiatric disorders as a percent of the total United States population were: schizophrenia, 0.5 to 3.0, manic-depressive psychosis, 0.3, neurosis (including other depressive disorders), 8.0 to 13.0, and personality disorders, 7.0.

UTILIZATION OF MENTAL HEALTH SERVICES

Data concerning the use of mental health services also tends to be somewhat unreliable. Definitive diagnoses are often not reported. Most data is from the public sector. In addition, since studies are not often based on enrolled populations, the denominator for determining utilization rates is elusive. However, federal reporting does provide information on admissions by disorder to mental health facilities as presented in Table 7–2.

From the available evidence (Table 7–3), women are slightly higher utilizers of mental health services than men; adolescent males use services more often than adolescent females (4). The response to symptoms and willingness to seek treatment vary within the population and affect utilization of services. For instance, adolescent males may act-out in a more visible manner than adolescent females and therefore be referred more often for care. Attitudes of society toward men or women seeking services may create a more comfortable climate for women to do so.

Psychologically oriented illness accounts for a significant proportion of ambulatory medical services and prescribed drugs. An estimated 54% of people suffering from mental disorders are seen by primary care physicians in an outpatient setting (Table 7–1). People with mental or emotional distress often seek care from their family physician, a hospital outpatient clinic, or an emergency room. Various studies of the prevalence of psychosomatic illnesses of patients with physical symptoms and no apparent organic explanation in primary care medical practices suggest that from 15 to 50% of visits are for such illnesses.

Substantial differences exist in utilization among racial and ethnic groups. The effect of client and organizational variables, such as patient socioeconomic status, the racial and cultural background of the therapist, and the organizational setting in which services are provided, on utilization of services has yet to be determined. Mexican-Americans have been shown to utilize mental health services when they are available in a community setting (5). Studies of the utilization of services in a community mental health center indicate that minorities are hospitalized more often than whites (6). Differences in the volume of services received by blacks, chicanos, and other minority groups as compared to whites have also been reported. For example, in a study of patients admitted to Los Angeles County General Hospital for psychiatric treatment, 11% of whites as compared to 3% of black patients had more than 10 visits per illness episode (7). White clients also received more psychotherapy services and minority clients, unlike whites, sometimes received medication but no therapy.

Rates of institutionalization, when correctional institutions are included, differ for whites and non-whites. In 1960, although mental hospitalization rates were only 20% higher for non-whites than for whites, non-whites were institutionalized primarily in correctional institutions and whites in medical care facilities. By 1970, the rate of institutionalization into correctional facilities was even greater for non-whites (8). The social nature of many mental illnesses raise questions as to whether these patterns reflect biases in society.

The use of private versus public facilities varies by income. Higher income people use private practitioners, predominantly, while lower income people rely more heavily on public sources of care. Race is also a factor, perhaps interacting with income, related to the location in which services are received. Approximately 36% of whites and 11% of non-whites in a recent national survey of mental health utilization received services in a private inpatient setting. This difference was moderated for outpatient services in which 32% of whites and 26% non-whites were treated in private facilities (8).

Minorities are more likely to be from lower economic groups, have less education, and perhaps also have a language barrier. Studies of blacks using mental health services refer to "black English" and report miscommunications between white therapists and black patients. Also, blacks are less likely to receive individual psychotheraphy which is often biased toward educated verbal clients from cultures similar to that of the therapists. Mexican-Americans and Native Americans encounter language, education, and economic stumbling blocks as well. Command of English and understanding how to access the formal mental health services system affect the type of treatment obtained. In response to these barriers and for traditional reasons, some people also rely on alternative sources of care within their own culture. For example, the Mexican-American may seek help from the Curandero and the Native American from the Medicine Man. The formal mental health system is slowly learning to view these alternative systems with respect and seek their advice in the treatment of people from different cultural backgrounds.

DEVELOPMENT OF THE MENTAL HEALTH SYSTEM IN THE UNITED STATES

EARLY MENTAL HEALTH SYSTEM

The development of American psychiatry in the nineteenth century was strongly influenced by Dr. Benjamin Rush, long considered the father of American psychiatry, who was also a pioneer in hospital reform. Prior to the nineteenth century, formal treatment centers were non-existent. Private physician services were available to those with money. The rest faced imprisonment or hospitalization, one being not much different from the other. The hospital reform spearheaded by Pinel in the late 1700s in France was paralleled in this country by Rush's activities. The American Psychiatric Association was started through the efforts of affiliated hospital superintendents who, like Rush, shared concern over hospital conditions. Even into the early twentieth century, treatment of mental illness occurred in state-supported hospitals, often located in remote areas and functioning as large human warehouses, and based on medical-clinical approaches.

TABLE 7–2. Number and Percent Distribution of Admissions to Selected Mental Health Facilities, by Mental Disorder, United States, 1975

Diagnosis	State and County Mental Hospital	Private Mental Hospital	General Hospital Psychiatric Inpatient Unit	Outpatient Psychiatric Services	Community Mental Health Centers	Total—All Facilities
Total	385,237	128,832	515,537	1,406,065	919,037	3,355,708
Alcohol disorders	106,615	10,827	35,932	53,125	89,338	295,837
Drug disorders	14,435	3,077	17,849	22,094	28,638	86,093
Organic brain syndromes	20,372	5,195	18,981	30,821	22,443	97,812
Depressive disorders	44,965	55,068	194,399	180,735	122,948	598,115
Schizophrenia	129,425	28,315	124,458	148,303	91,914	522,415
Childhood disorders	5,987	1,564	4,625	143,462	120,642	276,280
Social maladjustments	1,139	164	1,818	143,278	66,395	212,794
All other diagnoses	57,163	24,783	114,622	526,926	242,155	965,649
No mental disorder	5,136	839	2,853	157,321	134,564	300,713

Percent distribution by diagnosis

Total	100.0	100.0	100.0	100.0	100.0	100.0
Alcohol disorders	27.0	8.3	7.0	3.8	9.7	8.8
Drug disorders	3.7	2.4	3.5	1.6	3.1	2.6
Organic brain syndromes	5.3	4.0	3.7	2.2	2.4	2.9
Depressive disorders	11.7	42.5	37.7	12.9	13.4	17.8
Schizophrenia	33.6	21.8	24.1	10.5	10.0	15.6
Childhood disorders	1.6	1.2	0.9	10.2	13.1	8.2
Social maladjustments	0.3	0.1	0.4	10.2	7.2	6.3
All other diagnoses	14.8	19.1	22.1	37.4	26.6	28.8
No mental disorder	1.3	0.6	0.6	11.2	14.6	9.0

Source: President's Commission on Mental Health: *Final Report, Volume II, Task Panel Reports*. Washington, D.C., Government Printing Office, 1978, p. 102.

TABLE 7–3. Age-adjusted Admission Rates By Race, Sex and Type of Facility, Selected Mental Health Facilities, United States, 1975*

| Race and Sex | State and County Mental Hospitals | Private Mental Hospitals | Inpatient Psychiatric Services | | | Federally Funded CMHCs | Outpatient Psychiatric Services |
| | | | Non-federal General Hospitals | | | | |
			Total	Public	Nonpublic		
Total–all races	182	61	244	66	178	435	665
Male	245	55	209	70	139	427	611
Female	124	67	276	62	214	441	709
White	160	65	243	61	182	415	639
Male	213	57	206	64	142	404	588
Female	110	71	278	58	220	425	683
All other races	340	39	238	98	140	571	834
Male	477	40	219	108	111	593	747
Female	226	39	253	89	165	550	890

*Denominator is estimated 1975 United States population.

Source: President's Commission on Mental Health: *Final Report, Volume II, Task Panel Reports.* Washington, D.C., Government Printing Office, 1978, p. 103.

206

The disease concept of mental illness has implied that the patient can become "well" and generally assumes that the therapist, historically a psychiatrist, will diagnose the illness and define subsequent treatment. The Freudian model has lead to long-term and intensive psychotherapy, and therapeutic and personnel requirements that are beyond the resources available to the state hospitals. Mental illness was also highly stigmatized and subject to funding limitations by state legislatures, with the primary purposes being to provide public protection from "crazy people" rather than to provide a public good for people with psychiatric problems.

The National Mental Health Act of 1946 (P.L. 79-487) signified an increased federal interest in the plight of the mentally ill. The law created the National Institute of Mental Health, and increased appropriations for therapy and research. In addition, recognition of the psychological problems of soldiers during World War II motivated Veterans Administration hospitals to provide expanded mental health services.

DEVELOPMENT OF OUTPATIENT SERVICES

The development of psychopharmacology in the 1950s had a profound impact on the field of mental health. Psychotropic drugs led to dramatic breakthroughs in the treatment of mental illness and enabled thousands of patients previously considered incurable to be effectively treated on an outpatient basis. The use of these drugs also created a climate that encouraged the development of various innovative therapeutic approaches.

Prior to World War II, few outpatient mental health facilities existed. With growing federal interest, the number of outpatient facilities increased. At the same time, the prognosis for the thousands of patients in mental hospitals, many of whom suffered from schizophrenia, depression, and mania, remained dismal. However, the use of antipsychotic medications for schizophrenia, anti-depressants for depression and, more recently, lithium in the treatment of mania, rapidly improved the prognosis for these patients. With the development of psychotropic medications, medical-clinical models of treatment continued to be the major influence on hospital treatment of mental illness. Psychotropic drugs also led to a radical decline in hospital length-of-stays for patients with psychiatric diagnoses. Patients now could control their behavior through the use of these drugs and, it was hoped, could function in the community. Thus, a mental health system previously based primarily on inpatient facilities had to develop new approaches to providing services to patients who no longer needed to be hospitalized.

As mental health professionals continued to expand their understanding of mental and emotional disorders, the general public was still distrustful and misinformed about the nature of mental illness and there was little advocacy for improvement except from the mental health community. Nevertheless, there was a dramatic increase in outpatient clinics from 400 before World War II to 1,234 by 1954 (9). Finally, in 1955 the National Mental Health Study Act (P.L. 84-182) was passed which authorized $750,000 for a three year study of the entire mental health system. The result was the "Action for Mental Health Report," published in 1961. Although this report covered many issues in the provision of mental health services, the primary emphasis of the legislation that followed, during the Kennedy Administration, was on outpatient services. Concern was increasingly focused on providing comprehensive mental health services to people not requiring hospitalization as well as to those not previously having access to mental health services. The Mental Retardation Facilities and Community Mental Health Centers Construction Act of 1964 (P.L. 88-164) provided construction monies for community mental health centers which were to serve designated catchment areas of 75,000 to 200,000 people. The five basic services that the centers were required to provide included inpatient, outpatient, emergency, day treatment, and consultation and education services. Significantly, the legislation mandated that services be provided regardless of the patient's ability to pay.

Many centers were built with the newly available funding for construction, but money for staffing and operations continued to be scarce. Finally, in 1967, an amendment to the legislation provided the necessary operations money on a matching basis, with funding for each center declining over an eight year period. This was the "seed money" concept and it was hoped that the construction and development of a community mental health center would encourage the community to gradually assume financial responsibility for services. Since catchment areas varied in their ability to provide matching funds, the subsidy for services in different areas also varied considerably. And although there was an allowance for the poorer communities, the capability to readily obtain local matching funds was a distinct advantage for some centers. In retrospect, the whole notion of matching local funds ignored the inability of some communities to assume the associated financial burden, especially in areas of greatest "need." Since many centers faced closure or significant reduction in services, additional legislation (P.L. 94-63) was passed in 1975 which included provision for a one year distress grant at the end of the eight years of operational support if alternate funding was not obtained. This legislation was designed to overhaul the Community Mental Health Center network and also to increase the original five required services to twelve including care for drug abuse problems, children, the aged, and screening, followup, and community living services. In addition, the National Center for Prevention and Control of Rape was created. Planning and evaluation of local community mental health services was mandated; two percent of each Center's budget was to be used for these purposes.

Community Mental Health Centers are also required to operate under the authority of a Board of Directors which represents the local community. These Boards, however, are often composed of well-educated, upper-middle income people who are frequently health care providers despite the location of many mental health centers in lower income communities.

As a result of the failure of Community Mental Health Centers to provide comprehensive services, and the emergence of other community needs, alternate care sources have developed. These sources are often "grass roots" movements, funded on shoestring budgets, and organized by people who perceive unmet mental health needs. Examples include the over 2,000 hotlines, 200 houses for runaways, and 400 free clinics that operate throughout the nation (3).

MENTAL HEALTH PERSONNEL

PSYCHIATRISTS

Psychiatry, the medical specialty dealing with mental disorders, is firmly entrenched in the mental health services system and continues to promulgate primarily medical-clinical definitions of mental illness. However, social psychiatry is concerned with the environmental and societal phenomena involved in mental and emotional disorders and the use of social forces in the treatment of such disorders. Much of the scientific work of social psychiatry has been in the area of epidemiology and, particularly, estimating the incidence and prevalence of mental illness in community and hospital settings. Growing concern for the environment in large mental hospitals during and after World War II also added impetus to the social psychiatric movement and as early as 1946, the American Psychiatric Association adopted a strict set of standards for mental hospitals and appointed a Central Inspection Board for enforcement of these standards. Social psychiatry, in an effort to transform these large institutions from custodial care to treatment centers, developed the concept of the therapeutic community, the fundamental tenet of which is that patients can assist in their own rehabilitation as well as in the rehabilitation of other patients. Social psychiatry also includes transcultural and community psychiatry. Transcultural psychiatry addresses the study of the incidence and prevalence of mental disease across societies and the delineation of social forces that affect the manifestations of these illnesses. Community psychiatry has been described as "social psychiatry in action" (10) and is involved in the development, planning, and organization of community mental health programs and consultation to local agencies.

The number of psychiatrists in the United States has increased from approximately 7,000 in 1950 to over 27,000 today, including psychiatrists working primarily in administration (3). Psychiatrists are distributed approximately equally between private practice and public service in state mental hospitals and community facilities. Some psychiatrists work in both public and private settings.

PSYCHOLOGISTS

Psychiatrists have traditionally assumed clinical leadership roles but are now under attack from psychologists, psychiatric nurses, and social workers who seek more equal status with physicians. Psychology, which struggled to create its own professional identity in the early years of this century, has emphasized scientific research in academic settings. Beginning as a philosophy, psychology has become firmly established as a social science and psychologists have promoted and conducted research into the functioning of the human mind, especially through development of scientific testing instruments. Beginning in the early twentieth century, psychological testing began to be used in conjunction with psychiatric treatment. Research by psychologists in classical conditioning and behavioral theory also aided psychiatrists who still provided most therapeutic care.

During World War II, psychologists began to seek an expanded role in clinical practice. With the expansion of mental health services in the Veterans Administration hospitals, the training of clinical psychologists began in earnest. In 1946, the Veterans Administration (VA) in conjunction with the American Psychological Association, began the VA Psychology Training Program, still a major source of training for clinical and counseling psychology. The professional application of psychology received further endorsement in the American Psychological Association Vail Conference of 1973, which emphasized the continued training of clinicians and scientists in psychology.

Psychologists are licensed or certified in all states and the District of Columbia. In almost all states the training required for licensure is a doctoral degree although a few states allow limited licensure for graduates of master's degree programs though independent private practice is prohibited. Licensure is not required for practice in some settings, however, and unlicensed psychologists most often practice in school or community mental health facilities. In early 1977, the American Psychological Association reported a membership of 47,000 (11) although there may be as many as 70,000 master's and doctoral level psychologists (3).

SOCIAL WORKERS

The history of social work dates back to the late nineteenth century and the volunteer mothers who provided disadvantaged persons with charitable aid through the Charity Organization Societies. Social work began to develop as a profession during the early twentieth century. Reform minded women, struggling for equality, became social workers and began working in medical and psychiatric settings, schools and correctional institutions. The development of social psychiatry also prompted the formation of a professional identity for social workers. Adopting the Freudian psychoanalytical model of many psychiatrists, social workers struggled for increasing responsibility in the treatment of mental and emotional disorders. The practice of psychotherapy expanded the social worker's domain from providing charitable assistance to the poor to providing a therapy that was viewed as legitimate by middle and upper class people. Since psychoanalysis and psychotherapy remained medical specialties, social workers were not too successful in developing a separate professional identity and their practice continued in the shadow of psychiatry.

Social work continues to struggle for an independent identity and a more equal role in the delivery of mental health services. Training includes two year associate degree programs graduating human service workers, baccalaureate programs in social work, currently recognized as the beginning professional level, master's level degrees in social work, and doctoral programs. In addition to the basic training of the discipline, social work education offers specialized training in mental health and in human services administration. The National Association of Social Workers lists about 70,000 members but there may be as many as 300,000 social service workers (3). Social workers are licensed in 23 states and efforts toward social work licensure are underway in many other states.

PSYCHIATRIC NURSING

The professional training of nurses in this country began in the 1860s and consisted primarily of apprenticeships. The first training program that prepared nurses to care for the mentally ill was started in 1882 at McLean Hospital, a private psychiatric facility in Waverly, Massachusetts. Although there was a growing appreciation of nurses who received this type of training, poorly funded psychiatric hospitals continued to employ lesser trained aides at very low pay. Whatever nursing care did exist in these hospitals consisted mainly of custodial care focusing on the physical needs of the patient and the nurse continued to practice in a dependent relationship with a physician.

The development in the 1930s of somatic treatments for mental illness, such as insulin shock therapy, psychosurgery, and electroshock therapy, required the services of highly skilled nurses and established a more significant role for nurses in psychiatric treatment. The advent of the therapeutic community in psychiatric hospitals broadened the role of the nurse even further. As the 24-hour-care necessary for developing and maintaining the therapeutic milieu was recognized, nurses became a valuable member of the therapeutic team. The involvement of nurses in group psychotherapy after World War II resulted in federal appropriations for training nurses. However, despite the recognition of psychiatric nursing as a legitimate nursing role, vague notions remained as to the exact function of the nurse in mental health care.

Nursing education has become much more academically based over the past twenty years as the need for college level training programs and nursing research was recognized. Graduates of nursing schools obtained an increasingly strong professional and academic education, often training side-by-side with psychiatrists, psychologists, and social workers. Nurses who earned advanced degrees were often recruited for teaching, however, and the two year associate degree and diploma nurses were more prevalent in clinical practice. As nurses began to move into the role of psychotherapists, partially in response to the shortage of psychiatrists in most hospitals, interprofessional conflicts developed. But the exploding demand for psychotherapists further legitimized the nurse's role in therapy and, by the late 1960s, the clinical specialty of psychiatric nursing was firmly established. The first organization to certify clinical specialists in psychiatric nursing, in 1972, was the New Jersey State Nurses Association.

Nursing education includes training in psychiatric nursing at all academic levels. The associate degree nurse with two years of training in an academic program and the diploma nurse trained in a hospital program most often provide clinical services. The baccalaureate and master's level nurses often work in supervisory positions, or in teaching, and doctorate level nurses usually teach rather than provide clinical services. The majority of clinically active psychiatric nurses work in hospital settings.

Clinical psychiatric nurses have not been received with overwhelming enthusiasm by other mental health professionals, partially as a result of controversies over professional status and duties within the nursing profession itself. Nursing has yet to clearly define the appropriate roles of nurses and their relation to other mental health professionals. In addition, para-professionals such as mental health workers and psychiatric aides want nurses to perform supervision and management roles so as to leave a wider territory for their own struggle for psychotherapeutic practice rights. In community settings, social workers want to perform psychotherapy and have psychiatric nurses perform more in the tradition of the public health nurse. Currently, many psychiatric nurses in mental health settings do not have the specialized graduate-level training that the title implies. There are approximately 1,000,000 nurses in the United States (3); of the 177,000 nurses in the American Nurses Association, 29,000 are categorized as psychiatric nurses.

OTHER MENTAL HEALTH PERSONNEL CONCERNS

The roles of the various mental health service providers vary with the setting in which they practice. Inpatient psychiatric services are oriented toward the more traditional medical-clinical model with the psychiatrist assuming the primary role and nurses, psychologists, and social workers offering support services. The growth of community services provided some impetus for change toward a more egalitarian role for all mental health professionals, particularly in the Community Mental Health Centers which were intended to operate within the social and behavioral models of treatment. However, the more traditional therapies persist even in these centers and all professionals practice similarly. Differences in professional training are reflected more in incomes than in professional activity and most mental health professionals jockey for the same narrow therapeutic territory. Psychiatrists sometimes also assume consulting and supervisory roles in addition to providing care and supervising medications.

Administration in mental health has been largely performed by psychiatrists in mental hospitals. Community Mental Health Centers, although originally envisioned to have psychiatrists as directors, tend to utilize primarily psychologists and social workers as administrators. Since clinical skills alone are inadequate for administration, educational programs have been developed to offer some training in administration and management for mental health professionals, especially in social work and community psychiatry. In addition, there is a growing trend toward professionally trained mental health administrators without a clinical background.

Tables 7–4 and 7–5 present the supply and distribution among mental health facilities of personnel. The increase in personnel for the years 1950–1976 reflects the increase in mental health concerns and increased appropriations for training. Equally important to note is the increase in personnel with baccalaureate degree or lower levels of education.

The mental health system experienced a rapid explosion in the demand for practitioners as increased federal funding was authorized by the Congress. Table 7–5 shows the current level of positions in mental health settings. It does not include those in private practice. In addition to increased demand for psychiatrists, psychologists, social workers, and psychiatric nurses, a number of allied mental

TABLE 7–4. Estimated Number of Professional Mental Health Personnel, by Discipline, United States, Selected Years

Year	Psychiatrists	Psychologists	Social Workers	Registered Nurses
1950	7,100	7,300	NA*	NA
1955	10,600	13.500	20,000	NA
1960	14,100	18,200	26,200	504,000
1965	18,500	23,600	41,600	600,000
1970	23,200	30,800	49,600	722,000
1975	25,700	39,400	64,500	906,000
1976	26,500	42,000	69,600	961,000

*NA—not available.

Source: President's Commission on Mental Health: *Final Report, Volume II, Task Panel Reports*, Washington, D.C., Government Printing Office, 1978, p. 488.

TABLE 7–5. Full-Time Equivalent Positions, by Discipline, All Mental Health Facilities, United States, Selected Years

Discipline	Year			
	1968	1972	1974	1976
Psychiatrists	9,891	12,938	14,947	15,339
Other physicians	2,736	3,991	3,548	3,356
Psychologists	5,212	9,443	12,597	15,251
Social workers	9,755	17,687	22,147	25,887
Registered nurses	24,256	31,110	34,089	39,392
Other mental health professionals	12,136	17,514	29,325	34,249
Physical health	NA*	8,203	10,507	9,631
Total professional patient care staff	63,986	100,886	127,160	143,105
Licensed practical nurses	NA	19,616	17,193	15,337
Mental health workers	NA	120,753	128,529	130,021
Total patient care staff	NA	241,255	272,882	288,463
Administrative, clerical, maintenance	NA	134,719	130,142	134,795
Total	NA	375,974	403,024	423,258

*NA—not available.

Source: President's Commission on Mental Health: *Final Report, Volume II, Task Panel Reports*, Washington, D.C., Government Printing Office, 1978, p. 484.

health fields developed; these fields represent 12% of all mental health personnel (3).

Schools of education are training counselling and guidance personnel as well as special education teachers who work in schools and other settings. The special needs of people recovering from mental and emotional disabilities have been recognized by such professional groups as occupational and recreational therapists and vocational counselors. Practitioners in marriage counseling, art, music, and dance therapy, and religion provide counselling and therapy in many mental health settings. Training for these allied professionals varies tremendously and they serve in such positions as mental health workers, alcohol and drug abuse counselors, day-care workers, board and home care providers, foster parents, patient advocates, and hospital psychiatric aides. In some mental health centers, half of the positions are filled by these individuals.

Indigenous healers are rarely recognized by traditional mental health service providers but have an important role in caring for physical and emotional disturbances in many minority cultures. Community volunteers are also an important component of the mental health work force. Thousands of people offer their time and services, performing tasks ranging from assisting with clerical needs to working directly with patients.

Issues of access to care raise concerns over the racial and economic mix of mental health professionals and the predominance of male practitioners. Speculation about the capability of many providers to respond to different cultural groups, and especially the poor, fosters much of this concern, particularly since the poor and minorities often have lower utilization rates for mental health services. Psychiatry, in particular, includes few minority practitioners and foreign medical graduates often staff state and county hospitals. Foreign graduates may have difficulty adapting to the culture and language of their American clientele. Psychology also has few minority practitioners but graduate programs are now increasing the number of minority and women students. About 10% of graduate students currently are minorities and 33% of psychology doctorates in 1976 were awarded to women (3). Social work has long recognized the importance of training in different social and cultural systems, has many minority practitioners and, indeed, has traditionally been considered a woman's field. Men have now been increasingly entering social work and nursing.

THE ORGANIZATION OF SERVICES

FINANCING CARE

Many mental health services are provided in the public sector, funded by public money, and as a result are subject to the whims of legislatures and special interest groups. Unfortunately, advocacy for mental health has been weak and state legislatures generally have not placed high priority on these services. Public funding in mental health has been likened to a "floating crap game." The money "moves" from one priority to another depending upon popular therapies and modalities and the source of funds; provider agencies must try to stay ahead of the game. In addition to federal programs, state support has gradually increased but has remained inadequate. Local governments, through various taxing mechanisms, also provide some support. Reimbursement from private health insurance has provided only a small percentage of total revenue in public agencies but most of the revenue for private care. Philanthropy remains a negligible funding source.

Community mental health centers face a variety of cost problems. Some of the local money for services was to have come from resources no longer needed because of the deinstitutionalization of hospital patients. As patients moved from hospital to community care, it seemed that money no longer needed for their hospital care could be transferred to support community care. However, most state hospitals did not close as originally hoped would occur with the introduction of the wonderous new psychotropic medications. More and more, it is becoming evident that there is a group of people who simply cannot be supported by community resources and must remain in institutions. In addition, the dollars have not always followed the patient and those that have seem not to go as far. The centers are required to provide a wide range of services and do not qualify for reimbursement for all of them. Multiple funding sources also require multiple reporting and extra administrative effort. Demand for services has increased from both hospitalized patients and an increased number of people seeking care, not all of whom have the financial resources to do so. Centers are mandated to provide services to everyone, including the poor and working poor populations, regardless of ability to pay. As federal dollars become more scarce and states fail to fully replace federal funding, fewer resources must be spread more thinly.

Financing of services provided by private practitioners and private facilities is largely from third-party insurance or from out-of-pocket payments by patients. Most third party payers reimburse only psychiatrists although, in limited instances, some will reimburse psychologists and social workers.

INSURANCE COVERAGE FOR MENTAL HEALTH SERVICES

As discussed in Chapter 10, voluntary insurance coverage developed initially for acute care hospital services, and primarily for surgical care. Gradually, ancillary and outpatient services were added, although not to the extent that inpatient care was covered. Throughout this process, mental health services were simply not considered. Prior to World War II treatment for mental illness consisted primarily of removal from society and placement in state mental hospitals. With the exception of limited private psychiatric services, the state hospitals were the only source of care available and were not included in insurance plans.

Few incentives existed for insurers to add mental health benefits, especially since they were poorly defined, had few precise diagnoses, used controversial and changing therapies, and could not be demonstrated to have efficacious treatments.

Demand was not predictable and the users of services were unable to provide a strong advocacy. Mental health benefits are often considered low priority by people who do not feel that they are at potential risk. Mental illness has a stigma and is something that happens to "somebody else."

Eventually, some mental health benefits began to be included in insurance contracts. Short-term inpatient mental health services were covered initially, although not as extensively as inpatient medical and surgical services, and often had a high coinsurance provision (such as 50%), and a low total dollar benefit limitation. Outpatient benefits for mental health services are less comprehensive than for other types of ambulatory care and sometimes are nonexistent. The Federal Employees Health Insurance Plan was the first to experiment with comprehensive mental health benefits and reported high costs, lengthy treatment times, and questionable outcomes for psychoanalysis, the most commonly sought treatment. The United Auto Workers was the next major group to provide comprehensive coverage and experienced reasonable costs.

As Medicare and Medicaid were developed, they had limitations for mental health services despite the verbal support from federal officials for more comprehensive coverage. Medicare has dollar restrictions and coinsurance requirements. Medicaid, although originally intending to prohibit discrimination on the basis of diagnosis, required the states to specify mental health clinics as "providers" if mental health services were to be a covered benefit. Many states did not specify mental health clinics in their legislation and consequently do not provide benefits under Medicaid for mental health care.

Federally funded Health Maintenance Organizations are mandated to include mental health benefits but the emphasis is on short-term psychiatric intervention designed to stabilize and return the patient to work or other prior activity. Other prepaid group practice plans generally do not cover chronic mental illnesses or organic psychiatric problems. Often the terms of coverage specify that the mental illness must be amenable to short-term treatment with likelihood of significant improvement in the patient's condition. A study of utilization of mental health services in one large prepaid group practice plan indicated that the mental health visits for two-thirds of the patients were also the first exposure to any type of formal counseling for the patient. Diagnoses consisted primarily of acute crisis situations, marital maladjustment, or situational adjustment reactions and the enrolled population consisted primarily of stable middle class employees and their families (12). The average annual number of services per patient was 3.6, reflecting an orientation toward crisis intervention and short-term counseling.

SERVICES IN THE PRIVATE SECTOR

Services in the private sector include those provided by private psychiatric hospitals, psychiatric units in private acute care hospitals, private clinics offering outpatient services, and a proliferation of private practitioners operating in solo and group practice settings. Only very limited data is available on the providers and patients in private settings. An estimated 8,700 psychiatrists were in private practice in 1974. In a recent survey, nearly one-third of psychiatrists who responded indicated that their subspecialty was psychoanalysis, 10% child psychiatry, and 6% other subspecialties; the remaining 51% indicated no psychiatric subspecialty (13). The responding psychiatrists reported that 5% of patients were very mildly impaired, 18% mildly impaired, 50% moderately impaired, and 27% were considered severely impaired. Fifty percent of the patients of these private psychiatrists had at least some insurance coverage and most patients were from families with incomes in the $10,000—$30,000 range. In contrast, a study of patients seeking services in the public sector indicated that nearly all had incomes under $15,000.

Approximately 40% of patients seeking mental health services use the private sector, but their use represents only 15% of the total mental health visits in the country. This is explainable since 44% of those seeking services in the private sector are diagnosed and then referred for treatment elsewhere. In addition, private psychiatrists treat a much less diverse population than do community clinics and have little contact with alcoholic or drug abuse patients, or with children and the aged.

SERVICES IN THE PUBLIC SECTOR

A wide range of ambulatory public services are provided in outpatient psychiatric clinics, community mental health centers, halfway houses, "transitional" care facilities, and alternative care sources. Inpatient services include both state and county psychiatric hospitals, psychiatric units in public hospitals, and residential treatment centers for both children and adults. Other services are sought outside the mental health system. Psychological and emotional problems account for many visits to general medical facilities. Family service agencies provide mental health services as well as other social services. Limited mental health services can be obtained in school systems, colleges and universities.

Alternative services which have developed within the last 10 years address mental health, economic, environmental, and social issues. Hotlines, developed to handle crisis situations, offer anonymous and instant accessibility and have an up-to-date knowledge of the needs and problems of the communities they serve. Services for runaway young people started with little financial support beyond community philanthropy. Federal and state funding was later accepted by some but rejected by others due to confining mandated service requirements imposed by these sources. Other programs include long-term residential programs, pioneering programs offering women's mental health services, rape crisis centers, shelters for battered women, and service programs for older people. Many of the free clinics offering primary medical care also include social and psychological services. The holistic health clinics emphasize physical and mental illness, and "wellness," in a broader context than traditional medical and mental health services. Many of these alternative services utilize mental health providers and techniques, but often depend on "paraprofessionals" and lesser trained persons to provide care. These alternative services may appear and disappear overnight. They tend to be very responsive to immediate needs and often pave the way for innovation and change by more traditional providers. This care is considered by many to be equal, if not superior, to that offered by the more traditional mental health centers and is often much less expensive to provide (3).

ISSUES AND TRENDS IN MENTAL HEALTH

On February 17, 1977, Executive Order No. 11973 established the President's Commission on Mental Health. Public hearings were held across the country and many fact-finding task panels were created to review the mental health needs of the nation and recommend future courses for public policy. Recommendations of the Commission suggested more comprehensive, high quality care with special emphasis on underserved populations and greater responsiveness to the diverse racial and cultural backgrounds of people, more adequate financing of services, expanded personnel, and further research on the nature and treatment of mental disabilities. There was an emphasis on prevention and on protecting human rights and guaranteeing freedom of choice in the provision of care. These broad and challenging goals raise many current issues.

PROVIDING COMPREHENSIVE SERVICES

Numerous variables affect the utilization of mental health services. The recognition of psychological or emotional distress as a problem is necessary if people are to seek services voluntarily. What may be viewed as mental illness by professionals or family may not be viewed as such by the patient. Since mental illness is still stigmatized, patients may not acknowledge their problems to the extent of seeking services, or are deterred from doing so by family or friends concerned with the reaction of others. And as discussed above, what is "illness" to "society" or professionals may be acceptable behavior to the "mentally ill" person's social groups. The lack of accessible sources of care may preclude seeking services from the formal mental health "system."

Knowing where to seek care is essential. A study in Australia which compared a middle-class and a working-class neighborhood indicated that people from the higher socioeconomic group were more likely to know where to find help in time of stress (14). Often professionals themselves do not know all of the available resources. School and social welfare agency personnel, and mental health and other health care professionals may not know of each other's services nor have any formal communication channels to share information about resources.

COORDINATING SERVICES

Emotional problems do not exist in isolation. People may have several problems and need a variety of services. Many people may find themselves struggling to receive care within a system that addresses only a few of their problems and are unable to marshall services from diverse sources to meet all of their needs. People with multiple handicaps, such as physical and emotional disabilities, can face extraordinary problems in obtaining comprehensive care. Services received may depend on which problem is identified initially and referrals for multiple problems are often difficult. For example, emotionally disturbed mentally retarded people must utilize three separate "systems" for mental retardation, mental health, and rehabilitative services. Bureaucratic barriers exist for referring the client from one system to another; financial incentives encourage the provision of services for which reimbursement exists. Problems that are not within the realm of expertise available from a particular source of care may go unnoticed if they are not extremely evident.

Integration between mental health and educational programs is another excellent example of fragmentation. Children's services are not jointly funded between mental health and educational programs. Treatment for problems is often difficult or impossible to coordinate and even if there is a concern for coordination by the educator and the mental health professional, bureaucratic requirements may interfere.

BARRIERS TO SERVICE

Concern about financial barriers in mental health centers focused on federally mandated services which were to be provided regardless of the patient's ability to pay in Community Mental Health Centers. Access to and availability of care has encouraged the development of networks of outpatient facilities. The social status and racial or ethnic background of therapists as compared to patients, as noted previously, continues to be addressed by training professionals from diverse economic, racial, and cultural backgrounds. Education of the public about mental illness and sources of care helps to remove attitude and knowledge barriers. Research continues into the causes, treatments, and possible remedies for psychiatric and emotional problems. Yet many people still do not receive needed care.

Inpatient and outpatient mental health services are still more available in urban than rural areas. Funding for mental health is increasingly inadequate to meet the need for care. Although public services are available to moderate and low income people, they are not adequate to meet their needs. The concept of services to all people regardless of ability to pay is rendered less than effective by long waiting lists in many centers. If you can pay, you can buy services. If you can't, you may end up on a waiting list.

Outpatient services continue to be more heavily utilized by whites than by blacks and other minorities, while hospitalization rates for non-whites are higher. For example, in one study blacks were perceived as having more symptoms and complaints of persecution, suspiciousness, drug and alcohol abuse, and seizures than non-black patients (6); yet in this study, median length-of-stay was 16 days for blacks and 26 days for non-blacks. Only 25% of the black patients received individual psychotherapy compared with 80% of the non-black patients. Care may indeed differ, psychosocial variables modify how symptoms are perceived and recorded, and treatment may be influenced by provider attitudes, values, and administrative policy. Blacks use Community Mental Health Center services much the same as people of lower socioeconomic status use emergency rooms in general hospitals. They visit a community clinic in an emergency but do not continue in ongoing treatment once they are stabilized.

Services for the aged and children remain dismally lacking. Although many people below age 15 and over age 65 suffer from psychiatric and emotional disorders, most services are oriented toward young and middle-aged adults.

Deinstitutionalization has been an aim of federal legislation and of legal cases relating to a person's right to be treated in the least restrictive environment. In reality, few state hospitals have closed. New admissions to psychiatric hospitals have increased approximately 90% since 1950 and readmission rates have increased almost 600%. Average length-of-stay has declined from 20 years for psychoses and nine years for neuroses to an average overall length-of-stay of five months (15); censuses are lower but people are returning for readmission after they are discharged. The chronically mentally ill patient is still caught in a "revolving door," wandering in and out of the mental health system.

Despite efforts towards better case management for patients leaving the hospital and needing outpatient services, previously hospitalized people often "fall through the cracks" and do not again seek services until in crisis. Often this occurs as an emergency room visit at a general hospital. This has partially resulted in a significant increase in the availability of psychiatric services in acute care settings. Nursing homes also receive many previously hospitalized psychiatric patients. Discharges of state hospital patients to nursing homes has increased from 196 per 100,000 in 1950 to 456 per 100,000 in 1970 (15). Many patients leave the hospital, receive only occasional and fragmented services, and end up in communities of ex-hospital patients who are dependent upon other parts of the social welfare system for survival. Those patients who find their way into transitional care may end up in boarding house situations where few services are offered and continued dependence is fostered instead of integration into the community. Families may be ill equipped to deal with family members returning from the hospital and may have little or no support, either emotional or financial, in helping the ex-patient find a job, other housing, ongoing mental health care, or other necessary services.

MENTAL HEALTH LAW

Over the years the focus on laws relating to mental health has shifted along with changing attitudes, treatments, and services. In the past, public safety issues rather than patient rights were reflected in laws and legal decisions about mental health issues. As the dysfunctional effects of long-term institutionalization became more evident and a greater concern for individual rights was expressed, legislation began to recognize minimum criteria for treatment, alternatives to institutionalization, and a greater acknowledgment of patient rights. It is interesting to note that lawyers rather than mental health professionals led the way for patients' rights in the mental health field. Right to treatment, consent for treatment, and confidentiality are only some of the areas of litigation which bridge the judicial and mental health systems.

Right to treatment was first addressed in 1952 in civil commitment cases relating to sexual psychopaths. *Rouse* v. *Cameron* in 1966, based on arguments of cruel and unusual treatment and the right to due process, found that people judged criminally insane had the right to treatment (16). Since the early cases did not define criteria for treatment, but merely stated that some effort was required, there was little immediate impact. A decision by Judge Johnson of Alabama in 1972, based on a class action suit (*Wyatt* v. *Stickney*) related to conditions in state hospitals, required that right to treatment be enforced and implemented (17); various courts have subsequently specified minimum standards for treatment.

Other cases have addressed the right to the least restrictive environment for treatment. Donaldson, a patient in a Florida hospital for 14 years, sued for damages and demanded his release. The Supreme Court, in *Donaldson* v. *O'Conner,* ruled that patients cannot be confined in institutions against their will if they are not dangerous to society and themselves and have the necessary support to survive outside (18-19). A similar case went one step further when a federal court ordered the District of Columbia to create adequate facilities so that patients capable of treatment in a less restrictive community-based environment can be released from the hospital.

The right not to be treated raises often conflicting interests between the society, therapist and patient. The implications of behavior control through the use of behavior therapies, drug therapy, and psychosurgery create problems which have been addressed by the judicial system and by mental health professionals. State laws on involuntary treatment acts determine when a person can be involuntarily committed and use criteria such as dangerousness to self and to others. The term "gravely disabled," used in some state statutes for involuntary commitment, has not been clearly defined. Many people argue that dangerousness as a sole criterion for involuntary hospitalization deprives many mentally ill people of urgently needed protection and treatment. Relying solely on the "gravely disabled" criterion often means that a person is not hospitalized unless facing imminent danger from starvation or exposure. People in less extreme circumstances may need treatment but cannot be committed as "gravely disabled."

Even treatment with consent has been scrutinized due to the subtle pressures on the patient which may exist. A 1972 case, *Winters* v. *Miller,* recognized the potential for undue pressures to be placed on patients by their therapists and acknowledged the right not to be treated (20). Many other complex legal and ethical issues have yet to be adequately addressed.

PLANNING MENTAL HEALTH SERVICES

Planning in mental health has been largely nonexistent. Mental health services have expanded rapidly in the last decade and little or no attention has been directed toward the rational planning of that growth. As the funding for mental health care rapidly expanded, federal and state agencies took a second look and began to ask what they were paying for. They were aided in their information seeking efforts by electronic record-keeping. Accountability has become increasingly important in mental health and is measured by operational statistics such as numbers of patient visits and diagnostic categories. This reporting, a condition for continued funding in most cases, has come under considerable criticism for being insensitive to the true measure of what happens in human interactions. Activities such as those related to prevention become difficult to justify because they are not quantifiable. For example, how do you count the number of people who do not seek services as a result of prevention activities? As a result, the major focus of the mental health system in the public sector is on the treatment of mental illness rather than the maintenance of mental health.

Nonetheless, rapidly expanding technology provides an increasingly efficient means for mental health services to keep track of measurable activities such as the number and types of episodes of treatment. Accumulating, processing, and aggregating this data is a monumental task for federal, state, and county agencies who may not share information or coordinate activities with each other. Limited incidence and prevalence data and the inherent difficulties in measuring mental illness offer little data by which to measure or plan the activities of mental health facilities.

Planning mental health services is addressed by recent national health planning legislation (P.L. 94-641) discussed in Chapter 11. Members of planning agency boards may not include people knowledgeable about mental health care. Data bases used by these agencies for planning may not be suited to the reporting of mental health or mental retardation data and may not provide planners with meaningful data. Regional planning may be difficult if agency boundaries conflict with service areas for state mental hospitals and mental health and mental retardation centers, and state mental health planning regions. Cutting across these overlapping bureaucratic designations may prove at least difficult, if not impossible.

NATIONAL HEALTH INSURANCE

Expanded funding of mental health services through a national health insurance program could have a profoundly adverse effect if not based on enlightened and rational social policy. Programs for psychiatric services required as a result of involuntary commitment, rehabilitation services, job placement, and other services not recognized by even the more comprehensive insurance proposals will continue to need support. The scope of coverage of services will determine who will provide care. Reimbursing only certain providers, such as psychiatrists, will likely lead to increased numbers of those providers. If psychiatrists are the primary providers reimbursed, then a medical model of service will gain precedence. Recognition of the mental health center as a legitimate provider and allowing a broad background for professional therapists will emphasize yet another model of care. All of the current proposals vary in scope of coverage, nature of funding, and the degree of involvement of the insurance industry. All the comprehensive proposals provide some coverage for psychiatric inpatient and outpatient services but include restrictions through coinsurance, deductibles, and dollar and time limits.

Concerns have been expressed by the President's Commission on Mental Health and many professionals about planning mental health services to better meet the needs of underutilizers such as low-income and minority groups. There is a need to provide less fragmented services and to more clearly define and document the nature of mental illness, efficacious treatment, and potential remedies. Perhaps national financing will eventually provide further impetus to achieve these goals.

CONCLUSIONS

Our society is slowly working towards a better understanding of the nature of mental health. Much of what is currently known and believed is predicated on a mixture of fact and untested theory. Despite monumental efforts to incorporate the current knowledge and beliefs about the biological, sociological and environmental factors in mental illness, even the Community Mental Health Centers, touted as a giant step away from the medical model and psychoanalytic practices, continue to ramble along in the more traditional modes with only the provider of those traditional therapies varying. The mental health system works vigorously to catch up with current knowledge and philosophy but is warped by a confusing mixture of funding sources and mandates dictated more by special interests and budgetary concerns than by the efficacy of therapeutic practices.

Many people who seek services cannot pay for them, and even those who can afford to pay may not find comprehensive services in private psychiatric offices or facilities. Public services are structured by those agencies that pay for them and may not recognize the problems of those who might seek services. And in the current mental health system, where it is not clear who should be doing what to whom, there is little documented evidence as to which providers are better able to provide which services. With such a confusing and complex system, it is not surprising that many potential users become confused and either seek inappropriate services or none at all.

Despite the many problems that exist in the system, mental health professionals, citizen advocates, and consumers continue to labor toward better and more stable funding, better and more services, and less stigma for mental illness. Custodial treatment still exists. Many people do go unserved or inappropriately treated. But the problems of the mentally ill continue to receive attention and concern, and the mental health system continues to gain credence and legitimacy within the larger health care system.

REFERENCES

1. Shore JH, Kinzie JD, Hampson JD et al: Psychiatric epidemiology of an Indian village. *Psychiatry* **36**:70–81, 1973.
2. American Psychiatric Association, Taskforce on Nomenclature Statistics: *Diagnostic and Statistics Manual.* Washington, D.C., The Association, 1978.
3. President's Commission on Mental Health: *Final Report, Volume II, Task Panel Reports.* Washington, D.C., Government Printing Office, 1978.
4. Novack A, Bromet E, Neill T, et al: Children's mental health services in an inner city

neighborhood; 1. A 3-year epidemiological study. *American Journal of Public Health* **65**:133–138, 1975.

5. Heiman E, Kahn M: Mental health patterns in a barrio health center. *International Journal of Social Psychiatry* **21**:197–202, 1975.

6. Mayo J: The significance of sociocultural variables in the psychiatric treatment of black outpatients. *Comprehensive Psychiatry* **15**:471–482, 1974.

7. Cole J, Pilisuk M: Differences in the provision of mental health service by race. *American Journal of Orthopsychiatry* **46**:510–525, 1976.

8. Rosen B: Mental health and the poor: have the gaps between the poor and"nonpoor" narrowed in the last decade? *Medical Care* **15**:647–661, 1977.

9. Rumer R: Community mental health centers: politics and therapy. *Journal of Health Politics, Policy, and Law* **3**:531–558, 1978.

10. Schwartz DA: Community mental health in 1972, an assessment. In Barten HH, Bellak L, (eds): *Progress in Community Mental Health,* Volume II, New York, Grune and Stratton, 1972, pp. 3–34.

11. Letter from M. Brewster Smith, Ph.D., President and Officer of the American Psychological Association to Max Clelland, Administrator, Veterans Administration, Washington, D.C., October 18, 1978.

12. Spoerl OH: Treatment patterns in prepaid psychiatric care. *American Journal of Psychiatry* **131**:56–59, 1974.

13. Schiedemandel P: Utilization of psychiatric services. *Psychiatric Annals* **4**:58 –74, 1974.

14. Pemburton A, Witlock F, Wilson P: Knowledge about where to find help: a preliminary analysis. *Social Science and Medicine* **9**:433–439, 1975.

15. Redlich F, Kellert S: Trends in American mental health. *American Journal of Psychiatry* **135**:22–28, 1978.

16. *Rouse* v. *Cameron,* 373 F2d 451 (DC Cir 1966).

17. *Wyatt* v. *Stickney,* 344 F Supp 383 (MD Ala 1972).

18. *Donaldson* v. *O'Connor,* 493 F2d 507 (Stu Cir 1974).

19. *O'Connor* v. *Donaldson,* 43 USLW 4929 (1975).

20. *Winters* v. *Miller,* 466 F 2d 65 (1971).

Part Four
Resources
for Health Services

CHAPTER 8

Technological Resources for Health

Robert F. Rushmer

During the past 30 years, revolutionary changes have involved virtually every aspect of health services in this country. Many adaptations have been discussed in earlier chapters of this book. Some of the most dramatic changes involve new technological resources which are now available to detect and treat disease. These changes and their implications are the subject of this chapter which reviews the historical developments presaging modern technological achievements, their contributions to health care, and the unpredicted consequences and complications from their applications.

The most comprehensive basic medical research enterprise in the world has engaged the attention of faculties in Schools of Medicine, Public Health, Dentistry, Nursing, and allied fields. Sophisticated sensors and analytical techniques have been developed to provide objective and quantitative information. The functional characteristics of various organ systems can be assessed in health and disease with greater precision and more detail than could have been conceived even a few decades ago. Some of the basic research techniques have been converted into expanding arrays of diagnostic equipment, many of which are semi-automated, to provide information regarding the chemical and cellular composition of blood in remarkable detail. Microstructure of tissues and cellular components is revealed in amazing detail by the enormous magnification provided by electron microscopy. The size, shape, movement, and function of many internal organs are revealed by images produced by various forms of energy probes without pain, hazard, or disturbance to patients. Continuous measurement and display of vital functions can now be used to monitor the condition of patients in intensive care and during and after surgery or injury. Life support systems now permit surgeons to invade virtually any organ of the body to remove, repair, reconstruct, or replace components that have been distorted or destroyed by disease processes. Engineering

Supported in part by NIH Grant LM00010-01 from the National Library of Medicine.

technologies have been successfully employed to provide functional substitutes and supplements to many of the most important bodily functions.

The traditional family physician conducting medical practice out of a little black bag has been largely replaced by the highly trained specialists and new health professionals required to effectively utilize the increasingly complex equipment available for management of diseases of the various organ systems. Hospitals have assumed expanded roles as the institutions specifically designed and organized for ready access by patients and physicians to the many and varied health services that have become the essence of modern medicine and surgery. The government has become increasingly involved in the details of health care, not only in the support of the research enterprise, but also in the assurance of the safety and effectiveness of new devices (e.g., Food and Drug Administration), and in the financial support of health services for the military, veterans, the aged, the poor, and, potentially, the entire population under comprehensive national health insurance.

HISTORICAL HERITAGE OF HEALTH TECHNOLOGIES

At the beginning of this century, medical science was struggling for professional respectability, and rightly so. The methods of treatment of most medical problems were largely ineffectual with remarkably few exceptions (i.e., surgical removal or repair and certain effective drugs, minerals, and hormones). Otherwise, home remedies were virtually as effective as the ministrations of physicians. Medical schools were much more numerous than today. Most of them were diploma mills and even the best of them had little research activity. Basic medical research was very heavily oriented toward subjective descriptions of structure, function, and taxonomy. The mechanisms of function and control were mostly estimated on the basis of temporal relationships observed or recorded with crude mechanical devices and recording techniques. Quantitative measurements and dynamic analysis of functional relationships were extremely primitive, far outdistanced by the progress of 300 years in mathematics, chemistry, and physics. Most of the devices proposed and employed for diagnosis or treatment were outright fakes employed by charlatans. It has been estimated that at the turn of the century New York City contained some 20,000 quacks and only about 6,000 "regular" medical practitioners (1). The amazing variety of charms, amulets, and pseudoscientific gadgets with which health hucksters of the day engaged the gullible public defies imagination. The amazing but tragic diversity of devices "guaranteed" to cure long lists of unrelated ailments included impressive names such as Magneto Electric Device, Micro-dynamometer, Spectrochrome, Perkin's Patent Metallic Tractors, and Orgone Energy Accumulator. These devices were widely and persuasively advertised in newspapers, magazines, and even in the Sears Roebuck catalogue (2).

A full scale campaign was waged for many years against these excesses by Morris Fishbein as Editor of the *Journal of the American Medical Association* (3).

Reticence by modern medicine to adopt new technologies may stem in part from this colorful but shameful period.

The nation's basic medical research capacity became established with the reforms of medical schools following the Flexner Report of 1910 which critically assessed medical education in the United States (4). These changes formed the necessary foundation for both fundamental and clinical research in medical schools but the modern era of biomedical research was delayed until the period following World War II.

THE SURGE TOWARD SCIENTIFIC MEDICINE

The national commitment to large scale biomedical research and development did not originate from the medical community but instead was initiated by persuasive and persistent pressure by concerned citizens. This fascinating saga was detailed by Stephen Strickland (5).

The story begins with Matthew M. Nealey, Senator from West Virginia. In May of 1928, Senator Nealey made an impassioned speech to the Senate comparing cancer in its brutality to the guillotine and introduced legislation authorizing the National Academy of Sciences to investigate cancer and report to Congress on what the federal government could do to assist in coordinating cancer research, "conquering this most mysterious and destructive disease." Mary Lasker and her husband Albert, an advertising executive, were responsible for organizing an extremely effective "lay lobby" engaged in actively mobilizing the interest and support of key Congressional figures with whom they were personally acquainted. With patience and persuasion, the active support of powerful people like Senator Claude Pepper of Florida was attained. Public opinion was aroused by extensive use of press releases to newspapers and other communication channels. After extensive efforts, the Ransdel Act was signed into law in 1930 to establish a National Institute of Health (NIH) and to erect additional buildings to house a research activity as a Public Health Service. Dr. Roller E. Deider, Director of the original Institutes of Health, is reported to have indicated to the House Appropriations Subcommittee that the NIH would not be able to use any money beyond the $1,750,000 requested, and that the NIH leadership wanted to stay within that figure (5).

Since World War II, the NIH and the biomedical research enterprise of this country have soared to meteoric heights, both in scope and in expenditures. The enormous influence exerted by the lay lobbies and the voluntary health agencies (i.e., the American Cancer Society, the American Heart Association, and many others) have tended to place cancer and heart disease before the public as principal targets for both medical research and for the development of new and sophisticated technologies. The technical triumph of creating the atom bomb in a few short years by the Manhattan Project gave the mistaken impression that scientists could solve virtually any problem if provided with sufficient funds. This impression was reinforced by the rapid and successful series of dramatic moon landings by the National Aeronautics and Space Administration. The fundamental knowledge required for these impressive accomplishments was well established in advance and required only the solution of complex technical problems for which technologies were clearly attainable. There was widespread confidence in most quarters that by appropriating enough money for scientific research and development, virtually any problem could be solved.

The targets selected as highest priority were cancer and heart disease, based on the perception that they are the great "killers." Other "most favored" health problems were addressed in sequence as the various categorical Institutes of Health were established. There is little evidence that the principal participants gave serious consideration to the question of whether the fund of basic knowledge was an adequate foundation for the launching of major, definitive research programs to conquer cancer, cure heart disease, or overcome other disease categories. Many persistent problems have resisted the development of definitive therapy because their ultimate causation remains mysterious. It is difficult to devise a cure for a problem with unknown cause. To place this consideration in perspective, if President Kennedy had responded to the challenge of Sputnik by a declaration that America would *overcome gravity* instead of deciding to send a man to the Moon, the scientific community would have failed to achieve its goal. A great deal is known about gravity and its effects, but very little is known about its cause. An anti-gravity device cannot even be conceived at present because of a lack of knowledge of basic mechanisms. A corresponding situation pertains to the problems of most chronic diseases, conditions which persist as the most common hazards to the aging populations of modern societies as discussed in Chapters 1 and 2.

There are several theories regarding the causes of cancer, which include radiation, mutations, carcinogenic materials, viruses, and others. Similarly, there are several competing theories about the origins of the abnormal swellings in blood vessels known as atherosclerosis. However, the very existence of many conflicting theories is a sure sign that the actual cause is unknown. The same arguments can be advanced regarding the ultimate causes of chronic diseases of the lung, the kidney, the joints, and many other organs. For lack of specific causative targets, there is currently a major preoccupation with peripheral factors (i.e., risk factors). For example, there is little doubt that smoking is a contributing factor to both lung cancer and heart disease, but it is equally obvious that smoking is not the direct cause, because these diseases occur in people who do not smoke. With this historical perspective in mind, it is easier to understand and appreciate the factors responsible for the present priorities for research and development of medical techniques and technologies.

FACTORS FAVORING HEALTH-RELATED RESEARCH

Immediately following World War II, science and technology stood high in national esteem. The magnitude of the health problems of the country had been vividly exposed by the fact that some 30% of draftees were rejected for health-related reasons. There was widespread concern that a post-war depression might ensue. Programs to bolster the economy were sought, and health became an important one. Many counties in the country were lacking health services, and the importance of health as a "human right" emerged along with other social reform movements. Legislation in support of research and development for health rapidly became one of the most popular political issues of the period. The stage was set for a rapid build-up of the nation's health-related research capacity, centered for the most part in the various medical schools throughout the country.

THE BASIC MEDICAL RESEARCH ENTERPRISE

Dr. James Shannon was appointed director of the National Institutes of Health during the crucial period between August 1955 and September 1968, the "Golden Age of NIH." With the wholehearted support of leadership in both the House and Senate, the annual budgets for NIH expanded explosively at an unprecedented rate. Indeed, appropriations for NIH exceeded the administrative requests in all but four years during a span of about 15 years. Dr. Shannon was perceptive enough to realize that the state of biomedical knowledge with regard to function, control, and response to diseases by the various organ systems was not substantial enough to serve as the foundation for a broad scale attack on the major diseases affecting the population. He convinced his backers in Congress and many of his scientific colleagues of the absolute necessity for mounting major programs in fundamental research. As a consequence, large and growing projects and programs in basic medical research rapidly emerged throughout medical schools, in both basic medical science departments (e.g., Anatomy, Biochemistry, Physiology) and clinical departments. In a few short years, the United States could justifiably boast of the most comprehensive and advanced biomedical research enterprise in the world.

INITIAL SUCCESS STORIES

During the immediate post-war period, technical developments of great importance appeared to confirm the exalted expectations from medical research. The "sulfa" drugs and antibiotics emerged just before and during the war and quickly demonstrated enormous effectiveness in combating many diverse infections. Rheumatic fever, a common and dreaded cause of heart disease in children, came under control through prophylactic use of these antibiotics. Improved life support systems which sustained respiratory and circulatory function during surgery inside the chest provided opportunities to surgically alleviate or correct a wide variety of congenital and acquired defects in the valves and walls of the heart chambers. As these surgical techniques became perfected, the need for more definite and quantitative diagnostic techniques emerged. For this purpose, techniques involving cardiac catheterization were developed for measuring the pressures, oxygen content, and dye concentration in blood by inserting long hollow tubes through veins (or arteries) into the chambers of the heart. A surge of progress resulted in the rapid accumulation of knowledge regarding the function of the heart and lungs in health and disease. The anatomical location and severity of the defects were elucidated by shadows cast on x-ray plates by radio-opaque dyes coursing through the channels and chambers of the heart and circulation (angiocardiography).

Many of the conditions which had previously been regarded as degenerative changes due to aging were reconsidered and classified as diseases for which cures might reasonably be sought. For example, the association of high levels of fatty materials in the blood with the development of atherosclerosis caused it to be regarded for the first time as a metabolic disease which might be treatable just as diabetes or other metabolic diseases could be managed. A similar change in attitude occurred with respect to other chronic diseases such as arthritis and cancer. A major search for chemical agents capable of destroying cancer cells while sparing normal cells was launched by generous funding of a massive cancer chemotherapy program. The original promise of rich rewards from medical research appeared to be developing in accordance with advanced expectations.

By 1960, the NIH received a half-billion dollar budget and spent over half of it on more than 11,500 projects devoted to a broad spectrum of research endeavors. About 90% of all federally supported projects were initiated in the nation's universities and medical schools. The benevolent extravagance of Congress had produced such reckless expansion of the biomedical research enterprise that few were surprised when Congressman Fountain and his committee began to discover evidence of weaknesses in mechanisms of awarding, monitoring, and accounting for these vast sums of money (5). The inevitable criticisms and concerns of critical Congressmen grew and gradually contributed to mounting pressures for *results*. The momentum favoring continued research and development persisted for some years despite the growing criticism. Total federal expenditures for health research mounted from $550,000,000 in 1960 to more than $3,000,000,000 in 1974, as indicated in Table 8–1. The distribution of these funds among the various agencies of government has strongly favored the National Institutes of Health as displayed in Figure 8–1. However, despite continued growth in dollar amounts, the appropriations for NIH reached a plateau in the mid-1960s when corrections are applied to account for inflation.

TABLE 8–1. The Growth in Expenditures for Health Related Research and Development, 1960–1974

Source of Funds	Expenditures in Millions of Dollars							
	1960	1962	1964	1966	1968	1970	1972	1974
Total	$932	$1,372	$1,730	$2,147	$2,600	$2,856	$3,515	$4,452
Government	558	901	1,180	1,471	1,754	1,868	2,387	3,038
Federal	448	782	1,049	1,316	1,582	1,667	2,147	2,754
State	110	119	131	155	172	201	240	284
Industry	253	336	400	510	661	795	925	1,187
Private nonprofit	121	135	150	166	185	193	203	227
Foundations	40	40	43	44	49	47	53	54
Voluntary health agencies	36	38	42	47	57	61	63	84
Other	45	57	65	75	79	85	87	89

Source: National Institutes of Health. Basic Data Relating to the National Institutes of Health, Washington, D.C., 1976.

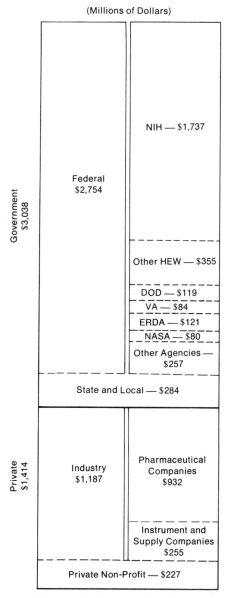

(Millions of Dollars)

NIH — $1,737

Federal
$2,754

Government
$3,038

Other HEW — $355

DOD — $119
VA — $84
ERDA — $121
NASA — $80

Other Agencies —
$257

State and Local — $284

Private
$1,414

Industry
$1,187

Pharmaceutical
Companies
$932

Instrument and
Supply Companies
$255

Private Non-Profit — $227

Figure 8–1. Distribution of biomedical research and development funds by source of expenditures, United States, 1974. (*Source:* Office of Technology Assessment, United States Congress. *Opportunities for Assessment.* Washington, D.C., 1976.)

PRESSURES FOR PAY-OFF

Along with continued financial support of research, there developed a growing and urgent expectation for tangible health benefits from the decades of generous support of biomedical research. Despite a veritable deluge of new and important basic information regarding the structure, function, and control of organs and their responses to disease, the primary targets, the "great killers," were not succumbing to the onslaught of research as rapidly as expected. Indeed, certain kinds of cancer, heart disease, chronic lung disease, and various resistant infections were gaining in prevalence.

In response to the mounting pressures for pay-off, at least three main trends emerged more or less simultaneously. First, risk factors were explored by large-scale epidemiological studies to seek clues with regard to the causes of major diseases. For example, the contributions of smoking, diet, and lack of exercise became the targets for major campaigns exhorting the public to contribute to their own health by individual health maintenance. By concentrating attention on the public propensity for engaging in unhealthy habits, the responsibility for relatively slow progress in conquering killers was subtly shifted from the medical community to the public at large. Second, the rapid development of sophisticated technologies for basic and clinical research was converted into a growing array of diagnostic methods—developing a "diagnostic imperative." And third, substitutes and supplements for function of various organs were developed "to treat" chronic disabilities lacking effective or definitive therapy.

The technological developments for health care were greatly influenced in this direction by the latter two trends. Intensive campaigns against smoking, drinking, and dietary indiscretions have affected behavior to varying degrees. The medical research community has been exposed to powerful pressures for pay-offs to greatly expand the diagnostic capability and to develop technical substitutes or supplements for various organ functions.

DEVELOPMENT OF DIAGNOSTIC TECHNOLOGIES

At the turn of the century, physicians were still highly dependent upon their own subjective senses for gathering diagnostic data. They were aided by the newly developed x-ray machines, the electrocardiogram, and a few laboratory tests on blood and urine. During the first half of this century, technical progress was remarkably slow. There appeared to be far more technical progress in the appliances added to the average kitchen than in the typical doctor's office. Many modern diagnostic devices have been developed by modifying and refining research tools originally intended for basic medical research.

BASIC MEDICAL RESEARCH TECHNOLOGIES

The traditional approaches to basic medical research were leisurely and scholarly, largely dependent upon subjective observations, leading to descriptions, classifications, and concepts of functional cause and effect, based mainly on time relationships. Structure was investigated by microscopy, composition by manual chemical analysis, and function by relatively crude recordings using mechanical levers and smoked drums (Fig. 8–2).

Revolutionary changes ensued following World War II. The explosive expansion of basic medical research required whole new arrays of tools and analytical techniques. Quantum jumps in magnification were attained by means of electron microscopes, ultimately coupled with sophisticated technologies for image analysis. The diversity, accuracy, and speed of chemical analyses were all enormously enhanced by spectrophotometers, ultracentrifuges, chromatographs, and fluorescence techniques. A variety of new sensors were developed to provide accurate information regarding the mechanical function of internal organs. For example, tiny devices for continuously measuring the changing pressures, dimensions, and

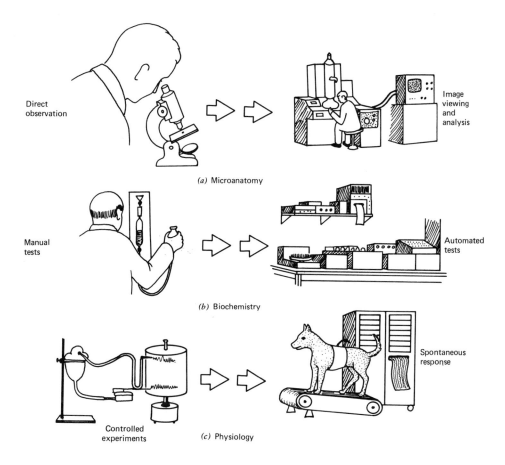

Figure 8–2. Changing technologies for biomedical research. *Note:* Prior to World War II, biomedical research was generally conducted using relatively primitive tools for observation and measurement; since then technologies have become increasingly sophisticated with such commercially available equipment as electron microscopes, elegant and sometimes automated chemical analyses, and new sensors capable of continuously monitoring the performance of internal organs in comprehensive and quantitative scales.

blood flow in the heart and major blood vessels could be implanted for investigating functions in healthy, active animals under both spontaneous and experimentally induced conditions (6). Such techniques provided comprehensive analyses of the function of this hydraulic system in much the same terms as engineers employ for analyzing the performance of mechanical systems. The few examples in Figure 8–2 are representative of an enormous expansion of the basic medical research capacity, a major advance toward the "science" of medicine which had progressed so slowly in earlier centuries.

CLINICAL CONVERSION OF BASIC TECHNOLOGIES

The newly developed tools of basic research were readily converted into diagnostic devices. They greatly expanded the diagnostic capacity of clinical medicine and at the same time represented tangible rewards for research support. For example, the electron microscope has opened new vistas in the study of subcellular elements in both fundamental and clinical investigation of virus infestations, cancer, genetic disturbances, and many other central issues. The growing diversity of laboratory tests for the chemical and cellular composition of blood, body fluids, and tissue samples have completely transformed laboratory procedures. Automation of testing sequences allows batch processing of small samples to provide multiple simultaneous test results (as many as 24 tests from single samples). Today, larger hospital laboratories provide a selection of more than 300 tests in contrast with only one or two dozen different types of chemical tests thirty years ago. The unit cost for each test has been greatly reduced but the volume has increased enormously. The physical measurements of pressures, electrical activity, and other characteristics of vital organs are now widely used for diagnosis and for monitoring the condition of patients during intensive care (e.g., during and after surgery or in life-threatening situations).

Diagnostic testing technologies can be conveniently considered in three categories (Fig. 8–3). The analysis of samples (e.g., blood, body fluids, and tissues) has been expanded and speeded by automation, particularly in testing chemical composition. Spectroscopy, chromatography, flame photometry, and other techniques commonly employed in academic and industrial applications have proved extremely valuable for clinical diagnosis. In addition, the number and types of blood cells are routinely tallied semiautomatically. Pathological changes in cells and tissues are accentuated by special staining and microscopic techniques. The use of automation in processing samples for the study of tissues and bacteria has been much slower and less effective than the use of automation in chemical analysis, where great strides have been taken.

INTRINSIC ENERGY SOURCES

The traditional methods of clinical diagnosis have always relied heavily on detecting and assessing changes in energy sources produced within the body. For example, excitable tissues produce recordable electrical potentials as a byproduct

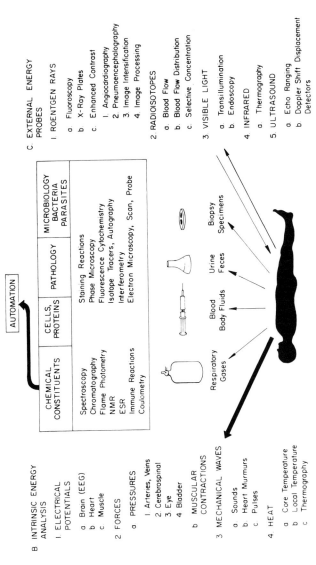

Figure 8–3. Three primary categories of diagnostic technologies currently available. *Notes:* (A). The chemical and cellular constituents of blood and body fluids can now be characterized by a large and growing selection of procedures, many of which have been automated to provide multiple simultaneous values from a single small sample. Techniques for eliciting information from other samples of fluids and tissues involve histological examination with various types of staining procedures and culturing techniques for identifying microorganisms. (B). Traditional components of the physical examination included subjective observations of intrinsic energy sources such as electrical potentials, pressures, sounds, and temperature. Electronic devices supplement subjective senses by recording such items as electrical potentials, pressures, sounds, pulses, and temperature. (C). External energy probes elicit valuable information regarding the size, shape, location, movement, and function of internal organs by means of beams of energy directed into the body and analyzing the energy coming out. The versatility of diagnostic x-rays is generally known. These are being extended by means of other wave energies such as guided light, infra-red, ultrasound, and atomic energies. (*Source:* Reprinted by permission from Rushmer RF, *Cardiovascular Dynamics,* ed. 4, Philadelphia, W. B. Saunders Co., 1976.)

of their functional activity. These can be routinely recorded from the brain (electroencephalography), heart (electrocardiography), and muscles (myography). Similarly, changes in pressures within the fluid-filled spaces of the body can be recorded from arteries, veins, heart chambers, the spinal canal, the eye, the bladder, and elsewhere. Mechanical waves are produced by the heart (pulses and heart sounds) and have attracted physicians' attention for many centuries. The heat produced by the metabolic activity and its regulation are reflected in body temperature. These traditional sources of information are still widely employed and the technologies have been refined, but not greatly advanced.

EXTERNAL ENERGY PROBES

Highly significant progress in diagnostic technologies have resulted from the many and varied applications of energy beams to probe the structure and function of internal organs. The development of advanced optics and fiberoptics have provided long flexible light guides for direct vision of the inner walls of virtually all the hollow organs of the body (e.g., bronchi, stomach, bowel, bladder, uterus, and abdominal cavity). Light will penetrate the tissues of the body but is so badly scattered that the eye cannot observe internal organs through the skin. The interaction between different wave bands of energy and tissues have provided a whole new spectrum of methods for extending the human senses beyond the normal range. For example, x-rays penetrate the body tissues with much less scattering than light and are absorbed to varying degrees by tissues such as lungs or bones. The images on fluorescent screens or x-ray plates provide valuable information regarding the size, shape, position, and displacement of many internal organs (Fig. 8–4).

The enormous potential of x-rays as diagnostic probes is being realized as a prototype for developments using other promising wave energies. By inserting or injecting appropriate radio-opaque substances, the functional characteristics of certain organs can be explored. For example, fluid mixtures containing barium can be observed traversing the stomach and intestines. Certain functions of the kidneys and liver can be observed on sequential x-rays following injection of appropriate materials into the bloodstream as they become concentrated in the gall bladder or urinary passages. By injecting radio-opaque materials into the bloodstream, the distribution of blood in various organs can be visualized. High speed computers can derive the shapes of some organs in three dimensions from simultaneous exposures in two planes. Monochromatic x-ray beams are a potentially useful analytical tool for painlessly exploring the composition of tissues (e.g., the iodine content of the thyroid gland or constituents of bone).

COMPUTERIZED AXIAL TOMOGRAPHY (CAT SCANNERS)

Tomography is a term applied to the development of x-ray images of various planes in the body by specialized techniques. For example, an x-ray tube programmed to move in one direction while the x-ray plate is transported in the opposite direction

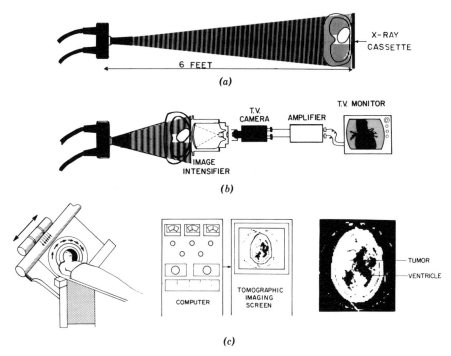

Figure 8–4. Examples of X-Ray energy probes for collecting diagnostic information. (*a*) Teleroentgenography. (*b*) Image intensifier. (*c*) Computerized Axial Tomography. (*Source:* Reprinted by permission from Rushmer RF, *Cardiovascular Dynamics,* ed. 4, Philadelphia, W. B. Saunders Co. 1976.)

will produce an image of a single plane which effectively remains stationary and unblurred by the movement. The application of high speed computers to this relatively simple mechanical process has produced costly but versatile instruments that have attracted the attention of physicians and the public alike. The basic principle has been recognized since 1917 that a two-dimensional image can be reconstructed from a large set of individual projections. Using a very narrow beam of x-ray penetrating the body from many different angles and positions, an enormous amount of data can be collected and processed to reconstruct an image of a plane transecting the body perpendicular to its long axis (7). This process provides an infinite number of views of the body that cannot be obtained using directly penetrating beams in the traditional manner. The process is illustrated schematically in Figure 8–4. An x-ray tube is mounted on one side of a large housing and a sensitive x-ray detector is positioned on the opposite side and coupled to the x-ray tube so that they move together. The tube and detector scan steadily back and forth across the portion of the body positioned within the circular orifice. The intensity of the x-rays that reach the detector is recorded at each of 160 positions along each scan. The housing then rotates one degree and another series of scans ensue. The process is repeated 180 times to produce 28,000 values for x-ray intensities of beams penetrating from all these positions and angles. They are stored and analyzed in the computer and reproduced as an image of some 6,400 to 25,000 tiny areas (pixels) in the plane of the scan. Very subtle differences in x-ray absorption are recorded to delineate both normal and pathological structures with different radio-intensity. The original devices were designed for scanning the brain, but rapid progress has led to devices for producing images of virtually any transverse plane of the body with increasing speed and definition. The many useful applications of x-rays represent revealing prototypes for future developments in a number of other forms of wave energy (8, 9).

DIAGNOSTIC ULTRASOUND

The normal hearing range extends to only about 20,000 Hertz (cycles per second). Very high frequency sounds can be readily generated by electrically pulsing certain types of ceramic crystals at frequencies in excess of 1 megahertz (1 million cycles per second). Relatively narrow beams of such ultrasound have proved extremely useful in detecting the location and distance of ships and underwater objects by a device commonly known as sonar. Such beams penetrate the tissues with nearly the same ease as water and are absorbed and scattered by tissues to different degrees than are x-rays. Thus, ultrasound can be employed to extract entirely different information from the internal organs than is revealed by x-ray techniques. A common example is the application of sonar techniques to measure the time required for pulses to traverse the brain substance and be reflected from a midline structure and the far side of the skull. A displacement of midline structure of the brain may indicate a developing brain tumor.

Ultrasonic images can be derived by scanning techniques corresponding to those described above for x-rays. By moving the source and receiver of ultrasound through positions and angles, an image of internal organs can be effectively painted on the surface of a television-like screen. Detailed transverse images can now be obtained of the brain, eye, abdomen, uterus, and other organs. The process promises to be rendered more effective and faster by current developments in arrays of ultrasound transducers and receivers coupled to high speed computers to improve both resolution and efficiency.

Ultrasound has unusual and valuable backscattering properties which provide extremely valuable information. For example, a beam of ultrasound traversing the heart (Fig. 8–5) is backscattered (reflected) from the walls of the chambers and from the valve leaflets. The movements of these various internal structures of the heart can be continuously observed on the face of an oscilloscope (A scan) or recorded on moving paper (B scan) for future analysis. Abnormal positions or dynamic movements of the various structures of the heart can be detected by such mechanisms. Ultrasound is also backscattered from blood cells providing a means of registering changes in blood flow velocity by the Doppler shift principle, the physical mechanism which causes a change in pitch of a whistle on a moving train as it passes by. The changing velocity of blood ejected from the heart can be continuously indicated by placing an ultrasonic probe at a strategic location just above the sternum or breast bone (see Fig. 8–5).

A combination of ultrasonic imaging and flow detection provides a means of obtaining information regarding the blood flow velocity directly on the corresponding location in the body, as indicated in Figure 8–5. It is even possible to produce

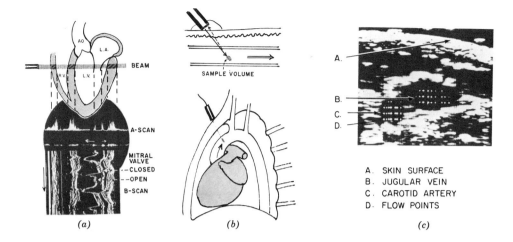

Figure 8–5. Ultrasonic imaging and flow detection to determine blood flow velocity (*a*) Ultrasonic scans (A and B). (*b*) Pulsed Doppler. (*c*) Duplex scan. (*Source:* Reprinted by permission from Rushmer RF, *Cardiovascular Dynamics,* ed. 4, Philadelphia, W. B. Saunders Co., 1976.)

an image representing the places where blood is flowing faster than some predetermined velocity when this is of interest. The many and varied applications of diagnostic ultrasound are being increasingly exploited in clinical laboratories providing a whole new spectrum of clinically useful information.

RADIOISOTOPES

The energy emitted by radioisotopes contributes additional information of value to the diagnosis of certain ailments. Injected intravenously, certain isotopes accumulate selectively in specific organs (e.g., iodine in the thyroid) as an indicator of function. The distribution of concentrations can be employed to indicate the blood flow in various internal organs. Arrays of isotope sensors (gamma camera) can produce images illustrating the geometrical distribution of isotopes in specific locations or organs and can be interpreted to indicate the position of blocked blood vessels in the lung or heart.

THERMOGRAPHY

Infra-red cameras commonly employed to display geographical characteristics of the ground from high flying aircraft or satellites can also be employed to record the temperature distribution over the surface of the body. Such thermographs have excited some enthusiasm as a means of detecting pathological processes (cancer or infection) under the surface of the skin. The expected promise of effectiveness has not yet been fully realized.

Other forms of energy are also potentially useful as diagnostic probes. For example, microwaves might have value in exploring the changes in the air-containing portions of the lung under various conditions.

This brief survey of the rapidly developing fields of diagnostic energies will suffice to indicate the dramatic advances in technologies by which more objective and quantitative information can be elicited using increasingly sophisticated equipment. The enthusiasm with which these new technologies are adopted should be tempered by important economic considerations.

EFFECTS OF ENERGY PROBES ON HEALTH CARE COSTS

The practice of "scientific" medicine necessarily entails the accurate identification of the disease or disabilities of each patient. The diagnostic wave energy techniques described above all have the common attribute of deriving large quantities of potentially relevant information from patients with minimal disturbance, discomfort, or hazard to the patient. Computerized axial tomography has attained a very high level of sophistication which has greatly increased the versatility and definition of its applications. The potential for providing additional information from the other wave energies is as great or greater than that for x-ray. Thus, the economic impact of CAT scanning can be used as a prototype to explore the potential economic impact of the large scale commercial development of new technologies.

CAT scanners have experienced rapid technological change with the development of three generations of models since the early 1970s. The enthusiasm with which the equipment was adopted produced a demand that outran the supply. With each new generation, the older versions became obsolete. A report by the Institute of Medicine indicated that purchase price and installation charges range from $300,000 to $700,000 and annual operating costs range from $259,000 to $371,000, averaging about $285,000 (8). These high costs can be amortized only through high volume use of the equipment (i.e., 2,500 patient examinations per year as a minimum). The enthusiasm with which hospitals aspired to obtain this equipment exceeded reasonable bounds so restraints are being considered or imposed by health planning agencies. Since the clinical effectiveness of these devices is not yet fully established, the uninhibited demand for these devices is decidedly premature. Furthermore, these is a growing conviction that the CAT scanner is being used primarily as an "add on" to supplement the traditional diagnostic procedures and therefore is not effectively utilizing its favorable properties to reduce the need for other traditional tests.

The estimated increases in health costs of $1,000,000,000 per year due to the expansion of CAT scanning is serious enough. Exactly the same arguments can be advanced for correspondingly costly and sophisticated developments employing other diagnostic wave energies such as ultrasound. They provide entirely different categories of information beyond those from x-rays (9).

EXPANDING ELECTRONICS INDUSTRY

The development of sophisticated diagnostic equipment has spurred the growth of a huge medical electronics industry. The early examples began at the turn of the century with electrocardiographs and x-ray systems, but the major advances became prominent only after 1950 with the advent of large-scale cardiac monitoring, cardiac catheterization, scintillation cameras (gamma cameras), medical computers, and other complicated equipment (Fig. 8–6). The domestic market for diagnostic, therapeutic, and monitoring medical electronic equipment reached $840,000,000 in 1974 and was estimated to exceed $1,400,000,000 in 1979. The growing ability to obtain ever more comprehensive and reliable information for purposes of diagnosis is generally regarded as a technical triumph of unquestioned value to the public, the profession, and society as a whole. However, consideration must be given to the "price of progress" in terms of two central issues. The first is that the ability to gather clinical data has proceeded so rapidly that it has outdistanced the ability to treat many of the conditions which can now be recognized with confidence. The second is the major contribution of diagnostic technologies to the soaring costs of health care, due in part to pervasive pressures toward overuse and inadequate incentives for restraint on the part of either the physician or patient.

DIAGNOSTIC IMPERATIVE

The role of the physician has been greatly affected by a growing dependence on advanced technologies for diagnosis; no longer is the doctor-patient relationship a process limited to personal encounters. The physician must select those health services which are appropriate to the conditions presented by the patient. A major new function is the role of the physician as "professional purchasing agent" for the patient through the ordering of tests, consultations, and therapeutic options. Both the patient and the physician's peers expect a full utilization of all available resources for diagnosis and treatment. A traditional criterion of the quality medical care is thoroughness and comprehensive consideration of the probable alternatives. The constant threat of malpractice that could result from any short-cuts or restraints is a powerful incentive to cover all contingencies, particularly in situations where third-party payment mechanisms are paying for all or most of the costs. Economic incentives also promote utilization of technologies. Consider the time and effort involved in a complete history and physical examination that might require 45 minutes and for which charges are $40. In contrast, the time required to order and interpret an electrocardiogram or x-rays may be only ten minutes and charges are $25 or $30. The objectivity of the tests and the permanence of the records also add to the attractiveness of technology. The same considerations apply to the generous use of the many tests which can be quickly ordered in various combinations from clinical and chemical laboratories. The patient and the physician tend to derive benefits in the form of reassurance from these diagnostic efforts. Restraints to utilization are often weak or absent.

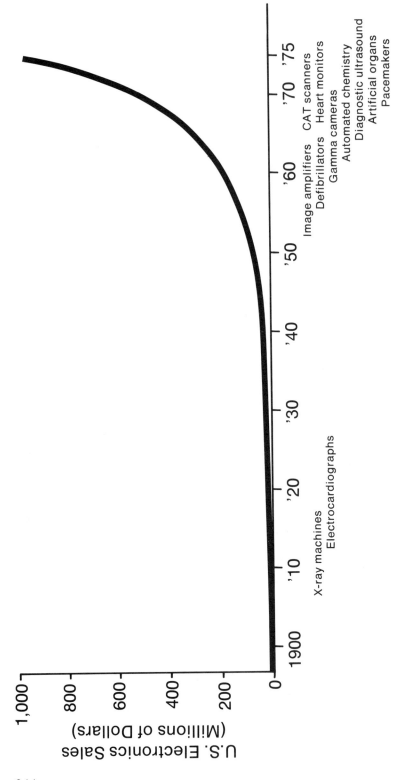

Figure 8–6. The expanding production of electronics for application in medicine. *Note:* The meteoric rise in expenditures for medical electronics began in the late 1940s and now exceeds one billion dollars annually. A number of the different technical developments that contributed to this industrial expansion are indicated at the bottom of the graph.

There is a growing awareness that semi-automatic or routine applications or diagnostic testing may yield little information or even provide unwarranted reassurance. For example, an x-ray of the skull is virtually routine in the case of head injury, without much regard for severity. Evaluation of the consequences of omitting this examination has disclosed relatively minor benefits to patients from the rather large expenditures involved. Yet both patient and physician may feel uneasy at the thought of dispensing with this semi-automatic ritual.

MONITORING METHODS

Techniques for continuously displaying the electrocardiogram, arterial pressures, and other vital signs have been incorporated into equipment for monitoring the conditions of patients requiring intensive care. Such equipment is now widely used during and following high risk surgical operations (e.g., intracardiac surgery). Similar systems are also employed in the care of patients following heart attacks in the familiar Coronary Care Units. Such sophisticated facilities, involving continuous surveillance by highly trained personnel, have been enthusiastically incorporated into hospitals of virtually all sizes. There is now an oversupply of coronary care beds and experience has demonstrated that the quality of care tends to be diminished in underutilized facilities. Cooperative activities in sophisticated settings requires an unremitting and continuous flow of patients to maintain optimal performance. An evaluation of the supply of coronary care units in Massachusetts was carried out using definitive criteria such as a maximum of 30 minutes travel time and 95% chance of obtaining a bed in the geographically closest unit (10). It was estimated that the contemporary 94 coronary care units in the state comprising 446 beds could be effectively reduced to 39 units and only 336 beds with both dollar savings and improved performance.

EMERGENCY MEDICAL SERVICES

The Emergency Medical Services Systems Act of 1972 provided aid to states and localities to establish coordinated, cost effective, area-wide Emergency Medical Service systems. This act was a response to the established fact that the most common hazards to life and health between the ages of 1 and 35 years are due to injuries from accidental or intentional violence. In recent years, an enviable record of performance has been achieved by dedicated Emergency Medical Technicians, appropriately trained and using modern equipment. Specifically, many metropolitan areas are served by integrated systems of mobile units capable of responding rapidly to the types of emergencies that can beset citizens in modern society. The developing communication-transportation networks have attained the present level of performance by combining highly concentrated special training with appropriate equipment. For example, the successful management of acute heart attacks is heavily dependent upon having sophisticated portable defibrillation equipment incorporating methods for monitoring heart rhythms. In addition, respiratory assist devices, appropriate selection of drugs, and effective communication with physicians in emergency centers all combine to afford a very successful application of technology. Indeed, most doctors will concede that patients are probably more effectively treated by experienced Emergency Medical Technicians for heart attacks, drowning, traffic accidents, physical violence, or other similar hazards than by physicians. Very few physicians have such broad and concentrated experience with these particular kinds of threats to life and health.

In some communities large proportions of the population have received training in Cardio-Pulmonary Resuscitation (CPR) for immediate life support during those critical minutes after a heart attack. For example, heart attack victims are probably better off in Seattle, where the CPR training extends to more than 20% of the population, than in many other cities. The success of civilian support is again highly dependent upon the back-up of appropriately equipped emergency personnel but it represents a vivid example of a growing trend toward public participation in health care for serious illness. Another prime example is the home care of patients with chronic kidney failure by means of sophisticated dialysis machines.

THERAPEUTIC TECHNOLOGIES

The application of engineering to clinical care has produced some spectacular achievements widely recognized by the general public as a result of extensive coverage by the mass media. Increasingly sophisticated technologies embodied in the artificial heart-lung machines support open heart surgery. Credible visions of bionic man have been produced by implantable heart pacemakers, the artificial kidneys, powered prostheses for amputees, and the prospects of an implantable artificial heart. These notable achievements have tended to obscure rather disappointing progress toward the control, cure, or prevention of many of the most important health hazards and disease states that the American public must confront.

Advances in therapeutic capability from symptomatic management through various steps toward cure, prevention, and elimination of diseases is illustrated schematically in Figure 8–7. The length of the arrow indicates the extent of progress and the thickness indicates the current prevalence of the various ailments.

Great strides have been taken toward the control, cure, or even elimination of many infectious diseases that formerly attained epidemic proportions (e.g., cholera, plague, smallpox, typhoid fever, malaria). Many infections persist to plague the public, particularly viruses responsible for colds, influenza, hepatitis, gonorrhea, and other resistant organisms. These are now the most common infections and progress toward their elimination is relatively limited as indicated in Figure 8–7.

Advances in nutrition and endocrinology have gone far toward prevention of

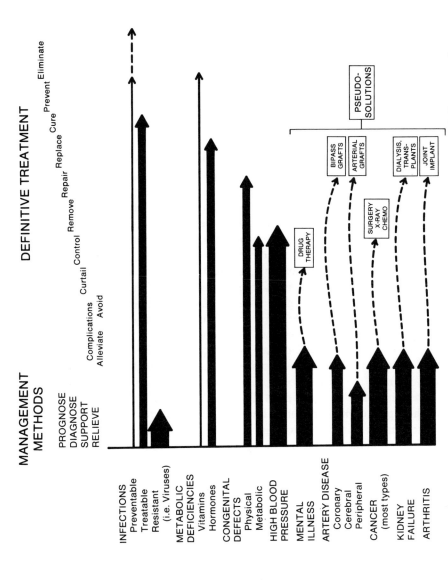

Figure 8–7. Advances in medical technology. *Note:* Progress in providing effective therapy differs widely for different conditions. For example, prevention, cure, and control has been attained for many infections. Many congenital malformations can be corrected by surgery and high blood pressure can be effectively controlled. For conditions lacking definitive therapy, sophisticated technologies have been developed to replace or supplement the structure and function of affected organs. These technical triumphs should be regarded as pseudosolutions of value to current patients but not really directed toward the underlying causes and cures that must ultimately be developed for the benefit of future generations.

vitamin deficiencies (e.g., ricketts, scurvy, beri-beri) and other deficiency diseases. The notable achievements in surgical correction of congenital heart disease have converted many impending tragedies into prospects of normal life spans. The development of drugs and procedures for controlling blood pressure has undoubtedly reduced the immediate threat of this condition, but it is uncertain whether the control of the hypertension adequately avoids the underlying processes leading to changes in arterial walls.

The most prevalent "killer disease" is atherosclerosis, or "hardening of the arteries," which is the uncontested leading cause of death. The current campaigns against excess consumption of fat and cigarettes represents a smokescreen obscuring the fact that these are but peripheral factors and the direct causes of the thickening of arterial walls remains controversial and mysterious. During the past thirty years a whole series of surgical operations have been touted in succession as means of supplying improved blood supply to the heart muscle when the coronary arteries are obstructed. These include methods of producing scar tissue on the surface of the heart by sprinkling talcum powder, roughening the heart surface with sandpaper, and inserting the cut ends of the arteries into the wall of the heart. Although none of these procedures have physiological validity, their advocates initially claimed high rates of success. Each has now fallen into disuse and they are replaced by a much more logical approach, the coronary bypass operation.

Bypass procedures utilize techniques of delicate vascular surgery that now permit skilled surgeons to install an accessory channel from the aorta (the main artery emerging from the heart) to a point beyond an obstruction with widely reported success in relief of chest pain. There is little doubt that this operation relieves the chest pain in many patients, but the overall effectiveness in prolonging useful life is still under critical evaluation by controlled studies. Even before these studies have been completed, the coronary bypass operation has become one of the most common operations in this country (some 70,000 in 1977 at an average cost of about $12,000 each). The unbridled enthusiasm for this surgical approach has been dampened in the minds of conservative physicians, but the enthusiasm of the surgical advocates remains intense. A provocative evaluation of this situation has been presented by Thomas Preston (11). It is interesting to note the widely varied rates of performance of the operation in different parts of the world (Table 8–2).

Critical evaluation of the outcome of coronary bypass surgery has indicated: 1) excessive zeal exhibited by the most vigorous proponents of the operations; and 2) persistent doubts regarding outcomes of surgery with respect to the potential for extending the lives of the patients as well as relieving the chest pain that is such a prominent problem for many patients. The controversy regarding long-term outcome discloses a fundamental weakness in current approaches to assessment of the modern medical technologies. The data in support of the beneficial effects of the operation are being assembled by a select few of the leading surgeons in the most prestigious institutions that are the most fully equipped and staffed in the country. It seems optimistic in the extreme to extrapolate these data to the wide spectrum of professional personnel and institutions across the country.

Pacemakers for the heart represent another major technical advance. The heart is provided with a built-in electrical ignition system that initiates each heartbeat in a regular fashion. When the conduction system of the heart is interrupted by

TABLE 8–2. Coronary Bypass Surgery Rates in Selected Locations

Location	Rate (operations/100,000 population)
Sweden, England, Finland	2*
Prepaid plans in United States	4*
Average for the United States	28*
Western Washington State	45†
Eastern Washington State	90†
Spokane, Washington	116†

*From Thomas Preston (11).

†From Guidelines for Heart Surgery Programs, Washington State Medical Association, 1977.

disease, the heart rate may become dangerously low. An artificial ignition system can now be installed under the skin with wires leading to the heart muscle to maintain the heart rate at appropriate levels. The need for replacing these devices after two or three years is being alleviated by the development of nuclear powered devices with much longer life expectancy. While the coronary bypass operation represents the installation of a structural element, an accessory blood channel, the pacemaker represents an electromechanical substitute for a vital function.

Another functional supplement or substitute is the "artificial kidney," a major technical achievement. In earlier days, patients whose kidney function became insufficient to clear the blood of wastes were doomed to death. During World War II an artificial kidney was developed by Wilem Kolff from a used washing machine that was capable of sustaining life for a few days or weeks in patients with temporary kidney failure. Advances in biomaterials provided the essential tubing that could shunt blood from artery to vein outside the body and provide access to the circulation so that the blood could be cleansed of wastes for months, years, or even indefinitely. Applications of engineering technologies have provided a steady series of improvements in artificial kidney design. The dialysis machines are now so reliable that patients and their families can perform the necessary meticulous processes of this potentially life-threatening treatment several times a week at home after an intensive training period of only about three weeks. Current research and development efforts have attained miniaturization to the point that the dialysis devices may become portable, perhaps the size of a thermos bottle.

STRUCTURAL SUBSTITUTES

The various tissues of the body have characteristics that are extremely difficult to duplicate. For example, the search for a substitute for skin to replace this vital covering when lost through damage, disease, or destruction (e.g., burns) has not yielded material that even approximate its protective properties. Surgeons in burn centers are still dependent largely on sources of mammalian skin from humans (or pigs). In other instances, substantial progress can be recognized. The problem is not new since artificial teeth have been known since antiquity. Arthritis is an extremely common disease resulting in destruction of joint surfaces that can render movement excruciatingly painful. The development of artificial joints has provided an alternative to this kind of suffering. Indeed, the installation of these artificial bone-joint combinations has become one of the most common orthopedic procedures at present.

Newly developed materials are now becoming widely used for a variety of purposes, including artificial heart valves, and artificial ducts or channels which substitute for the esophagus, bile ducts, and arteries. Structural elements include bone implants, cartilage replacements (ear, nose, or joint), artificial tendons and cosmetic implants to improve external appearance.

Artificial extremities of widely varying complexity have been developed for amputees. Sophisticated controlled and powered hands and arms are fully developed but have not been widely accepted because of preference for the rather simple mechanical versions that remain dominant in present use.

PSEUDO-SOLUTIONS

The functional and structural supplements and substitutes mentioned above are identified as "pseudo-solutions" in Figure 8–7 because they appear to represent attractive solutions to complications of diseases but do not deal with the underlying disease process. Excessive enthusiasm over successful relief of symptoms by means of structural and functional substitutes can divert essential attention and resources from the more important tasks of identifying the underlying causes of these diseases and disabilities which could lead to ultimate prevention and cure in the future. Considerations applicable to most of these technologies can be illustrated by a specific example.

The dialysis machines which support the lives of patients with inadequate kidney function are recognized as technical triumphs of vital importance to the patients who are dependent upon them. Congress has included financial coverage for patients requiring dialysis under Medicare to cover costs too great for most individuals to sustain. In 1976, this program provided care for 21,500 eligible patients at a cost of $448,000,000. The cost is expected to reach $1,000,000,000 by 1984 and perhaps cost $1,700,000,000 by 1990, covering some 70,000 patients (12). There is no question of withdrawing this kind of support from patients who would die without it. However, it seems desirable to query what alternatives are being neglected by virtue of this large allocation of resources for the benefit of a relatively small number of patients. For example, kidney transplants are recognized as preferable to continued enslavement to dialysis machines. The common rejection of kidney transplants can be avoided only by greater understanding of the underlying immune reactions. Our policymakers must carefully consider whether the huge expenditures for dialysis are diverting efforts away from solving the immune reaction problem or developing a basic understanding of kidney disease processes. The potential benefits of the much preferred treatment, cure, or prevention of kidney disease for future generations could be sacrificed in exchange for limited benefits for a relatively small number of patients today. These consid-erations apply to all of the present pseudo-solutions but is perhaps best exemplified by the artificial heart.

TOTALLY IMPLANTABLE MECHANICAL HEART

The concept of substituting an artificial pumping device for the heart appeared realizable in 1939 when John Gibbon succeeded in keeping cats alive for nearly three hours with a mechanical apparatus that substituted for both the heart and lungs. The life support systems that opened the thorax and the heart chambers to surgical repair and reconstruction were the direct result. By the late 1950s heart "assist" devices had reached a stage that encouraged some investigators to push for a totally implantable heart. Congress earmarked appropriations for such a devel-opment in 1965. Most of the technologies, essential materials, and successful implantable pump systems have been developed. Animals have been kept alive for weeks with implanted pumps and external power sources. Methods of meeting the power requirements remain elusive. The original projections were for the manu-facture of sufficient devices to serve extremely large numbers of patients (as many as 200,000 per year). Growing concerns over the ultimate consequences of technical success stimulated the convening of a special interdisciplinary panel to consider the personal, social, and cultural implications of successful development of such hearts (13). This survey constituted one of the first and foremost assessments of the overall impact of technologies in the field of health care.

TECHNOLOGY ASSESSMENT: THE BROAD VIEW

Most of the pressing problems of modern society can be traced to unpredicted consequences of technological triumphs (e.g., population explosion, urbanization, pollution). This realization has prompted a growing interest in developing tech-niques for evaluating, in advance, the potential and probable impacts of new technologies while development is still in progress. The kinds of considerations that emerge are represented by issues encountered in the technology assessment of the totally implantable artificial heart.

Advances to date indicate that successful prototypes could be ready for implantation in man within a decade. Estimated numbers now are in the range of 17,000 to 50,000 people per year, although, judging by the popularity of coronary bypass operations, this estimate seems extremely conservative. The implications for various components of society include the following examples (12).

PATIENTS

Recipients of artificial hearts could be expected to lead a fairly active life but the anxieties and uncertainties of treatment could have serious psychological effects. Monitoring of patients may be required to keep track of the radioactive materials incorporated into the nuclear power package. This could lead to some loss of freedom. The commonly quick and relatively painless death from heart disease may be relinquished in favor of a more prolonged and lingering existence.

PATIENTS' FAMILIES

The benefits to the family may be significant, particularly if the patient is the breadwinner. The cost must be born by some third party, otherwise the family's financial stability would be permanently jeopardized. The personal and psychological impacts on the family are difficult to evaluate.

SOCIETY

Many of the candidates for implant will be elderly. This will further increase the number and relative proportion of the older age group in the population. The natural tendency for society to preserve lives of individuals at "any cost" indicates that the government must become the source of funding. The demand may well become so great that sufficient numbers cannot reasonably be produced to meet all the requirements. Under these conditions, the rationing of such life-sustaining equipment becomes a difficult or impossible task for the government of a democratic society.

LEGAL SYSTEM

The court system would undoubtedly be involved whenever there were insufficient numbers of artificial hearts to satisfy the real or perceived demand. Liability for failure would fall on the manufacturers, physicians, and perhaps government.

HEALTH SERVICES SYSTEM

The requirements for extensive and expensive surgical facilities for implantation of hearts would need to be supplemented by many adjunct services including intensive care, monitoring stations, and social and psychological counseling services.

The total cost of each implant would probably be about $25,000, not counting all of the ancillary services required. The diversion of major financial resources toward heart implants would necessarily deplete funds required for many other types of health services.

ECONOMIC IMPLICATIONS

The minimum expected costs of artificial hearts would be at least $500,000,-000 per year, based on 20,000 eligible recipients. This figure neglects the enormous potential costs from ancillary services or much greater demand for artificial hearts than can currently be visualized. It is worth noting that the annual costs of artificial kidneys already exceeds that figure by a substantial margin.

The time has come when these and many related considerations must be explored in relation to the ultimate impact of current pseudo-solutions and the new ones that are emerging every year. For example, the same kinds of analyses are urgently needed to assess the efficacy, economy, and outcome benefits from such sophisticated diagnostic equipment as CAT scanners.

FUTURE FORECASTS

Health care technologies have induced revolutionary changes in the practice of medicine and surgery during the past twenty-five years. The original emphasis on basic medical research during the Golden Age of NIH has been reduced and diverted toward more tangible health benefits by pressures for short term pay-offs by the public and their representatives in Congress. Both attention and resources need to be restored for the elucidation of the fundamental causes of the most common and critical diseases as the essential ingredient for more definitive diagnosis and therapy of persistent health problems.

Greatly expanded research is needed for such central issues as virology, immunology, genetics, and related subjects which are fundamental to many of the diseases affecting mankind (e.g., cancer, atherosclerosis, arthritis, and allergies). In addition, the mechanisms which are directly involved in the production of specific lesions need to be explored in-depth before definitive diagnosis and therapy can be developed to optimal levels. Diagnostic equipment has greatly expanded in diversity, objectivity, and relevance. Ideally, a definitive diagnostic test can indicate the nature and severity of an ailment from a single quantitative value. Some of the infectious diseases can be diagnosed with this degree of certainty and, in general, their causes are known. Despite enormous progress in both basic and clinical medicine, the causes of most other common persistent disease problems remain uncertain. Continued commitment to basic medical research should progressively elucidate the causes of a growing list of diseases, creating opportunities for definitive and quantitative diagnoses. Continued pressures for pay-off will insure that the fruits of basic research technologies will be promptly converted into diagnostic methods.

The current trends toward the development of extremely costly substitutes for definitive therapy, technical pseudo-solutions, is likely to continue at the peril of the economic stability of the country. The need for multi-disciplinary evaluation of the ultimate impact of health technologies is just now becoming more widely apparent. Technology assessment is a concept whose time has come, perhaps too late to avoid the mistakes of the past but absolutely essential for the avoidance of even worse problems in the future.

The impact of health care technology has affected all components of both the health services system and the general public's relation to it. Health care professionals have become increasingly dependent upon these technologies and have assumed the role of professional purchasing agent for the patient in selecting appropriate health services. One consequence has been the progressive specialization of physicians and other professionals. A corresponding decrease in general practitioners has depleted the ranks of primary care physicians. The sophistication of health technologies has increased the dependence of the public on the health professionals to the point that they assume a helpless stance in treating even trivial health problems. The average citizen must become more responsible for health maintenance and for the management of the most common self-limited ailments through aided self-care. The well established technologies of communication and transportation must be mobilized into readily accessed networks by which the citizen can assume these responsibilities with confidence and with appropriate protection against complications.

There is growing evidence that advances in health technologies have developed too far, too fast, and with exuberant enthusiasm by health professionals. The outcome for the public in terms of their actual health status has been recognized in the improved management of life-threatening ailments. The common malfunctions and chronic complaints that depress the quality of life for many people have gone essentially unchallenged. A realignment of priorities seems timely in support of the health status of the productive population between 16 and 55 years of age, even if this requires a reduction in the relative resources devoted to prolonging life and postponing death in the aging population. The process of technology assessment must be developed and progressively refined to permit such crucial evaluation of current and future priorities. The single most important requirement for effective technology assessment is the broad consideration of interdisciplinary impacts on the social, economic, legal, and political aspects of modern society.

The need for long-range health planning on a national scale has been recognized for years. The excessive duplication of costly technologies is one of the most pressing problems to be resolved. The crucial first step, the development of national health goals, policies, strategies, and criteria for evaluation, has not been taken. However, there is awakening interest in these needs as evidenced by increasing statutory requirements in legislation.

The ramifications of these issues are vast. They fundamentally affect every facility and service discussed in the previous chapters of this book. They are also driving forces that are intimately influencing the quantity and form of the resources devoted to health care and the means through which our nation controls those resources.

REFERENCES

1. Maple E: *Magic, Medicine and Quackery.* London, Robert Hale, 1968.
2. Ray C: *Medical Engineering.* Chicago, Year Book Medical Publishers, Inc., 1975.
3. Fishbein M: *Fads and Quackery in Healing.* New York, Covici, Friede, Publishers, 1932.
4. Duffy J: *The Healers; The Rise of the Medical Establishment.* New York, McGraw-Hill Book Company, 1976.
5. Strickland SP: *Politics, Science, and Dread Disease; A Short History of the United States Medical Research Policy.* Cambridge, Harvard University Press, 1972.
6. Rushmer RF: *Cardiovascular Dynamics,* ed. 4. Philadelphia, W. B. Saunders Company, 1976.
7. Gordon R, Herman GT, Johnson SA: Image reconstruction from projections. *Scientific American* 233(4):56–71, 1975.
8. Institute of Medicine: *Computed Tomographic Scanning: A Policy Statement.* Washington, D.C., National Academy of Science, 1977.
9. Rushmer RF: *Medical Engineering: Projections for Health Care Delivery.* New York, Academic Press, 1972.
10. Bloom BS, Peterson OL: Patient needs and medical-care planning: the coronary-care unit as a model. *New England Journal of Medicine* 290:1171–1177, 1974.
11. Preston T: *Coronary Artery Surgery: A Critical Review.* New York, Raven Press, 1977.
12. United States Congress: *Development of Medical Technology: Opportunities for Assessment.* Washington, D.C., Office of Technology Assessment, 1976.
13. National Heart and Lung Institute: *The Totally Implantable Heart.* Report of the Artificial Heart Assessment Panel, National Institutes of Health, Department of Health, Education, and Welfare, Washington, D.C., 1973.

CHAPTER 9

Health
Care
Personnel

Paul R. Torrens
Charles E. Lewis

Health services are provided by people for other people. Those with health "needs" (a commonly used term which is seldom defined with precision) present these needs to others. In the process, those providing the services are also engaged in meeting their own needs, primarily related to job and personal satisfaction. These need meeting encounters between consumers and provider occur within a system— the personal health system—that determines whose "needs" shall be met by whom, with what degree of provider training, in what settings, at what cost, and at whose expense.

The focus of this chapter is on health personnel — the numbers, types, and functions of people who represent the human capital investment in the health care system — and the factors that enable them to deliver the services needed by the nation. It will also deal with certain factors and forces that limit their numbers, functions, and abilities to provide services, and special issues and policy concerns of national importance.

The literature on health care personnel is enormous and endlessly varied. The chapter presents the major principles, trends and pressures involved so that by understanding the underlying principles, made more apparent by illustrative examples, the reader will have an effective analytical framework for assessing all aspects of health care personnel.

It should first be pointed out that health care personnel must be considered in the broader context of the total health care system since personnel issues are shaped by exactly the same forces and pressures that affect other aspects of the system. Only when personnel "sub-policies" are derived from an overall national health policy can there be any hope of rational solutions to personnel (and other) problems. Thus, as with all other chapters of this book, there are important and extensive interdependencies between the various discussions of the component parts of the system.

TRENDS IN HEALTH CARE PERSONNEL IN THE TWENTIETH CENTURY

The most important trend in health care personnel during the last twenty five years has been the extraordinary growth in the number of individuals working in the health sector (Table 9–1). From 1950 to 1975, the total number of persons in the United States work force increased from 63,000,000 to 91,000,000, a gain of 44%. During the same period, however, the number of people employed in the health care system increased by 215% from 1,530,000 to 4,600,000, and by 1975 they comprised more than 5% of the total U.S. work force (1, 2). As a result, the health care industry is the largest single employer of people among the approximately 150 specific industries monitored by the U.S. Department of Labor (3). Since approximately 70% of the jobs in health care are held by women, the health care industry is also the largest single employer of women, providing more than 7% of all jobs held by women in this country (4).

The second significant trend in health care personnel is the increased specialization of personnel and the longer period of training required to enter one of the health professions. This change involves not only an increasingly narrow definition of the scope of practice of an individual (for example, for physicians, from general practitioner to pediatrician to pediatric cardiologist to research pediatric cardiologist), but also proliferation of types of personnel providing care. Prior to 1940, there were fewer than 40 primary or alternate job titles in health care identified by the U.S. Department of Labor; by 1975 the number of individually identifiable positions had risen to 665 (2). This increase in specialization has been forced by the incredible growth in scientific knowledge, as well as by the remarkable expansion in sophisticated diagnostic and therapeutic techniques available for use in patient care as discussed in Chapter 8. The extent to which this specialization has accelerated the expectations of the American public is not known, but it most assuredly has had a major influence on the orientations and expectations of students in the health professions, encouraging their interest in professional fields which are increasingly narrow in scope but deep in detail.

Paralleling the increasing number of identifiable health professions, there has also been remarkable growth in efforts to certify, license, or otherwise delineate the boundaries, qualifications, and standards of each particular professional area. Of the 665 primary or alternate job titles in health care that could be identified by the Department of Labor in 1975, more than 150 of them were subject to separate certification or professional designation by various professional organizations or agencies(2). The majority of these certification efforts have been initiated by the professional groups themselves and continue to be controlled by them, with relatively little influence by persons outside of the profession. This has the positive

TABLE 9-1. Estimated Number of Persons in Certain Occupations in the Health Field, United States, 1950–1980

Occupation	1950	1960	1970	1973	1975	1950–1975 (Percent increase)	1980 (Estimated)
Physicians	209,000	247,300	311,200	337,000	364,500	74	444,000
Dentists	79,200	91,100	102,200	107,300	112,000	41	126,200
Registered Nurses	316,200	527,000	750,000	857,000	961,000	204	1,152,000
Dental Hygienists	7,000	12,500	16,000	21,000	23,500	235	NA*
Dental Assistants	55,200	82,500	92,500	116,000	120,000	118	NA
Dietetic and Nutritional Services	22,900	25,000	47,000	68,000	75,000	227	NA
Licensed Practical Nurses	146,000	245,000	400,000	459,000	477,000	226	NA
Nurse Practitioners	NA	NA	500	2,000	5,000	NA	NA
Occupational Therapy	2,000	8,000	12,800	13,700	13,700	585	NA
Physical Therapy	4,600	9,000	24,000	24,600	26,100	467	NA
Physicians' Assistants	NA	NA	NA	1,100	2,000	NA	NA
Social Workers	6,200	11,900	29,800	33,800	40,000	545	NA
All Health Workers	1,525,100	2,266,800	4,273,700	4,425,800	4,855,501	218	NA

*NA—not available or not applicable.

Source: U.S. Department of Health, Education, and Welfare, Public Health Service, Bureau of Health Manpower: A Report to the President and Congress on the Status of Health Professions Personnel in the United States. DHEW Publication No. (HRA) 78-93, Washington, D.C., Government Printing Office, August 1978. 1980 estimates from Stambler, H: Heath Manpower for the Nation—A look ahead at the supply and the requirements. *Public Health Reports*, 94:3–10, 1979.

effect of ensuring higher standards of quality and performance, but also the possibly negative effects of restricting entrance into the profession and of possibly conducting the profession with complete disregard for the felt needs of the public. These issues are also discussed further in later chapters.

THE QUESTION OF SUPPLY: SHORTAGE OR SUFFICIENCY?

One of the key questions concerning health care personnel relates to supply: are there enough professionals in all categories? Unfortunately, our definitions of "enough" are not very specific and the answer to the question may vary from decade to decade and place to place. The supply of physicians and our evaluation of its adequacy illustrates this point very well.

At the turn of the century, medical education was a somewhat informal non-scientific affair carried out in rather rudimentary proprietary institutions of somewhat dubious standards. There were large numbers of these schools, 14 in Chicago alone in 1910, and 10 each in Missouri and Tennessee, and they produced great numbers of physicians.

In 1908, Abraham Flexner undertook a study of medical education in the United States for the Rockefeller Foundation and his report, *Medical Education in the United States and Canada,* recommended that the training of physicians be a university function based on a firm scientific foundation. As a result, large numbers of medical schools closed, medical training expanded in length and complexity, and fewer physicians emerged into practice. Obviously Flexner (and others) thought that there were more than enough physicians in 1908.

By 1928, the situation seemed to have changed, or at least the public's perception of it was different, as reflected by the statement of the National Grange at the annual meeting of the American Medical Association for that year:

According to the findings of a survey made for the General Education Board by Lewis Mayers and Leonard V. Harrison published in 1924, there were approximately 33,000 physicians in places of 1,000 inhabitants or less in the United States in 1906. In 1924, according to this report, this number had been reduced to 27,000 showing an actual loss of 6,000 rural physicians in 18 years. More recent investigation shows that almost two-thirds of the towns of 1,000 or less throughout the United States which had physicians in 1914 had none in 1925. The average age of rural doctors throughout the country in 1925 was 52 years. Since the average age at death of American physicians is 62 years, it will be seen at a glance that the present generation of country doctors will have practically disappeared in another ten years. Notwithstanding this situation, we find that the Commission on Medical Education which is now studying the subject reports that with the medical school capacity we have in the country at the present time, and their graduates averaging 27 years of age, the number of physicians in practice is actually decreasing and their number will not regain its present size of 130,000 until 1965. In the meantime, the population of the country, the Commission estimates will have increased from 115 millions to 165 millions.(5)

Obviously, the Grange felt that there was a shortage of physicians in the country, at least in the rural areas, in 1925.

By 1933, however, concern had shifted to the problem of our possibly having too many doctors. In the annual presidential address to the American Medical Association (AMA) that year, Lewis suggested that "There is apparently an overproduction of doctors . . . . Careful studies indicate that there are in the United States 25,000 more physicians than are required"(6). One of his suggested remedies was to restrict the number of foreign medical graduates (FMGs) who came to the United States after graduation abroad.

The pendulum began to swing back, however, and by 1953 the President of the AMA for that year was suggesting that there was a shortage of physicians and the number of medical schools should be expanded. By 1961, the AMA was editorially calling for the use of federal funds in the construction of new medical schools to alleviate shortages in medical personnel.

The federal effort began in 1963 with the passage of the Health Professions Education Assistance Act (P.L. 88-129), followed in 1965 by further amendments (P.L. 89-290). These were amplified by the Health Manpower Act of 1968 (P.L. 90-490) and by a special physician augmentation program in 1969. As reflected in Table 9–2 these legislative efforts have had their impact, with the number of U.S. medical schools increasing 31% from 87 in 1963 to 114 in 1974 and the number of graduates of U.S. schools increasing 59% from 7,264 in 1963 to 11,613 in 1974 and to 14,393 in 1978(7).

Finally, in the mid 1970s, the cycle turned once more and increasingly the projections predict that there will be an oversupply of physicians in 1990, both in individual states and in the country as a whole (1, 8, 9, 10). Concerns have been expressed that perhaps the medical schools have expanded too far and too rapidly, and at least one group of sophisticated commentators suggest that "If anything, there may be a doctor glut over the next decade"(8).

Reviewing the experience with physician supply since 1900, it is clear that the nation does not have good operative indices of "shortage" or adequacy of supply, at least for physicians, and that our ability to forecast physician supply accurately has been rather poor. It is also clear that to determine whether there are "enough" physicians (or any other health personnel), it is necessary to know more about the way in which practitioners actually use their professional talents, where they locate geographically, what access patients have to their services, and what impact the services are having on people's health. With this information perhaps the supply of physicians and other health resources can be more accurately planned. Thus, the factors that determine how many physicians, dentists, nurses, and other personnel are "needed" or are "optimal" are exceedingly complex, encompassing issues discussed in all of the chapters of this book.

TREES HIDDEN BY THE FOREST: SUB-GROUPS OF HEALTH PROFESSIONALS

Information about health professionals is often presented as if all members of that professional group were exactly alike and worked in the same way at the same task and with similar results. Unfortunately, nothing could be farther from the

**TABLE 9–2. Medical School Students and Graduates,
United States, 1963–1978**

Year	Number of Schools	Total Enrollment	Graduates
1940–1941	77	21,379	5,275
1945–1946	77	23,216	5,826
1950–1951	79	26,186	6,135
1955–1956	82	28,839	6,845
1956–1957	85	29,130	6,796
1957–1958	85	29,473	6,861
1958–1959	85	29,614	6,860
1959–1960	85	30,084	7,081
1960–1961	86	30,288	6,994
1961–1962	87	31,078	7,168
1962–1963	87	31,491	7,264
1963–1964	87	32,001	7,336
1964–1965	88	32,428	7,409
1965–1966	88	32,835	7,574
1966–1967	89	33,423	7,743
1967–1968	94	34,538	7,973
1968–1969	99	35,833	8,059
1969–1970	101	37,669	8,367
1970–1971	103	40,487	8,974
1971–1972	108	43,650	9,551
1972–1973	112	47,546	10,391
1973–1974	114	50,886	11,613
1975–1976	114	56,244	13,561
1976–1977	116	58,266	13,607
1977–1978	122	60,456	14,393

Source: Medical Education in the United States, *JAMA* Special
Edition, Dec 22–29, 1978, Vol. 240, No. 26, p. 2822.

truth. Very often, the grouping of all members of a particular health profession into a single descriptive category will obscure certain important differences among sub-groups within the larger whole. Again, the medical profession presents a good example of this phenomenon.

In 1976, there were 404,338 Medical Doctors in the United States, giving the country a ratio of 190 physicians per 100,000 population, or one physician for every 527 people(11). These ratios were among the best in the world and would generally suggest to the casual observer that there are adequate numbers of physicians.

Unfortunately, as shown in Table 9–3 these figures do not necessarily mean that all 404,338 physicians were readily available to care for all of the people in this country for the full range of their problems. Instead, it means that groups of physicians serve specific groups or areas of population and frequently provide services for only a limited range of concerns.

For example, although there were over 404,000 physicians in the country in 1976, 25,787 or 6% were employed by the Federal government to provide a

Table 9–3.   Physicians by Type of Practice, United States, 1976

Type of Practice	Number of Physicians
Total physicians	404,338
Non-federal	318,089
Patient care	292,152
Office-based	213,117
General practice	45,503
Other full-time primary specialty	167,614
Hospital-based practice	79,035
Training programs	58,482
Full-time hospital staff	20,553
Other professional activity	25,787
Federal	25,937
Patient care	22,086
Office-based practice	1,652
General practice	519
Other full-time primary specialty	1,133
Hospital-based practice	20,434
Training programs	3,934
Full-time hospital staff	16,500
Other professional activity	3,701
Inactive	22,024
Not cassified	29,681
Unknown	8,757

Source: AMA Center for Health Services Research and Development: *Physician Distribution and Medical Licensure in the U.S., 1976,* Chicago, Illinois, American Medical Association, 1975. Reprinted with permission.

specific range of services for selected populations such as the military or veterans, as discussed in Chapter 1, and to American Indians on reservations and inmates of federal prisons. As a result, the pool of active physicians with known professional activities to serve the non-Federal population was only 318,089. Concentrating on the 318,089 physicians in non-Federal service, it will be noted that only 292,152 (2% of all the U.S. physicians) were engaged in "patient care" activities. Of these only 213,117 (3% of all U.S. physicians) were engaged in office-based practice (as opposed to hospital-based practice). And of these 213,117 in "office-based practice," 45,503 are listed as "general practitioners" (that is, they have no stated medical specialty) and 167,614 are listed as specialists, including primary care specialties.

If one were interested in knowing how many physicians are available for some type of office-based general practice in a community, for example, the important figures would be the 45,503 physicians without a stated specialty and the 167,614 physicians in office-based specialty practice (of whom at least some would be available for general practice). This combined figure of 213,117 physicians available for service is quite different from the 404,338 physicians first mentioned and provides quite different perspectives than does the original figure.

In the same fashion, one might again examine the number (404,338) of physicians in the United States in 1976 and feel quite comfortable with the great abundance of physicians available to care for the needs of the country. However, a total of 62,416 physicians, or 15% of all U.S. physicians, are in training programs of one kind or another (Table 9–3). While these physicians obviously provide considerable patient care, they are also very much involved in the learning process and are not necessarily available full-time in communities that need more office-based physicians.

Further, simply because a physician's site of practice may be known does not necessarily reveal anything about the actual services being provided. For example, Table 9–4 reflects that there were 343,876 physicians active in 1976 whose areas of specialty were known, suggesting that there should be sufficient numbers of physicians to meet the general health needs of the country. Further examination of the data, however, would show that 97,416 of these physicians (32% of the total) were surgical specialists and were primarily available only for the care of patients with very specific surgical needs(11). While one might be heartened by the country's more than 300,000 physicians available in 1976, it might also be very disheartening to discover, on closer examination, that nearly one out of every three doctors in the country was a surgeon!

Finally, the knowledge of physicians' specialty interests does not reveal much at all about the number of patients that are seen, the specific problems that are handled, and (most important) the impact that these services have on the patients. Indeed, so little is really known about what transpires in a physician's office, as noted in Chapter 4, and the interaction is so critical, that it seems almost ludicrous to use the gross personnel figures for planning purposes. Thus, the gross accumulation of information about health professionals in large unitary groupings frequently conceals many important sub-groupings that are critical for any pertinent evaluation of the use of professional resources and any accurate forecasting of the future need for these professionals.

THE DISTRIBUTION OF HEALTH PERSONNEL: HOW DO YOU GET PEOPLE WHERE THEY ARE NEEDED?

One of the perplexing problems facing those who would forecast the future supply of health care personnel is an almost total inability to influence the geographic distribution of personnel throughout the country, and in many instances the type of work or setting in which health care professionals practice. While the country may have available to it many hundreds of thousands of personnel of a particular kind, it is difficult to predict and influence where those thousands of individuals will eventually settle and practice. Again, the situation with regard to physicians illustrates the point very well.

It is generally agreed that this country now has approximately enough physicians in terms of total numbers, and may soon have many more physicians

TABLE 9–4. Type of Practice and Primary Specialty of Active Non-Federal and Federal Physicians, United States, 1976*

Primary Specialty	Total Active
Professionally active physicians	343,876
Primary care	134,051
General practice	54,631
Internal medicine	57,312
Pediatrics	22,108
Other medical specialties	18,702
Dermatology	4,755
Pediatric allergy	469
Pediatric cardiology	537
Internal medicine subspecialties	12,941
Surgical specialties	97,416
General surgery	31,899
Neurological surgery	2,959
Obstetrics and gynecology	21,908
Ophthalmology	11,326
Orthopedic surgery	11,689
Otolaryngology	5,788
Plastic surgery	2,337
Colon and rectal surgery	667
Thoracic surgery	2,020
Urology	6,823
Other specialties	93,707
Anesthesiology	13,074
Neurology	4,374
Pathology	11,815
Forensic pathology	203
Psychiatry	24,196
Child psychiatry	2,618
Physical medicine and rehabilitation	1,665
Radiology	11,627
Diagnostic radiology	3,794
Therapeutic radiology	1,202
Miscellaneous	19,139

*M.D.s only.

Source: Goodman J; AMA Center for Health Services Research and Development: *Physician Distribution and Medical Licensure in the U.S., 1976.* Chicago, Illinois, American Medical Association, 1977. Reprinted with permission.

than are needed. At the same time, it is also generally agreed that there are not enough physicians in primary care and that there is a relative shortage of physicians in rural areas. As presented in Table 9–5, for example, the overall ratio of physicians to population was one physician per 768 people for the entire country in 1973. At the same time, however, the ratio of physicians to population varied from a low of one physician per 511 people in the most central metropolitan areas to a high of one physician per 2,512 people, a five-fold difference, in the most rural areas. Disregarding the overabundance of physicians in the metropolitan areas, possibly caused by physician clustering around large hospitals, the supply of physicians in most rural areas is nowhere near sufficient to meet the health needs of rural people as reflected in comparatively lower utilization rates (Chapter3).

Yet very little has been done, and perhaps can be done, to affect this problem, short of some form of coercion. A variety of voluntary, incentive-based programs have been attempted which involve loan-forgiveness (in exchange for an agreement to work in rural areas), salaried financial support for the first few years of practice (such as provided by the National Health Service Corps), and low-interest loans or outright grants to purchase equipment or facilities (as made possible by various private foundations), all with comparatively little success. Physicians still tend to cluster in the larger metropolitan areas, where the hospital facilities are better, where there is a larger pool of potential patients, and where living conditions are more congenial for the physician's family. Although it might be desirable for physicians to distribute themselves on the more ideal basis of the health care needs of the nation's population, in reality they are distributed on the more practical bases of income potential, compatible living conditions, and accessability to superior hospital facilities and specialist colleagues.

In the same vein, for many years there was great concern expressed about the apparently dwindling supply of physicians in general practice, family practice, and

TABLE 9–5. Physician-Population Ratios by Size of County, United States, 1973

Demographic County Classification	Population per Physician
Total	768
Nonmetropolitan Areas	
Less than 10,000 inhabitants	2,512
10,000 to 24,999 inhabitants	2,040
25,000 to 49,999 inhabitants	1,432
50,000 or more inhabitants	1,100
Metropolitan Areas	
Potential metropolitan	1,095
50,000 to 499,999 inhabitants	835
500,000 to 999,999 inhabitants	747
1,000,000 to 4,999,999 inhabitants	623
5,000,000 or more inhabitants	511

Source: AMA Center for Health Services Research and Development: *Distribution of Physicians in the U.S., 1973.* Chicago, Illinois, American Medical Association, 1974.

primary care. Whether these fears were real or imagined, various steps were taken to influence the situation. These included increasing the number of primary care residencies from 3,974 first year residencies in 1960 to 8,016 first year residencies in 1974 (12), insisting that medical schools establish Departments of Family Practice, establishing a medical specialty board for family medicine in 1969, and other measures which made these areas of medical practice more attractive to physicians and easier to enter and to obtain appropriate post-graduate training. Recent evidence suggests that these efforts have been so effective that many states will find themselves with a potential over-supply of family or primary-care physicians by the end of this century (1, 8, 9, 10). The evidence also suggests, however, that the current shortage in the supply of such physicians in rural areas will not be affected at all by the increase in the overall supply, with most of the increase accruing to non-rural areas, just as at the present time (13).

Thus, the mere presence of a large pool of professional talent does not necessarily mean that it will be distributed evenly or in any relationship to the needs of a particular population for services. The distribution will more likely be controlled by the individual needs of the professionals doing the serving, rather than by the people being served. For the present, it would seem that our society is reduced to utilizing indirect measures of influence in trying to affect this distribution, since more direct and pertinent measures are either not available or are not politically acceptable; other related issues of regulating system performance are discussed in Chapter 11.

THE MORE THINGS STAY THE SAME, THE MORE THEY CHANGE: PHARMACISTS AND DENTISTS

In reviewing the third and fourth largest groups of health care personnel, pharmacists and dentists, one is confronted with many of the same issues that affect all other health care personnel. There are some issues, however, which are quite different and deserve specific comment.

Since 1950, although the numbers of pharmacists and dentists have increased somewhat, the ratio of pharmacists and dentists to the population hardly changed at all; indeed, for pharmacists, it has decreased. In 1950, there were 75,310 active dentists in the United States, or 48.9 dentists per 100,000 population. Twenty five-years later, there were 35% more civilian dentists, 106,740, but the dentist to population ratio was still only 51.4 (14).

There were 101,630 pharmacists in 1951, yielding a ratio of 68 pharmacists per 100,000. By 1973, the number of pharmacists had increased 30% to 132,899, but because of the parallel greater increase in the U.S. population, the ratio of pharmacists to population had actually dropped to 63 per 100,000 (15).

Nevertheless, the productivity of both of these groups has increased markedly and the output of patient services provided directly or supervised by pharmacists and dentists has risen sharply. This increased productivity seems to be directly related to increased use of auxiliary personnel and the availability of more efficient and easily utilized materials and equipment.

Although the numbers of dentists and their proportions to the population have not changed at all, there has been an explosive growth in the numbers of dental auxiliary personnel. In 1973, there were an estimated 22,540 practicing dental hygienists, an increase of approximately 14,000 (200%) since 1960. In 1973, there were an estimated 118,000 dental assistants in the country, an increase of approximately 74,000 (59%) over 1960 (2). The greatly increased utilization of dental hygienists and dental assistants by practicing dentists over the last 20 years is shown in Table 9–6.

With regard to pharmacists, although there has been an increase in various assistant personnel, there is nowhere near the rapid growth in auxiliary personnel that there has been in dentistry. Indeed, there is not even a pharmacist auxiliary personnel category that is as well-defined and numerous as the dental hygienist or dental assistant.

On the other hand, the pharmacist's basic equipment and materials have changed markedly, so that there is no longer the need for the individual pharmacist to compound pharmaceuticals or medications as was the custom in the past. Now, with the continuous availability of pre-packaged medications, of specific-dose packages, and of carefully-designed dispensing systems, and with the wide variety of innovations in the packaging and delivery of the basic materials, pharmacists are freer to direct their attention to more productive services. Indeed, one of the most striking features of the pharmacist's professional activities has been the fairly significant change in the tasks performed today as compared with the past. The pharmacist today spends much more time counselling physicians and patients on proper medication usage and spends comparatively less time in actual preparation

TABLE 9–6. Percent of Independent Dentists Who Employ Auxiliaries: Selected Years, United States, 1955–1975

	Percent of Dentists Employing:		
Year	Dental Hygienists	Dental Auxiliaries	All Types of Auxiliaries
1955	10.3	70.7	77.1
1958	14.0	75.5	81.8
1961	15.0	76.7	82.6
1964	20.2	82.4	89.9
1967	25.2	86.6	92.4
1970	30.8	85.6	89.9
1972	36.9	90.2	93.6
1975	41.3	92.5	96.1

Source: American Dental Association, Bureau of Economic Research and Statistics: The 1975 Survey of Dental Practice. In *A Report to the President and Congress on the Status of Health Professions Personnel in the United States.* Bureau of Health Manpower, United States Department of Health, Education, and Welfare, DHEW Publication No. (HRA) 78–93, August 1978.

of medications. A much greater proportion of time is spent reviewing the patient records, checking for possible harmful interaction effects from multiple drug prescriptions, and teaching other health professionals about the uses and abuses of medications than was ever the case in the past. The pharmacist's role as educator, counsellor, and monitor of patient care has increased, while some of the more traditional roles have receded or disappeared entirely.

Thus, dentists and pharmacists demonstrate that the numbers of professionals available do not have to change at all for there to be a considerable increase in services if there is a parallel increase in some of the auxiliary personnel at the same time. Also, because of the changes in some of the basic features of the equipment and materials of the professional, the role and tasks of that professional may change accordingly. They may still have the same name they did previously, but other aspects of the professional role may have changed in very significant ways.

NURSING: THE DIFFICULTIES OF WOMEN IN THE HEALTH CARE WORK FORCE

In 1978, there were more than 5,000,000 people employed in health-related occupations. One half of these were in nursing (or related services) and they comprised the largest single group of health professionals in the country. Their large numbers and their absolutely essential position in any program of patient care would lead one to expect that the nursing profession would be vigorously optimistic and flourishing. Unfortunately, this is not always the case, and nursing personnel have had significant problems, most of them directly parallel to the difficulties of other women in the U.S. work-force.

In 1972, a total of 1,127,657 Registered Nurses were included in an inventory of nurses conducted by the American Nurses Association in cooperation with the state boards of nursing. Of these, it was known that 778,470 (69% of the total) were actively employed in nursing and 316,611 (28%) were not employed in nursing at all (16). A repeat survey in 1974 by the Interagency Conference on Nursing Statistics did not attempt to identify the total pool of all registered nurses, but did determine that there were 857,000 actively employed nurses, an increase of approximately 78,000 over the 1972 figures (17). As shown in Table 9–7, the 1974 survey also revealed that only 608,000 of the 857,000 active nurses were employed full time, while another 249,000 were employed part-time. Using the 1972 figure of 1,127,657 as a rough indicator the number of nurses potentially available for full time employment, it is apparent that less than one-half of the potentially employable nurses in the country are actually working full-time in nursing.

Nursing remains a largely hospital-based profession, as demonstrated by Table 9–8. Of the 780,000 nurses employed in 1972, more than 74% were employed in hospitals and nursing homes, with approximately 13% working in private physician's offices and similar activities. The various categories of nurses based on training is presented in Table 9–9.

In 1974 there were 492,000 employed practical nurses in the country, an increase of 33,000 over the prior year (Table 9–10). The increase in numbers of

TABLE 9–7. Number of Registered Nurses and Ratio to Population, United States, Selected Years

Year	Number of Nurses in Practice			Number per 100,000 Population
	Total	Full-time	Part-time	
1960	504,000	414,000	90,000	282
1962	550,000	433,000	117,000	298
1964	582,000	450,000	132,000	306
1966	621,000	466,000	155,000	319
1967	643,000	476,000	167,000	327
1968	667,000	489,000	178,000	335
1969	694,000	503,000	191,000	345
1970	722,000	519,000	203,000	356
1971	750,000	534,000	216,000	366
1972	780,000	548,000	232,000	376
1973	815,000	578,000	237,000	390
1974	857,000	608,000	249,000	407

Source: National Center for Health Statistics: *Health Resources Statistics: 1975.* United States Department of Health, Education, and Welfare, DHEW Publication No. (HRA) 76–1509, 1976.

licensed practical nurses has been rapid, from 137,500 in 1950 and 206,000 in 1960 and to the 1974 figure of 492,000 (18). The great majority of licensed practical nurses work in hospitals (65%), nursing homes (20%), and other inpatient facilities (7%).

Although the actual numbers of both registered nurses and licensed practical nurses have been increasing steadily, and the ratio of nurses to population has

TABLE 9–8. Place of Employment of Registered Nurses, United States, 1972

Place of Employment	Number of Nurses	Percent of Total
Total	780,000	100
Hospitals and nursing homes	578,000	74.1
Public health and schools	54,800	7.0
Nursing education	28,400	3.6
Occupational health	20,000	2.6
Private duty, doctor's office, and other fields	98,800	12.7

Source: National Center for Health Statistics: *Health Resources Statistics: 1975.* United States Department of Health, Education, and Welfare, DHEW Publication No. (HRA) 76-1509, 1976.

TABLE 9–9. Major Types of Nurse Training Programs in the United States

Program Category	Length of Training	Degree or Diploma
Practical nurse	1 year in vocational school, hospital, junior college	No degree or diploma
Diploma nurse	3 years in hospital	Diploma–eligible for R.N.
Associate degree nurse	2 years in junior college	Associate degree eligible for R.N.
Baccalaureate nurse	4 years in college/university	B.A./B.S.; eligible for R.N.
Advanced degree nurses	1 to 4 more years beyond B.A./B.S.	Masters and doctoral degrees

improved markedly as well, the situation with regards to nurses is exactly the same as with physicians: the mere increase in numbers does not necessarily mean that these personnel are distributed evenly or in any direct relation to actual need. The ratio of nurses to population varies widely across the country. In 1972, the overall ratio was 380 nurses per 100,000 population, but this varied from a low of 190 nurses per 100,000 population in Arkansas to a high of 649 nurses per 100,000 in Massachusetts (16). The projections of the future supply of nurses are also very similar to those for physicians, with a steady increase in both absolute numbers and nurse to population ratios through the end of this century, with many experts suggesting a possible over-supply of nurses in many parts of the country.

At the same time, hospitals all over the country repeatedly report great difficulties in obtaining adequate numbers of nurses, considerable turnover, sometimes averaging 50% of the nursing staff annually, and a resulting impairment in

TABLE 9–10. Licensed Practical Nurses in Relation to Population, United States, Selected Years

Year	Number of Practical Nurses in Practice	Number of Practical Nurses per 100,000 Population
1950	137,000	1,101
1960	206,000	868
1962	225,000	820
1964	250,000	760
1966	282,000	690
1968	320,000	621
1970	370,000	548
1971	400,000	513
1972	427,000	486
1973	459,000	456
1974	492,000	428

Source: U.S. Department of Health, Education, and Welfare: *Health, United States,* 1975. DHEW Publication No. (HRA) 76-1232, Washington, D.C., Government Printing Office, 1976.

patient care. This seeming incongruity between substantial total numbers of nurses (and perhaps gross oversupply) and the inability of hospitals in many areas to hire adequate numbers of nurses requires careful examination.

Although a large number of persons have at one time been trained as nurses, a significant percentage of them (perhaps as many as half) do not practice the profession full time and are thus mostly unavailable to the active work force. The abundance of nursing personnel, therefore, does not translate into an equal supply of labor resources for health care.

As shown in Table 9–11, both male and female graduates of nursing schools have high rates of employment (both in the 92–96% range) immediately following graduation. After age 25, female graduates begin to show a steady reduction in the percentage of nurses actually employed, as the women begin to marry, bear children, and become involved in family life. Male nursing graduates, however, not being forced to make this choice between work and child-bearing and child-rearing, continue to be employed in nursing at higher rates throughout all age groups (19).

The dilemma between work and child-rearing is reflected in various opinion surveys of currently employed nurses about their work situations. Although salary and working conditions are cited as being important, far more stress is placed on the need for child care assistance and more flexible work schedules to allow for family needs. Surveys of inactive nurses that attempt to determine prerequisites for returning to work repeatedly list more flexible choice of working hours, assistance with child care, and need for refresher training. (20).

The United States has made great efforts to produce adequate numbers of trained nurses and has been quite successful in doing so. Graduates are pouring out of nursing schools in increasing abundance every year. Unfortunately, hospitals have not been very successful in coping with the particular needs of their women

TABLE 9–11. Registered Nurses by Sex, Age Group, and Employment Status, United States, 1972

Age	Total	Male		Female	
		Number	Percent Employed in Nursing	Number	Percent Employed in Nursing
All ages	1,127,657	14,625	86.0	1,111,206	70.9
Under 25	73,396	657	96.5	72,696	91.5
25–29	164,926	2,076	91.9	162,774	77.1
30–34	143,914	2,144	91.1	141,692	65.5
35–39	129,075	1,679	89.0	127,334	66.0
40–44	117,181	1,465	88.2	115,620	70.8
45–49	124,706	1,206	87.8	123,365	73.9
50–54	99,969	1,013	83.6	98,823	74.1
55–59	76,978	908	76.0	75,963	71.9
60–64	66,213	557	70.8	75,529	66.4
65+	59,953	541	49.3	59,223	43.2
Age not reported	71,347	2,379	83.2	68,187	71.9

Source: *Facts About Nursing, 1972–1973.* Kansas City, Missouri, American Nurses Association, 1973.

nurse-employees, with the result that many trained nurses rapidly leave the nursing field and never return.

In addition to the dilemma of work versus child-bearing and child-rearing, there is an additional problem that has caused some dissatisfaction among nurses and has most certainly given rise to some of the departures from active nursing. Repeatedly one hears from nurses, particularly the best and brightest of the profession, that they are trained to know and do more than they are ever actually allowed to carry out in clinical practice. The feeling in many instances is one of marked frustration among a professional group that feels that they are not allowed to use the full range of talents they worked very hard to obtain through years of training. Although there have been significant efforts in recent years to open new avenues for more creative and independent nursing practice, the over-riding sense of frustration is still a very real concern. These and related issues of the changing role of nurses will be discussed further later in this chapter.

SPECIAL ISSUES FOR HEALTH PERSONNEL

IMPORTED LABOR: THE FOREIGN MEDICAL GRADUATE

During the 1800s, physicians in this country who wanted the best training in medicine went to London and Edinburgh for their education. Later on, from 1900 to the advent of World War II, physicians seeking the best of training were just as likely to go to Vienna or Berlin. Following the end of World War II, the tide turned and instead of the American physician going abroad to study, it was now the turn of the foreign physician to come here. And come they have, in ever increasing numbers, until by 1978 there were approximately 80,000 foreign medical graduates in the United States, or approximately one-fifth of all physicians in the country. The exodus of foreign physicians to the United States differed in one major respect from the previous departures of American physicians to study abroad. While American physicians returned to their native land after the completion of their studies, most of the foreign physicians entering the United States for medical training have stayed permanently.

During 1966, 6,628 foreign medical graduates (FMGs) came to the United States for the first time. That year, foreign medical graduates comprised 18.5% of all newly licensed physicians in the country (Table 9–12). This percentage continued to increase until by 1972 foreign medical graduates comprised an incredible 46% of all newly licensed physicians in the country. By 1973, this phenomenon started to taper off and by 1975, foreign medical graduates received *only* 35% of all new medical licenses in the country (1).

In view of the continuously increasing numbers of physicians being produced by American medical schools and the country's relatively excellent physician to population ratio (at least compared to the rest of the world), one might wonder

TABLE 9–12. Foreign Medical Graduates (FMGs) as a Percent of New
Licentiates, Filled Residencies, and Numbers of New Entry FMG Aliens,
United States, Selected Years

Year	FMGs as Percent of New Licentiates	FMGs as a Percent of Total Filled Residencies	Total New FMG Entries to U.S.	U.S. Medical Graduates
1966	18.5	30	6,628	7,574
1967	22.9	32	8,115	7,743
1968	22.4	32	8,405	7,973
1969	23.1	33	6,939	8,059
1970	27.3	33	7,630	8,367
1971	35.2	32	7,879	8,974
1972	46.0	32	7,024	9,551
1973	44.4	30	8,123	10,391
1974	40.0	29	8,352	11,588
1975	35.0	NA*	7,316	12,714

*NA—not available.

Source: Manpower Analysis Branch: *A Report to the President and Congress on the
Status of Health Professions Personnel in the United States.* Bureau of Health
Manpower, United States Department of Health, Education, and Welfare, DHEW
Publication No. (HRA) 78–93, August 1978.

why there has been such a need for this continuing influx of foreign medical
graduates. The answer is relatively simple: the foreign medical graduates are used
to fill those apparently less desirable training and work situations for which
American-trained physicians cannot be obtained. In general, these are concentrated
very heavily in house-staff training positions in city-county hospitals, staff positions
with state and local health departments, staff positions in nursing homes, and the
like. Although there is a general abundance of American-trained physicians (and a
prediction of an even greater abundance in the future as noted above), it is still
difficult for some hospitals and other health care institutions to obtain enough
American medical graduates to fill their needs, and so they turn to foreign medical
graduates instead.

In spite of this apparent demand for FMGs, there has been considerable
controversy about these physicians. Much of the controversy is related to the
quality of care provided by FMGs and it has been suggested that many are trained
in medical schools which are inferior to those in the United States, that they have
language and cultural barriers, and that they are not familiar with many of the
more advanced technologies utilized in this country. While there may be some
validity to these arguments, competition for entry to medical school is often more
rigorous abroad and in many instances any training deficiencies can be alleviated by
additional training in this country. Although studies have suggested some differences in the quality of care provided by FMGs as compared to U.S. graduates,
there is little conclusive evidence on the subject (21).

Quite aside from the incongruity of the most affluent country in the world
being forced to turn to other, less fortunate, countries to meet its needs for

physicians, this situation raises certain moral and ethical questions as well. By 1978, approximately 80,000 physicians in this country were graduates of medical schools in other countries. Large numbers of these physicians were originally educated in countries that could scarcely afford to lose such valuable national resources through emigration to the United States. In 1975, 10,410 of these physicians were from the Philippines, 8,559 were from India (which that year had a physician to population ratio of one physician per 4,820 people), 3,479 were from South Korea, 2,362 were from Iran, 1,015 from Pakistan, and 1,408 from Thailand (Table 9–13) (22).

The situation with regard to nurses and many other health personnel seems to be only slightly less serious than that for physicians, but the data is less readily available for analysis. In a number of large American cities, the public and voluntary hospitals depend heavily on foreign nursing graduates to staff their wards and it is not unusual to have one-third to one-half of a hospital's nursing staff from other countries.

The American health care system apparently cannot meet its needs with domestically trained personnel and has chosen to go outside the country for solutions rather than trying to find answers closer to home. At a time when the nation had the capacity of producing more and more physicians, certainly enough to meet our needs and considerably over that *if personnel were deployed in a more efficient and appropriate manner,* it seems inordinately wasteful and immoral to have needed to depend upon the scarce health resources of other countries. At the same time, high incomes and other factors have attracted many professionals to this country, expecially during those years when entry was relatively easy.

In recent years, the Congress of the United States has realized some of these

TABLE 9–13. Principal Sources of Foreign Medical Graduates in the United States, By Country of Graduation, 1975

Country	Total	Country	Total
Argentina	1,743	Ireland	1,068
Australia	430	Italy	3,584
Austria	1,576	Japan	903
Bangladesh	367	Mexico	2,556
China	655	Pakistan	1,015
Colombia	1,251	Philippines	10,410
Cuba	3,200	South Korea	3,479
Dominican Republic	795	Spain	2,357
Greece	1,007	Switzerland	2,516
Haiti	439	Taiwan	1,888
India	8,559	Thailand	1,408
Iran	2,362	Turkey	1,014
		United Arab Republic	1,198
		United Kingdom	2,811
		West Germany	3,365

Source: Center for Health Services Research and Development. *Medical School Alumni, 1973, Professional Characteristics of U.S. Physicians by Medical School and Year of Graduation.* American Medical Association, Chicago, 1975.

incongruities and has begun to take steps to reverse some of these trends. Public Law 94-484 declares that "there is no longer an insufficient number of physicians and surgeons in the United States such that there is no further need for affording preference to alien physicians and surgeons in admission to the United States under the Immigration and Nationality Act." The full implementation of this Congressional intent was delayed five years until 1978, and it is now being put into effect. Perhaps partially closing the door to an easy "outside" answer to some of our health personnel problems will force the American health care system to review more carefully how it utilizes "home-grown" graduates.

EDUCATIONAL PATHWAYS AND PROFESSIONAL SOCIALIZATION

While foreign medical graduates raise many questions, there has also been concern expressed about many aspects of the training of health personnel, and especially physicians and nurses, in the United States. These concerns include the nature and effects of the educational pathways to professional careers and the content of the training programs themselves.

Education for health professions assumes many forms and differs substantially between fields. In all instances, however, the potential professional follows a "pathway" leading from one educational level to another and eventually to practice in the community. For physicians, this pathway includes high school, college, medical school, residency, fellowship, and other specialized training programs. For nurses, pharmacists and many other professionals, the pathway includes high school and college level education and, in some instances, formal education in hospital-based training programs or in technical schools.

Concern has been expressed about the effect of the educational pathway from a number of perspectives. The often extensive preparation required and the highly competitive nature of entrance into many educational programs such as medicine and dentistry increases the difficulty of entry for some population groups. As a result, many minorities, for example, have been underrepresented in some of these professions. In medicine and other fields there have been attempts to bolster opportunities for these individuals by special programs which offer tutoring or other additional instruction to aid the student after entry into the professional school. Other programs have attempted to provide special instruction prior to admission. However, the severe competition and rapid pace of instruction in many of these schools, combined with inadequate prior education, sometimes places these students in a Catch-22 situation. Failure of society to adequately educate them in their earlier years results in difficulty in meeting the demands for performance in professional programs that strain even the best of students.

As a result of the difficulty of training large numbers of minorities today, and of the biases of many professional schools against accepting them in the past, blacks, chicanos, American Indians, and other groups in the population continue to be underrepresented in medical and many other professional schools and in the total pool of these specialized health personnel. These issues are discussed in further detail as they relate to the specific concerns of mental health professionals in Chapter 7 and remain a pressing problem which society must cope with.

In addition to discrimination against minorities, medical, dental, veterinary, and other health professions schools have also been adverse to accepting women in past years. Many had argued, for example, that women, due to child-rearing, were not professionally active during much of their career and, therefore, societal resources should be directed toward men. Recent evidence suggests that either these beliefs were never valid or that they no longer are applicable (23). As a result of these policies, women are underrepresented in many fields. Programs to increase the number of women in professional schools have been successful, but women still constitute a smaller proportion of enrollments than total national population and biases in some professions remain strong. And minority and low income women have had to face especially severe constraints. Women have, however, had greater access to some professions such as nursing, largely as the result of traditional roles in our society. Indeed, many women interested in medicine and other fields entered nursing because of the prevailing societal attitudes. These situations are changing now but many constraints remain, as discussed elsewhere in this chapter.

For all health professions and all pathways, there is a socialization process that occurs during training. Individuals are taught "how" to think, are instilled with certain perspectives and beliefs, and are exposed to various role models while they obtain their technical knowledge and skills. As a result of this process, there is a certain orientation or value system that frequently is instilled in new entrants into professions. Physicians gain clinical skills but also learn to view patients and other professionals in certain ways. Nurses identify certain roles and relationships that seem appropriate to their field. As each professional gains these beliefs and orientations, they also tend to become more focused on their own profession. The result is that each individual tends to think in terms of his/her own interests, background, and training rather than in terms of the larger health care system. Health teams have been developed to create environments in which people from different disciplines can work together but they have been only partially successful. One of the problems that has yet to be solved in the area of health personnel is increasing the cooperation between various professions and better integrating multidisciplinary skills, something that is quite related to the issue of professional mobility discussed elsewhere in this chapter and to the identification and perform-ance of appropriate professional roles.

NEW HEALTH PRACTITIONERS

Over the years, the perception that there was a shortage of health care providers, and especially physicians, has resulted in the development of programs to train new types of providers that could perform many of the functions of the more highly trained personnel. These training programs have been developed for nurse-practitioners, MEDEX, physician assistants and others in medicine as well as dental hygienists, dental assistants, and health personnel in a number of other fields. The training of these individuals differs substantially but generally involves one to two or more years of specialized education, often combined with field experience through a supervised preceptorship. In some programs, such as nurse-practitioner training, the specialized curriculum requires the previous completion of an undergraduate or equivalent degree in nursing or another field. In others, such as the MEDEX program, originally developed to retrain military corpsman returning from active duty for civilian employment, no specific educational degree is required. Each of these "new" fields has developed its own measures of achievement such as certification, licensure, and specialization (e.g., nurse-practitioner programs in adult medicine, pediatrics, or women's health care).

Overall, programs for training new types of practitioners, such as those discussed above, have been remarkably successful. Graduates have generally performed quite well and those trained have often filled gaps in health resources, especially in rural areas (24). The quality of care and the ability of these people to independently provide care to patients, as well as patient satisfaction with them, has exceeded expectations and suggests that there is an important role for such individuals in the provision of services. For the most part, these providers are concentrated in primary care areas and are adequately trained to deal with the routine needs of patients, provided that they have access to technical advice.

While these providers have successfully performed primary care and other health services roles, they have also raised a number of important issues. Indeed, the success of the training programs and of the patient care roles of these practitioners has been so great that they have prompted concerns that may not have been originally anticipated when the programs were initiated. Most of these concerns center around professional roles and role conflicts.

ROLE CONFLICTS IN HEALTH SERVICES

As new provider roles are developed, and especially as the number of health care providers expands beyond current needs, there is an increasing concern about the proper roles for each professional. For example, many physicians believe that nurse-practitioners should function only under the direct supervision of the physician while some nurse-practitioners believe that they can provide care relatively independently of the physician with backup consultation advice when needed. Many of the arguments related to professional roles result from a protectionist approach to professional "turf" with each professional field seeking to carve out a defined part of the health care practice for itself. The result is a conflict in roles which manifests itself in the political process and in the provider's office. Politically, each professional group seeks to encourage the enactment of legislation that defines its privileges and roles as broadly as possible. For example, nurses often lobby legislatures for the enactment of nurse practice acts that will broaden the scope of care that the nurse can provide (such as the prescription of certain drugs by nurse-practitioners or the independent office practice of nurses). Dental hygienists argue at times that they can perform certain functions adequately without being in the employ of dentists. These role conflicts will continue to broaden in scope and perhaps in magnitude as each of the newer professional categories expands its professionalization and seeks a larger role in the provision of services without as extensive subservience to other professionals as has occurred in the past. The outcome of these struggles will affect many other factors such as the extent of interprofessional mobility, as discussed elsewhere in this chapter.

The definition of professional roles which is now occurring also relates to some fundamental issues concerning the optimal allocation of resources in health care. These center around determining which types of services should be provided by which professionals and how patients can be matched with the level of service and practitioner they require, as discussed in Chapter 4. The increasing use of other types of providers requires that the health services system define the appropriate role of each individual, such as nurses (25), and develop effective mechanisms for allocating specific patient care tasks to each (26). As tasks are increasingly performed by providers who did not function in these roles in the past, it is necessary to alter the distribution of roles and relationships between more traditional providers and the new practitioners. For example, as nurse-practitioners, physician assistants, and others assume more of the burden of certain types of care, physicians will have to at least partially change their own roles and traditional ways of thinking about nurses and other co-workers (27). These changes might include concentrating on more severe cases while the nurse-practitioner or physician assistant provides routine, less complicated, care. Indeed, many physicians have complained that their work-day becomes especially difficult and grueling when this process occurs because they are left with only the difficult problems. In addition, there is an increased importance to the supervising and consulting roles when other providers are utilized. There are also strains from decreased control over practice patterns, and perhaps less identification with individual patients as physicians, dentists, or other professionals yield an increasing proportion of patient contact to other practitioners.

Although there is considerable discussion and an expanding literature on these topics, there is still little agreement on the optimal mix of providers and services. The substitution of different types and levels of practitioners for providing patient care has been addressed (28), but the ideal or optimal mixes have not been determined as discussed earlier for physicians. These optimal mixes will be heavily dependent on the types of patients in a practice, on the ability and willingness of all providers to work together, and on the acceptance by patients of these new roles. The new providers have demonstrated their abilities to provide high quality care and especially to address the caring function of health services.

Finally, professional role conflicts are also evident in other areas of health services. The Doctor of Osteopathy has traditionally strived to compete with the Doctor of Medicine for many of the same patients and care functions. Osteopathy traditionally is based on somewhat different tenets than allopathic medicine but now provides similar training, including specialty residency programs in many fields, as that received by the Doctor of Medicine. Osteopathy has also traditionally sought an extensive primary care role and has provided services in rural and other underserved areas. However, osteopathy often operates separate hospitals from allopathic medicine and there continues to be conflict between the two with far less interaction than might be desirable.

Many other areas of health services also evidence role conflicts and struggles for shares of the health services marketplace by different professionals. Examples include competition for vision care services by ophthalmologists, optometrists, and opticians; and expanded foot care services by podiatrists in competition with orthopedic surgeons and others.

THE CHANGING ROLE OF NURSES

As new types of practitioners have developed, the traditional role of the nurse has been increasingly subject to debate. The role of nursing has largely emerged out of the hospital's needs for individuals who could perform certain functions as discussed above and in Chapter 5.

The relationship of the nurse to the physician has especially been the target of discussion and controversy (29). The nurse has traditionally performed a circumscribed set of tasks at the direction of the physician while decisionmaking and responsibility ostensibly rested with the physician. In reality, the nurse assumed considerable responsibility for the ongoing care of patients and for clinical decisionmaking but without the reimbursement and prestige of the physician. In particular, much of the caring function of medicine and the "routine" tasks for actually providing care were the province of the nurse.

As new health practitioners have developed and as a general awakening has occurred among all health personnel, nurses have increasingly questioned their roles and responsibilities in health care. This is in part related to their relationships with physicians, but is also part of a broader reassessment of the function of the nurse in health care and the constraints of the system (such as those related to scheduling flexibility and professional mobility as discussed previously). This includes the appropriateness of various training programs (e.g., diploma versus degree programs) and the distribution of responsibilities between different types of nurses (e.g., R.N.s and L.P.N.s). The strengths of nursing education are needed in health care, especially as they relate to the caring function and to the assurance of adequate care on a day-to-day basis for both institutionalized and ambulatory patients. The degree to which nurses can assume an expanded patient care role has yet to be determined and will be based on the outcome of a variety of political and clinical developments. The relationship between registered nurses and those with more advanced training such as nurse-practitioners, also remains to be determined. Finally, the role of nurses is inextricably interrelated to many of the other issues and trends discussed throughout this book such as insurance coverage for care provided by a wide range of professionals, the implications of technological change for professional roles, licensure and regulation of the performance of personnel, and the range of health services needed by society.

OPTIMIZING HEALTH CARE PERSONNEL RESOURCES

IS THERE SUCH A THING AS A "POOL" OF HEALTH CARE PERSONNEL?

At the beginning of this chapter it was mentioned that the health care "industry" employs approximately 5,000,000 people at the present time, probably more than any other industry in the country. At the same time, the impression might well have been left that these 5,000,000 people form some sort of "pool" of health care personnel, with the unstated assumption that it is possible to move within the "pool" from one area of professional work to another. It is important to correct that possible mistaken assumption and to point out that there really is no "pool" of health care personnel. Instead there is a series of very separate and very isolated ponds and puddles, with relatively limited movement between them.

For example, although there is significant commonality among the basic science backgrounds for many of the health care professions, if a person were to leave one profession and attempt to enter into another, very little credit would be given for prior training or experience. The new candidate would have to start at the beginning of training just as any neophyte entering health care work for the first time.

Not only is movement from one professional group to another difficult, movement upward *within* a particular group is equally difficult. Simply because a person is employed as a dental hygienist or a dental assistant does not mean that this individual has an inside track on becoming a dentist. Just because a person becomes a physician's assistant does not necessarily mean that the path to medical school is any easier. Thus, what may first appear as a large "pool" of 5,000,000 health care personnel ready to flow back and forth between needed professional areas is really a series of separate and isolated pockets of personnel, each with its own carefully delineated boundaries and protective entry requirements.

Why is this so? Why is there little movement between the different health personnel groupings and within the groupings, from lower ranks to higher ones? What are the barriers that hinder movement of health care personnel and continue to isolate one professional group from all others?

There are a number of reasons for this restricted movement among the health professions, probably the foremost of which is the desire of the individual professional groups themselves to preserve the integrity of their professional "turfs." Many professional groups have worked hard over the years to upgrade the competence of their members and the prestige of their particular professions and view any attempt to "open up" their profession as an infringement on their "rights" and as a potential dilution of what they have worked so hard to attain. Protectionism toward the quality and integrity of a professional group often is expressed through rigid training requirements and necessary successful completion of certification examinations and tests. While the general intent of the improved movement of personnel between professional areas may be a general social good, the more specific individual good of a protected professional enclave becomes more important.

Much of the professional desire to develop high standards is further re-enforced by various licensing laws instituted by state governments in an attempt to protect the public from unqualified professionals. Since most of the licensing efforts are controlled, either directly or indirectly, by the health professions being licensed, they usually represent further extension of the profession's own certification or approval processes. This is discussed further in Chapter 12.

Another force which has inadvertently helped to limit movement between professional groups, or at least any experimentation in the development of new professional roles and relationships, has been the threat of malpractice. Many professional groups might well be interested in testing new methods of training or practice which involve easier movement from one professional area to another or broader professional roles, but they hesitate for fear of possible legal action if something untoward happens to a patient. The specter of being forced to appear in front of a plaintiff's attorney and be asked, "Did this professional have the usual and customary training for your profession before beginning a professional career?" is frequently enough to discourage any attempt at improved professional mobility.

Restrictions on health insurance reimbursement under which only specific health professionals may receive payment (i.e. physicians and not nurses) has tended to discourage experimentation with new roles and settings for providing care. Although this barrier is being lowered in some instances, it is still customary for insurance programs to reimburse for a particular service when provided by one type of health professional but not reimburse for exactly the same service delivered in exactly the same fashion by another professional.

Finally, underlying all of these barriers is the public's desire for the "best" care. In practice, this means the public would like to have services provided by the most highly trained, most highly qualified, and usually most highly certified health professionals available. The mere suggestion that a particular task could be done by someone with lesser qualifications, lesser training, or different certifications very frequently is met with suspicion if not outright hostility on the part of the public. The result is frequently a reluctance to initiate new programs of training or education which might be seen by the public as lessening the quality or ability of the major professional group.

This country is wasting a tremendous amount of potential skill and intelligence by limiting flexibility in the personnel pool and movement between the health professions. While there may have been good reasons in the past for developing the highly compartmentalized and rigid structure that now exists, it is clearly in the public interest to develop personnel policies and strategies that allow greater individual opportunity for advancement and for developing and applying expanded capabilities into new professional roles. This might save money and training time and, more important, would enable the country to take complete advantage of the skills and experience of the health personnel "pool." Finally, such a strategy would allow for personal career enhancement, increased job satisfaction, and more flexibility in utilizing people's talents beyond today's narrowly defined and often arbitrary professional roles.

PRODUCTIVITY

Improving movement between professional fields to achieve increased flexible and more effective use of skills is one aspect of increasing productivity. Productivity is a complex concept but relates fundamentally to the efficient and effective use of resources. Thus, providing organizational settings which facilitate the effective use of people's time, such as well-designed operating rooms, can promote productivity. So too can appropriately trained support personnel, high quality equipment, and efficient scheduling of patient and provider time. Examples of the effects of increased productivity for dentists and pharmacists were discussed earlier in this chapter. Increasing the extent to which existing people are utilized to the fullest extent of their abilities through whatever mechanisms possible can increase their productivity, reduce health care costs, increase access to care, and promote satisfaction with employment by health professionals.

NEEDS FOR HEALTH PERSONNEL

Determining the optimal number of each type of health care provider that the country needs is not easy as noted earlier. A variety of attempts have been directed toward this effort (30, 31, 32, 33, 34), yet not all are fully satisfying. This difficulty is in large measure attributable to the many uncertainties in medicine including technological developments, changing roles, evolving institutional settings, changes in productivity, and so forth. One of the major challenges facing health services is how to optimize the pool of human resources so important to providing care. An important related question is who will make these decisions.

WHO SHOULD CONTROL THE HEALTH PROFESSIONS: THE PROFESSIONALS OR THE PUBLIC?

A key question to be asked about health care personnel is, "Who should control the health professions: the professionals or the public?" It is, unfortunately, a question that our society has not asked itself until rather recently and even now is uneasy about posing.

At the present time, the individual professions control their own standards and methods of entry into the various fields, control (or influence very heavily) the certification and licensing processes, and set the standards and guidelines for the actual conduct of the professions. The numbers of professionals produced by the nation's training programs are very heavily influenced by the professions themselves, and the way in which the professionals are eventually distributed throughout the country and throughout the various specialties within the professions are largely a matter of individual choice.

In recent times, it has become apparent that there are some inherent problems in leaving such important matters solely in the hands of the professions themselves. There are certain interests of the public that simply are not well served by a series of individual, random decisions that are not subject to any review by society. This is examplified by the long-standing problem of obtaining enough physicians and other health professions in the rural areas of the country. Another frequently discussed example has been the inadequate number of primary care and family practice physicians and the overabundance of surgeons. It has been pointed out that movement between the various professions is difficult and is often actively discouraged by the individual professions themselves. There seems to be little that the nation can do to change these situations since the decisions that created the problems were made by the professions and not the public.

And yet, it is now becoming increasingly apparent that the public not only gives the professions their social license and mandate to exist but also provides the greater proportion of the financing to make their existence possible. During 1974, for example, the federal government alone spent $1,600,000,000 in training funds and assistance for construction of educational institutions (35). In 1972–73, the medical schools of this country received $964,362,000 in federal funds for one purpose or another, which was 44.8% of their total income. Public medical schools received an additional $316,410,000 in state government funds which accounted for another 32.3% of their income (36). In 1972–73, there were $70,480,103 in loans made to medical students to help finance their education, of which $30,-470,861 (43.2%) were from federal funds (36). With regards to the post-graduate training of physicians in 1973–74, fully 62% of all internships and residencies were taken in governmental hospitals, 50% of them in city, county, or state hospitals and 12% in federal hospitals, primarily those operated by the Veterans Administration. Indeed, it can be estimated that approximately three-fourths of all medical education and post-graduate training of physicians is directly supported by tax-generated funds of one kind or another. Without this support, it would be virtually impossible for new physicians to be added to the ranks of those already in practice.

This is not to suggest that physicians are the only health professionals to benefit from public support of education and training activities. As shown in Tables 9–14 and 9–15, virtually all health professions have received support from tax-generated funds and virtually all depend heavily on these funds for their continued existence and once in practice, most health personnel receive all or part of their incomes either directly or indirectly from governmental sources.

Thus, society creates the environment that allows health professionals to work. It gives them license and social approval, it finances their education and training, and it pays for their services once training is finished. At the same time, it is clear that the public is dependent upon these health professionals to make the health care system work. Without the individual health professionals (and particularly without a few key ones such as physicians and nurses), it would be impossible to operate a health care system.

TABLE 9–14. Federal Outlays for Training and Related Construction by Type of Training, United States, 1974

Purpose of Funding	Amount (Thousands of Dollars)
Total	$1,596,561
Training	1,385,397
Research personnel	184,867
Physicians	407,172
Dentists	81,720
Nurses	127,243
Other health professionals	291,268
Non-degree training	293,127
Construction	211,164

Source: Russell L, Bourque BB, Bourque DP: *Federal Health Spending, 1969–74.* Washington, D.C., National Planning Association, 1974.

TABLE 9–15. Students and Trainees Receiving Federal Educational or Training Support, United States, 1974

Personnel Category	Support Received
Research personnel	20,956
Pre-doctoral training grants	9,608
Post-doctoral training grants	5,618
Research fellowships	2,420
Research career awards	1,158
General research support programs	2,252
Medicine and osteopathy	22,595
Medical students receiving loans	12,196
Medical students receiving scholarships	8,431
Osteopathy students receiving loans	1,120
Osteopathy students receiving scholarships	848
Dentists	9,855
Dental students receiving loans	5,967
Dental students receiving scholarships	3,888
Nurses	49,500
Nursing students receiving loans	30,000
Nursing students receiving scholarships	19,500
Optometry	1,926
Optometry students receiving loans	1,171
Optometry students receiving scholarships	755
Pharmacy	9,515
Pharmacy students receiving loans	4,500
Pharmacy students receiving scholarships	5,015
Podiatry	773
Podiatry students receiving loans	497
Podiatry students receiving scholarships	276
Veterinary	2,701
Veterinary students receiving loans	1,549
Veterinary students receiving scholarships	1,152

Source: Russell L, Bourque BB, Bourque DP: *Federal Health Spending, 1969–74.* Washington, D.C., National Planning Association, 1974.

The health professionals and the public, therefore, are in a uniquely important relationship with one another, and yet the guidelines and the rules for that relationship have never been made explicit. The time seems to be at hand when the terms of their relationship need to be reviewed with clearer and stronger social controls to ensure that the interests of the public are well-served. Any resulting decisions must be made within the context of overall national health policy and in recognition of the complex and changing nature of health services.

REFERENCES

1. Manpower Analysis Branch: *A Report to the President and Congress on the Status of Health Professions Personnel in the United States,* Bureau of Health Manpower, United States Department of Health, Education, and Welfare, DHEW Publication No. (HRA) 78–93, August 1978.

2. National Center for Health Statistics: *Health Resources Statistics: 1975.* United States Department of Health, Education, and Welfare, DHEW Publication No. (HRA) 76-1509, 1976.

3. U.S. Bureau of Labor Statistics: Employment and Earnings, in *Statistical Abstract of the United States,* Washington, D.C., Government Printing Office, 1974.

4. U.S. Bureau of the Census: Detailed Characteristics, United States Summary 1974, in *Health, United States, 1975.* National Center for Health Statistics, Department of Health, Education, and Welfare, DHEW Publication No. (HRA) 76-1232, 1976.

5. McVey W: Shortage of doctors in rural communities. *Journal of the Kansas Medical Society* 29:312–314, 1928.

6. Lewis D: The place of the clinic in medical practice, President's address. *Journal of the American Medical Association* 100:1905–1910,1933.

7. Medical Education in the United States, Special Edition, *Journal of the American Medical Association* No. 26, **240**: 2803-2928, December 22-29, 1978.

8. Lave JR, Lave LB, Leinhardt S: *Medical Manpower Models: Need, Demand, and Supply.* Rand Corporation Report R-1481-CHD, Santa Monica, California, Rand Corporation, March 1974.

9. *Report of the Governor's Special Committee on Health Costs.* Sacramento, California, State of California, January 1975.

10. Reinhart U: *Physician Productivity and the Demand for Health Manpower.* Cambridge, Massachusetts, Ballinger Publishing Company, 1975.

11. Goodman, LJ: *Physician Distribution and Medical Licensure in the U.S., 1976.* Chicago, Illinois, American Medical Association, 1977.

12. Bureau of Health Manpower, Department of Health, Education, and Welfare: Supply and Distribution of Physicians and Physician Extenders. In *A Report to the President and Congress on the Status of Health Professions Personnel in the United States, op. cit.*

13. Institute of Medicine: *A Manpower Policy for Primary Health Care. Report of a study.* Washington, D.C., National Academy of Sciences, May 1978.

14. Health Resources Administration, Bureau of Health Manpower, Division of Dentistry, based on data from the American Dental Association, Bureau of Economic Research and Statistics. In *A Report to the President and Congress on the Status of Health Professions Personnel in the United States, op. cit.*

15. National Association of Boards of Pharmacy: 1973 Proceedings of the National Association of Boards of Pharmacy. Licensure Statistics and Census of Pharmacy. In *Health Resources Statistics: 1975, op. cit.*

16. *The Nation's Nurses: 1972 Inventory of Registered Nurses.* Publication No. D-43, Kansas City, Missouri, American Nurses Association, 1974.
17. Interagency Conference on Nursing Statistics. In *Health Resources Statistics: 1975, op. cit.*
18. U.S. Public Health Service, Division of Nursing. In *Health, United States, 1975, op. cit.*
19. *Facts About Nursing, 1972–73.* Kansas City, Missouri, American Nurses Association, 1973.
20. White C, Mahan P: A Study of Recruitment of Registered Nurses by California Hospitals and Nursing Homes. Mimeo, California Hospital Association, June 1978.
21. Williams K., Brook R: Foreign medical graduates and their effects on the quality of medical care in the United States. The Rand Corporation, Santa Monica, California, Report Number R-1698-HEW, January 1976.
22. AMA Center for Health Services Research and Development: *Medical School Alumni, 1973, Professional Characteristics of U.S. Physicians by Medical School and Year of Graduation.* Chicago, American Medical Association, 1975.
23. Heins M, Smock S, Martindale L et al: Comparison of the productivity of women and men physicians. *Journal of the American Medical Association* 237:2514–2517, 1977.
24. Lawrence D, Wilson W, Castle CH: Employment of MEDEX graduates and trainees. *Journal of the American Medical Association* 234:174–177, 1975.
25. Starfield B, Sharp E: Ambulatory pediatric care: the role of the nurse. *Medical Care* 6:507–515, 1968.
26. Kehrer B, Intriligator M: Task delegation in physician office practice. *Inquiry* 11:292–299, 1974.
27. Steinwachs D, Shapiro S, Yaffe R et al: The role of new health practitioners in a prepaid group practice: changes in the distribution of ambulatory care between physician and nonphysician providers of care. *Medical Care* 14:95–120, 1976.
28. Reinhardt U: Manpower substitution and productivity in medical practice: review of research. *Health Services Research* 8:200–227, 1973.
29. Bates B: Doctor and nurse: changing roles and relations. *New England Journal of Medicine* 283:129–134, 1970.
30. Fahs I, Choi T, Barchas K et al: Indicators of need for health care personnel: the concept of need, alternative measures employed to determine need, and a suggested model. *Medical Care* 9:144–151, 1971.
31. Schonfeld H, Heston J, Falk I: Numbers of physicians required for primary medical care. *New England Journal of Medicine* 286:571–576, 1972.
32. Scitovsky A, McCall N: A method of estimating physician requirements. *Milbank Memorial Fund Quarterly* 54:299–320, 1976.
33. Lave JR, Lave LB, Leinhardt S: Medical manpower models: need, demand and supply. *Inquiry* 12:97–125, 1975.
34. Kriesberg H, Wu J, Hollander E et al: Methodological approaches for determining health manpower supply and requirements. Volume 1, Analytical perspective. Rockville, Maryland, National Health Planning Information Center, U.S. Department of Health, Education, and Welfare, DHEW Publication No. (HRA) 76-14511, 1976.
35. Russell L, Bourque BB, Bourque DP: *Federal Health Spending, 1969-74.* Washington, D.C., National Planning Association, 1974.
36. Medical Education in the United States, 1974-1975, *JAMA* 75th Annual Report, *Journal of the American Medical Association,* Vol. 234, Supplement, December 1975.

CHAPTER 10

Financing Health Services

William C. Richardson

Financing of health services cannot be considered independently from the various other dimensions of the "system" that are presented in this book. For example, human resource development, medical care technology, health services utilization, and institutional arrangements all are affected by, and in turn affect, the economic aspects of the system. The purpose of this chapter is to describe and analyze health services financing from four perspectives: health service expenditures and trends in health care costs, financial arrangements and economic relationships in the health care market, organizations or institutions financing health services, and major financial issues and alternatives for the future.

HEALTH CARE EXPENDITURES

DISTRIBUTION AND SOURCES

The United States spent $863 per person for all health services during the year that ended September 30, 1977 (1). This total national expenditure of $192,000,-000,000 included money spent for hospital care, physicians' services, dentists' services, drugs, nursing home care, other personal health care, construction of hospital facilities, government funded research, and the cost of administering health insurance plans. By far the largest category of expenditure was for hospital care, which accounted for slightly under 40% of all health expenditures (Table 10–1). About four out of every five dollars spent for these services go to community hospitals. Community hospital expenditures are divided between inpatient services and outpatient services in a ratio of approximately nine to one.

287

TABLE 10–1. National Health Expenditures by Type of Care, United States, Fiscal Year 1977

Type of Care	Percentage
Hospital care	39.5
Physicians' services	18.3
Dentists' services	6.9
Drugs and drug sundries	7.9
Nursing home care	8.2
Other personal health care	6.5
Other health spending	12.7
Total	100.0

Source: Gibson RM: National health expenitures, 1978. *Health Care Financing Review* (Summer, 1979), p. 24.

The second largest category of expenditures is for physicians' services. Just under one-fifth (18.3%) of the dollars spent went to physicians. The professional services of dentists (6.9%), drugs (7.9%), nursing home care (8.2%), and other personal health care (6.5%) were of approximately equal magnitude. Somewhat over one-half of the drug expenditures are accounted for by prescription drugs. Only 2.6% of total expenditures were devoted to traditional public health activities. This proportion declined from a level of 3.1% in 1975, primarily as a result of more rapid increases in non-public-health expenditures.

The expenditure of $192,000,000,000 (9.1% of the Gross National Product), or $863 per person, is substantial by any standard. The distribution of expenditures across sources of financing, however, reflects the diffusion of these expenditures in such a manner as to lessen their visibility in the society and usually their obvious impact on individual families. Approximately 88% of total national health expenditures are accounted for by the cost of personal health care. And only 30% of personal health care costs were paid for directly by individuals or families in 1977. An additional 9%, representing various insurance premium payments paid for directly by individuals or families, results in a total of 39% of personal health care costs that were "out-of-pocket" expenses paid directly by consumers.

So as not to double count, consider only the 30% in direct payments to providers. Of the other 70% of payments for personal health care in 1977, 28% was financed through the federal government, 12% by state and local governments, 2% by charity and private industry, and the remaining 28% of personal health care expenditures was paid as a result of private health insurance benefits.

The dispersion of sources of health care financing is particularly pertinent in light of the uneven distribution of health care costs across the population. For example, in 1974 slightly over 1% of the population accounted for approximately 20% of national health care expenditures, or an average of $8,600 per capita (2).

Because of the high proportion of expense paid through governmental programs and voluntary health insurance, generally referred to as third parties, patient care decision-making in any particular illness is more likely to be influenced by the existence or availability of sophisticated medical resources than by the costs entailed. On the other hand, as discussed further later in this chapter the societal implications of both the uneven distribution of catastrophic illness expenses and their magnitude are very consequential.

Recent advances in medical technology (Chapter 8), including expensive equipment and large numbers of highly trained personnel, while important, account for only one-half of the expenditures of the so-called catastrophic population. The other half represent the 1,200,000 catastrophically ill individuals who are patients in long-term care institutions. As Birbaum points out, "[these] are persons for whose conditions there are no technological remedies yet who are no longer able to care for themselves. Thus, the levels of technology and know-how polarize catastrophic expenses. To a significant extent, catastrophic illness is a result of an absence of technology" (3).

TRENDS IN HEALTH CARE EXPENDITURES

Between 1950 and 1978 per capita health care expenditures in the United States have increased ten-fold. As presented in Table 10–2, the nation was devoting twice as large a proportion of the Gross National Product to health services in 1978 as in 1950 (9.1% versus 4.6%). During that same period, there was a dramatic shift in the sources of funds from the private sector to the public sector. For example, in 1950, and continuing until 1966, between 25 and 26% of national health expenditures were financed through governmental agencies. With the enactment of Titles XVIII and XIX of the Social Security Act (Medicare and Medicaid), the government share began to increase. This increase was dramatic in 1967 and 1968, and has been more gradual since those years. Estimates for 1975 through 1977 indicate a fairly stable proportion of expenditures financed through government ranging between 42 and 43% of the total.

TABLE 10–2. National Health Expenitures as Percent of GNP, United States, Selected Fiscal Years 1950–1977

Fiscal Year	Percent of Gross National Product
1950	4.6
1960	5.2
1965	5.9
1970	7.2
1975	8.5
1977	8.8

Source: Gibson RM: National health expenditures, 1978. *Health Care Financing Review* (Summer, 1979), p.3.

It is obvious from the increasing proportion of the Gross National Product (GNP) accounted for by health care expenditures that the rate of growth in this industry has been substantially higher than for the economy as a whole. The increases in total expenditures can be attributed to three principal factors: growth in the population, changes in the quantity and nature of the services consumed, and price inflation. With respect to the second factor, for example, and as noted in Chapter 3, there have been increases in the rate of hospital admissions per 1,000 population and in the number of doctor visits per person. There have also been increases in the numbers of tests and procedures performed, and, more generally, an increased intensity of medical care technology used in treating various conditions.

Table 10–3 presents the distribution of increases in expenditures attributable to these three factors for the periods 1950–1965, 1965–1971, 1971–1974, and 1974–1976 (4). The total increase over the 26-year period was $110,000,000,000, starting from a base national expenditure for personal health services of $23,-100,000,000 in 1950. The population growth factor has always been the smallest component of expenditure increases for health services. Further, over the years it has declined, accounting for one-fifth of the rise in total expenditures in 1950 compared to one-twentieth of the increase in expenditures in 1977.

From 1950 through the 1970s, an even more important factor in expenditure increases has been the change in the nature of the services provided. By the early 1970s, this element accounted for at least half of each year's increase. Furthermore, this factor may be understated relative to price increases due to the way in which consumer prices are measured.

An important aspect of changes in the type or intensity of services is that changes in technology, on balance, tend to be cost-raising rather than cost-saving. Such an assertion says nothing about the cost-effectiveness of new technology since the end result may reflect benefits that outweigh the increased cost, benefits that are less than the increased cost, or, indeed, no benefits at all.

A recent study by Scitovsky and McCall (5) of the treatment for several common conditions and the changes in services and associated costs over a 20-year period illustrates the impact in the intensity factor. For example, there has been a steady increase in the average number of diagnostic laboratory tests per case over the 20-year period. Similar results are evident for other procedures such as x-ray and

TABLE 10–3 Factors Contributing to the Increase in Personal Health Expenditures, Selected Periods, Fiscal Years 1950–1976

	Percent Distribution for Fiscal Years				
Factor	*1950–65*	*1965–71*	*1971–74*	*1974–76*	*(1950–76)*
Price	43.8	49.9	43.1	78.3	(54.6)
Population	21.0	8.9	7.9	5.8	(10.5)
Quantity and Quality increase	35.2	41.2	49.0	15.9	(34.9)
Total	100.0	100.0	100.0	100.0	(100.0)

Source: Gibson R, Mueller M: National Health Expenditures, Fiscal Year 1976. *Social Security Bulletin*, 40(4):13-22, 1977.

electrocardiogram (EKG). On the other hand, hospital lengths-of-stay declined quite consistently over the 20-year period, offsetting in some cases the increases in intensity. On balance, however, the changes in medical practice tended to be cost-raising rather than cost-saving. It is also not evident that there is a relationship between the decline in hospital lengths-of-stay and the increase in diagnostic and therapeutic procedures used. Thus, the latter may continue on into the future after the former has reached some apparently irreducible minimum.

Price increases, *per se*, have accounted for substantial increases in personal health expenditures in recent years. This is in part due to increased demand fostered by rising incomes and the greater prevalence of health insurance benefits, but also reflects a catchup phenomenon after the removal of controls under the Economic Stabilization Program of the early 1970s and subsequent higher rates of general inflation in the United States economy. Again, as is evident from the increasing proportion of the GNP accounted for by personal health care expenditures, resources devoted to this sector of the economy have outpaced most other items. Price increases are currently the dominant factor in rising expenditures and, as is evident from Table 10–4, have been outpacing price increases for other major necessities of life with the exception of fuel (6).

From the distribution of national health expenditures by type of service over time, it is evident that hospital care, including outpatient hospital services, has been accounting for an increasing share. For example, in 1929 hospital care was responsible for 18% of total expenditures, a figure which had increased to 31% by 1950, 33% by 1960, 37% by 1970, and stood at 39.5% for the year ending September 1977. On the other hand, the proportion of expenditures accounted for by physicians' services has been quite stable since 1950, declining slightly from 22.4% in that year to 18.3% in 1978. Most other categories of personal health care expenditures have declined as a proportion of the total, with drugs, eyeglasses, and appliances all accounting for substantially less. The other major category, in addition to hospital care, that has accounted for an increasing proportion of total expenditures is nursing home care. Nursing home costs, which are discussed in

TABLE 10–4. Consumer Price Increases, United States, Selected Years

Consumer Price Index (CPI) Item	Percentage Increase for Year		
	1975	1976	1977
CPI, all items	9.1	5.7	6.5
Medical care services	12.6	10.0	9.9
Housing	10.8	6.2	7.0
Fuel, oil and coal	9.6	6.6	13.0
Transportation	9.4	9.9	7.1
Apparel and upkeep	4.5	3.7	4.5

Source: Gibson RM, Fisher CR: National health expenditures, fiscal year 1977. *Social Security Bulletin* 41(7):3–20, 1978, p. 10.

detail in Chapter 6, have increased from less than one percent of national health expenditures in 1940 to 8.2% of all expenditures in 1978.

As was noted earlier, health care expenses fall unevenly on the population. As would be expected from the discussion of factors affecting utilization in Chapter 3, age is a major determinant of hospital, nursing home, physician, and other health care expenses. If age 65 is considered as the lower bound for the elderly segment of the population, per capita expenditures for the elderly in 1976 ($1,522) were three times higher than the per capita figure for younger persons. Further, the rate of increase in per capita expenditures for the elderly since the passage of Medicare has been greater than the rate of increase for the remainder of the population by approximately two percentage points (7). Somers points out that the cost experience of federal Medicare and Medicaid health financing programs has been so conspicuously unfavorable, with recent annual increases over 15%, as to be having a major impact on other federal programs. She cited Medicare and Medicaid, for example, as being major factors in "the continued postponement of national health insurance for the entire population, [as well as] preventing the extension of benefits to desperately needed long-term care services for the elderly . . . " (8).

The factors responsible for increases in health care expenditures for the elderly are somewhat different than for the remainder of the population. For example, population increases in this age category are far more substantial. In addition, women, who are heavier users of health services than men, are increasing as a proportion of the elderly population. Family social support seems also to be declining with the result that society can expect "a growing proportion of elderly persons who will be living without the traditional support of either a legal spouse or children" (9). Finally, Somers notes that the use and type of health services, as a component accounting for the increase in expenditures, is also different from the rest of the population. Even with the implementation of Medicare in the mid-1960s, there was no increase in the average number of physician visits per day by the elderly during the following decade, nor was there an increase in the number of days of hospital care per 1,000 older persons. Increases in admission rates were more than offset by a decline in lengths-of-stay. On the other hand, the services provided within these broader categories of utilization have changed. For example, surgery rates for the elderly more than doubled over the decade after the implementation of Medicare and there has been greater use of more complex, and therefore, more expensive, medical procedures and other services.

FINANCIAL ARRANGEMENTS AND ECONOMIC RELATIONSHIPS

The health care market has long been recognized as a "special case" in terms of financial arrangements, economic relationships, and the formulation of public policy. This is not to say that the familiar concepts of economics such as supply and demand, production functions, and so forth are not applicable or useful in analyzing health care financing. Rather, it is an indication that the health care market is a complex one, involving as it does third-party financing (governmental programs and voluntary underwriting), employers who pay a majority of the premiums for their employees, physicians who both provide care and act as the patient's agent in obtaining care, not-for-profit hospitals, assorted regulatory agencies, and so forth. Thus, no simple model will help to explain or predict behavior of the various participants, nor are there any simple solutions to the various problems found in the health care market.

PATIENT-PHYSICIAN RELATIONSHIPS

This section considers financial and other relationships between patients and non-institutional providers. The physician is used as the example throughout the section since the physician is the most prevalent and traditional provider relating to the patient. However, numerous other providers including, for example, dentists and optometrists, have similar relationships with patients and the discussion applies to them also.

The patient generally initiates the medical care process seeking to find out what is causing a physical or mental discomfort and what should be done about it, or less often simply seeking reassurance or possibly an examination in the absence of symptoms (a general checkup). It is important to recognize that faced with this initial contact, the physician has tremendous discretion in responding, and tremendous control over the subsequent medical care process. Patients cannot order tests, prescribe drugs, or admit themselves to the hospital. The physician on the other hand, while having substantial discretion within the bounds of professionally acceptable practice, may be limited by knowledge and availability of various services, local practice patterns, specialty orientation, and the professional referral network, including the hospital's medical staff organization (Chapter 5).

Financing is critical in determining the types of services available, the relative emphasis given to primary, secondary, and tertiary patient care, and the combinations of resources the physician uses to achieve various diagnostic or patient management objectives. The physician's role can be considered as consisting of three elements: entrepreneurial, technical, and professional. The entrepreneurial element includes choice of specialty, practice setting, and services to be provided directly by the practice. The technical element includes the physician's personal laying on of hands, and the professional element includes the critical role of acting as the patient's agent. These elements occur to varying degrees, depending on practice setting and the associated economic incentives. For the most part, however, the entrepreneurial element has been a major one, and the range of professionally acceptable options available to independent, fee-for-service physicians acting as the patient's agent have been substantial.

Before the advent of third-party insurance coverage for physicians' services, both the patient and the patient's agent, the physician, were necessarily concerned with the patient's ability and willingness to pay for various options. An analagous situation still exists today for the most part in dentistry where patients have the choice of more or less expensive types of restoration.

Indeed, the practice of medicine in the days when the patient paid the bill was not unlike dentistry today in the sense that the general practitioner was responsible for delivering most of the services within the context of the practice setting. Medicine has changed, however, so that a great deal of the care that is rendered, and particularly expensive care, is likely to be provided by a referral specialist or within an inpatient setting. In the entrepreneurial role, the physician has decided what services will be available within the practice, what patterns of referral will be established, and what other resources will be available (such as particular hospitals). The physician's technical role may be limited to a specialty or sub-specialty. Factors associated with both the entrepreneurial and technical roles will impinge upon the decisions made within the context of the professional role where the physician serves as the patient's agent.

In combining resources to serve the needs of any particular patient, the physician may draw on the practice for providing ancillary services such as diagnostic tests, may refer to another physician, typically a specialist, or may hospitalize the patient. In understanding the financing of health services and the economic relationships that exist, it is not sufficient to consider only whether or not the patient has third-party coverage for these various options, although this is important. In addition, the costs to the physician, in the entrepreneurial sense, of various choices, must be considered. A physician with a busy practice could only manage a limited number of very sick but potentially ambulatory patients if such management required instructing the family on how to care for the patient, being available for repeated consultation with the family when certain changes in the medical condition occurred, and arranging for the use of other professional services on an ambulatory basis. If, instead, the physician hospitalizes the patient all of these costly functions are carried out by appropriately trained professionals within the institutional setting. The physician need only be available for daily rounds and occasional consultation, and has only to order procedures and consultations available within the hospital through a note in the medical record. The point of this discussion is that the physician can handle a larger and more complex patient load through increased use of the hospital. Thus there are both professional and economic incentives to hospitalize; these incentives are especially strong since the physician does not have to pay for this service out of practice income either directly or indirectly because of the subsidization of hospitalization by third parties. This discussion assumes financing under a fee-for-service system, as well as independent office practice. There are a number of mechanisms for reimbursing the physician, some of which introduce other types of incentives.

PHYSICIAN REIMBURSEMENT

There are three principal mechanisms for paying for physicians' services. The first, which is the predominant method, is fee-for-service. Under this system the physician is reimbursed for each procedure or service. Services can be "small" and discreet, such as a follow-up office visit, a laboratory test, or the reading of an EKG; or they can be substantial and inclusive such as the comprehensive fee for normal delivery or for a major surgical procedure which would include prenatal or pre-operative care, the procedure itself, and some follow-up care. Relative value scales have been developed to reflect the relationship between procedures in terms of time and skill required to provide services.

One problem with fee-for-service is the definition of a particular service and what is included in it. The more general issue, however, is the incentive inherent in the fee-for-service approach. The physician's income depends upon the volume of services provided and the price of those services. Obviously, more services result in a higher income, as would the provision of more complex and therefore expensive services. In particular, technical procedures tend to be weighted more heavily, given the amount of time it takes to perform them, than physician time when the physician is providing patient counseling, consulting, or a history and physical examination, as noted in Chapter 8.

A second mechanism for reimbursing physicians is capitation. Capitation involves paying the physician a fixed amount per person per unit of time without regard to the volume of services provided. Thus, a physician may agree to take responsibility for a group of patients, called a panel, for a month or a year, and would agree to provide to those patients whatever was necessary within a previously agreed range of services (for example, primary care). The capitation method assumes that the physician is qualified to provide the agreed upon services and will be available to do so. Since the physician's income is determined by the number of individuals in the panel, rather than the number of services provided, there is an incentive to maximize the number of patients in the panel and to minimize the number of services provided to each patient. This method assumes an organization serving as a third party (the National Health Service in England and Wales, for example). The third party can limit panel size, and use various mechanisms to monitor the volume and mix of services being rendered. In addition, under such a system the patient would typically have a choice of physicians, and the opportunity to switch should there be concern about under-provision of care or any other unattractive facet of the doctor's practice.

The third method for reimbursement of physicians is salary, or payment per unit of time. As in other sectors of the economy, one observes salary used only in organized settings where various other mechanisms are employed to assess or encourage the type of care given and the level of productivity.

Each of the three methods has been described in terms of compensation for the individual practitioner. Fee-for-service and capitation reimbursement can also be used for groups of physicians. For example, under the capitation method, a multi-specialty group with broad responsibility for virtually all types of patient care can be paid on the basis of the number of persons enrolled with the group. The implicit incentives that apply to the individual practitioner can also be attributed to the group. However, payment of individual physicians by the group might be arranged on a salary or some other basis. Various related aspects of group practice are discussed further in Chapter 4.

HOSPITAL REIMBURSEMENT MECHANISMS

Next consider hospitals and their relationships to both physicians and third parties. The community general hospital, which accounts for the largest segment of the resources used for inpatient care in the United States, is the focus of this discussion. Other types of hospitals are discussed further in Chapter 5.

Community hospitals offer a wide range of services with the degree of technological complexity largely a function of the composition of the hospital's medical staff. The typical hospital's objectives would include providing as broad a range of services as can be supported by the community and to the largest feasible population. One way of achieving these objectives is through maximization of the quality of care as perceived by both physicians and prospective patients. Hospitals compete for patients indirectly by competing for physicians. Physicians in turn are attracted to hospitals by the status of members of the medical staff, the availability of those services needed in support of the physician's practice or, in economic parlance, the production function, and the ease of access to hospital services for the physician's patients.

These characteristics are not remarkable in and of themselves. It is only when they are coupled with third-party reimbursement that the system strays from a self-correcting economic model. In 1975, 80% of consumer expenditures for hospital care were paid through voluntary hospital insurance. All third-party payments, including those by government, to all kinds of hospitals in the same year added up to 94.8% of total expenditures for hospitals (10). Although precise data are not readily available, it is estimated that third parties accounted for over 90% of revenue derived by community general hospitals. The effective price facing many patients at the time services are delivered is a small fraction of the price charged by the hospital for the service. The difference, of course, is financed through the various third-party mechanisms, both voluntary and governmental.

As with physicians, hospitals can be reimbursed through a variety of mechanisms. The first, which is analogous to fee-for-service, is reimbursement for specific services. A related method is reimbursement on a per-case basis. Hospitals can also be reimbursed using the capitation method, under which the institution receives a fixed amount for each enrolled patient. A fourth approach is to reimburse the hospital a proportion of its budget, with the shares for which various third parties are responsible being determined by the amount that their enrollees use the hospital in a given year. Finally, and most common, the hospital may be reimbursed on the basis of a day of care. That is, the third party pays an amount for each day that one of its enrollees is hospitalized.

With the exception of payment for specific services, all of these methods assume a formal relationship between the hospital and a third party, whether it be state or federal government or a voluntary underwriter. Payment for specific services, on the other hand, is simply based on the hospital's charges. These charges may be inclusive as for the daily service charge (for bed, board, and nursing services), or for the use of special facilities such as the operating room (usually on a per minute basis after a minimum charge), or on an item-by-item basis as for laboratory and radiology procedures. Increasingly, hospital charges are directly related to the unit cost of producing the service. Where it is not, some of the revenue generated from one source may possibly subsidize other services. In addition to cross-subsidization, financial requirements of the institution generally require an inclusion of a component in charges for future growth and development. Considering all methods of payment, operating margins, or the difference between revenues and expenses, for community hospitals have been approximately 3 to 4% in recent years.

In some states, the schedule of charges established by hospitals are subject to approval by a state rate commission. Almost by definition, charges are established on a prospective basis and are derived from the anticipated budget of the hospital. Rate review mechanisms, therefore, generally concern themselves with the reasonableness of the proposed budget, including the projected cost of various services, the volume of use anticipated, and particularly the growth and development factor that arises from a projected positive operating margin.

Since each hospital charges for hundreds of different services, it is not feasible to determine the reasonableness of all charges. On the other hand, there are advantages to using charges for specific services as the basis for paying hospitals. First, it seems most equitable to determine the payment from each patient on the basis of those services actually used. This is in contrast to approaches which will be described below which tend to average payments across patients. Second, charges are a system well understood by the consumer since this is the approach used throughout the economy for most goods and services. Third, it is possible to introduce co-payments, where the patient has responsibility for a fraction of the charge, into the insurance system for those services for which patient or physician cost consciousness is considered particularly important. Finally, if a uniform system of charges were developed, it would enhance the buyer's ability to compare hospitals on the basis of price, whether the buyer were a patient, a voluntary underwriter, or a government.

All community general hospitals use charges as one method of obtaining payment. Patients with commercial insurance coverage, some Blue Cross patients, and others who are responsible for part or all of their bill (e.g., for days that are not covered by a third party) are charged on this basis. By far the most important source of revenue to hospitals, however, is derived from the *per diem* basis of reimbursement by which the hospital is paid for each day that a patient is in the hospital without regard to the particular service used. Most Blue Cross plans have used *per diem* reimbursement for many years. Further, when Medicare and Medicaid were adopted in the mid-1960s, these governmental programs adopted the Blue Cross approach to *per diem* hospital reimbursement.

Per diem reimbursement as used by Blue Cross and government has been based on retrospectively determined costs. The approach is to determine the hospital's total cost of delivering patient care for a year, and then to divide this amount by the total number of patient days of care rendered by the hospital during the same period. The resulting cost per day (*per diem*) then becomes the amount to which the hospital is entitled for each day of care rendered to a particular third-party's enrollees. For example, if a hospital's total costs were $20,000,000, and it had delivered 100,000 days of patient care in the course of the year, the resulting *per diem* costs would be $200. Thus, for each day that a Blue Cross or Medicare patient was in the hospital, the hospital could expect to receive this amount. In actual use, however, this method is far more complex.

Traditional *per diem* cost reimbursement, as noted above, is retrospective in nature. The actual periodic payments to hospitals by third parties are generally based on some interim estimate of *per diem* costs, since these are not known until the end of the period. This payment may be calculated as a function of charges, the previous year's *per diem* costs plus a factor for inflation, or some similar approach. It is important to re-emphasize, however, that after a year-end adjustment, the hospital will ultimately be paid its actual audited *per diem* costs under this mechanism.

Two major issues that have accompanied *per diem* cost reimbursement over the years are the definition of allowable costs and equity between classes of patients. The issue of which hospital costs should be subject to *per diem* reimbursement has been debated for decades. Accommodations were reached between hospitals and Blue Cross plans in a number of areas. For example, when costs are incurred in nonpatient-care areas where other sources of revenue are collected (e.g., gift shops and cafeterias), costs would be determined after deducting such revenue. In the patient care areas, teaching costs are considered allowable on the grounds that the teaching activity improves the quality of patient care. Research costs, however, are generally not allowable because they may benefit patients ultimately, but are not of direct benefit to a patient in the hospital at the time the research is conducted. Depreciation is allowed, usually on the historical cost basis. Bad debts are generally not allowed on the theory that cost reimbursement obviates bad debts for those patients subject to it. An exception is bad debts incurred in relation to deductibles and co-payments associated with Medicare.

More generally, the Social Security Administration in developing the regulations for implementation of the Medicare law followed the traditional Blue Cross pattern by and large in determining "reasonable" costs. Notable exceptions were the policy followed with respect to equity among classes of patients, and that part of hospitals' financial requirements needed for growth and development.

HOSPITAL REIMBURSEMENT, EQUITY, AND HOSPITAL GROWTH

Blue Cross plans have over the years endeavored to enroll a broad cross section of the community, and further, these plans historically were in close alliance with hospitals. Thus, in developing cost reimbursement arrangements, Blue Cross assumed that its subscribers reflected the mix of all patients that were hospitalized. Consequently, Blue Cross reimbursed hospitals an average amount per day, without regard to the particular services, or their costs, employed on behalf of their subscribers.

The adaptation of *per diem* cost reimbursement under Medicare did not follow this line of reasoning. Because the program was originally intended only for those age 65 and over, certain costs were disallowed outright, such as for maternity and pediatrics. More consequentially, however, it was asserted by the Social Security Administration that because of the extended lengths-of-stay experienced by those over age 65, the *per diem* cost for ancillary services, which tend to be concentrated in the earlier days of the hospital stay, should be lower on average than for those under age 65. Consequently, hospitals were reimbursed for ancillary service costs in proportion to the ratio of ancillary service charges for the elderly to ancillary service charges for those under age 65.

Hospitals argued that while ancillary service costs might be lower for the elderly on a *per diem* basis, nursing costs were higher. After several cost studies and some years, the Social Security Administration recognized the nursing differential. The point of this discussion is not to go into the details of cost reimbursement formulae, but rather to point out the difference between a *per diem* system that assumes that the patients of a particular third party are representative of all patients, versus one that recognizes ahead of time that its enrollees, or prospective patients, may be less expensive than average. Carried to its logical conclusion, the latter approach would result in reimbursement based on actual costs incurred by each patient, which is similar to a system based on charges, where charges are directly related to unit costs.

Both the issues of allowable costs and equity come into play in considering the growth and development factor that is allowed hospitals. Blue Cross plans have typically included a "plus factor" in *per diem* reimbursement. This factor has ranged from 2 to 8% depending on the Blue Cross plan. The Social Security Administration included a 2% plus factor in its original formulation, but this was discontinued early in the Nixon Administration. The plus factor is intended to recognize hospitals' financial requirements, and particularly the need for internally generated capital funds. On the other hand, it has been argued that the planning and development of community resources should not be tied to a particular hospital's ability to generate funds from depreciation, a plus factor, or a surplus from other sources. Some of the reservations that have been expressed about the growth and development factor relate more broadly to the incentives inherent in cost-plus reimbursement. In recent years, these concerns have led to a shift toward experimentation with prospective reimbursement.

PROSPECTIVE HOSPITAL REIMBURSEMENT

One approach to prospective rate setting has been discussed; that is, the situation in which hospitals are reimbursed on the basis of charges subject to prior approval. Such a system has been in operation in the state of Indiana for more than 20 years under agreements between hospitals and Blue Cross. More recently, this approach has been adopted by several states using state rate commissions. The other major approach to prospective reimbursement is a modification of *per diem* cost reimbursement.

Prospective cost reimbursement differs from retrospective cost reimbursement in that the *per diem* amount is established before the beginning of a year (and thus before the hospital's actual costs are known), rather than being adjusted to reflect the actual costs incurred for the previous year. Under prospective *per diem* reimbursement, if a hospital's actual costs exceed its approved costs, the hospital would suffer a loss. Thus there is an incentive for the hospital to keep its costs at or below the approved level. This is in sharp contrast to retrospective *per diem* cost reimbursement under which the hospital receives payment for whatever level of costs it incurs, and therefore is not subject to a loss should costs be higher than anticipated. With a plus factor, the hospital may actually benefit from higher costs. This benefit would carry forward to future years since the hospital would be starting from a higher cost base.

Under prospective *per diem* cost reimbursement, the incentives for keeping costs below the approved level are weak, if they exist at all. Even though the hospital may keep the difference between revenues derived from the prospectively approved *per diem* rate and the actual *per diem* costs, the institution has merely deferred expenditures to future years by carrying forward a surplus. In the process, the hospital risks obtaining a lower approved rate for future years by virtue of its lower base costs for the following period.

There are several approaches to establishing the prospective *per diem* rate. The two popular approaches, however, are based on a formula or on individual hospital-negotiated budgets. In the former, the rate setting agency, whether it be a voluntary prepayment plan such as Blue Cross or a state rate setting authority, would establish a formula which provides the basis for determining the percentage increase in *per diem* costs that will be allowed for the following period. The starting point is generally the hospital's *per diem* cost for the preceding period, adjusted upward for input cost increases of various types including labor costs, services, supplies, and so forth. The overall increase would generally be subject to a ceiling established for each category of hospital. The categories might be based on hospital size, for example. With a strict exception policy, this approach seems to have the greatest potential for holding down the rate of increase in hospital costs. On the other hand, because it starts with the hospital's current *per diem* costs, it does not necessarily reward the more efficient hospital, and as noted above there is some incentive to incur costs up to the allowed level. Further, since the unit of service is a day of care, there is an incentive for hospitals to place less pressure on the medical staff for reduced lengths-of-stay or, alternatively, to allow lengths-of-stay to increase somewhat in order to generate higher total revenues for the year. This tendency may offset savings that would otherwise accrue from a tight policy of allowable percentage increases in *per diem* costs. The rate setting agency must also consider the financial viability of the institutions whose costs it is attempting to regulate.

The other extreme is the approach which considers each hospital's budget individually. It would probably be more difficult for a rate setting agency to reduce the rate of increase in *per diem* costs under this system. Instead of a rather mechanistic formula where few exceptions are allowed, the third party or state regulator must consider the particular circumstances and financial viability of each institution. Hospitals can make persuasive cases in terms of their financial requirements for the coming period, and these may be difficult to ignore or refute in the rate setting process. The approach is also more difficult to administer since it involves individual consideration of large numbers of hospitals. On the other hand, this approach has the advantage of recognizing legitimate differences in hospitals and particularly year-to-year changes in growth, case-mix, and so forth. Standards would have to be developed to determine the reasonableness of those elements of cost that comprise each hospital's projected budget. There is a tendency toward uniform measurement of hospital costs and services, and considerable effort is being directed toward grouping of hospitals which may make the budget review process the more constructive approach in the long run.

The approaches to prospective rate setting described above are based on hospital costs. Some have argued that the connection between historical costs and prospective rates should be broken for purposes of establishing a cost containment strategy. An alternative approach would be to place limits on allowable increases in hospital revenue, without regard to costs. The hospital would then have to manage its resources so as to operate within such revenue caps. The obvious drawback to this approach is its potentially arbitrary nature, especially if hospitals' operating situations are not considered. That is, for a reasonable system to be implemented some account must be taken of the hospital's current and anticipated situation with respect to costs and volume of service. A cap on the percentage increase allowed for total revenues of an institution for a year, for example, would institutionalize existing differences between hospitals and not allow for the dynamic nature of hospital growth and development or, alternatively, of attrition.

A still further approach would be to regulate the revenue that could be generated on a per-case basis, with differentiation across types of admissions by diagnostic category. The incentives in such a system would be desirable in terms of cost containment behavior by hospitals with respect to both resource use and length-of-stay. But, this approach would introduce incentives to modify case-mix, which would be difficult to predict in terms of their result on medical management in the aggregate.

In summary, hospital reimbursement as it has been developed over several decades has led to a heavy emphasis on cost-plus reimbursement which in turn has enabled, and indeed encouraged, the diffusion of technology, the elaboration of hospital services, and an increase in the amenity level in most institutions. Since hospitals compete for physicians, and indirectly for patients, and would seem to have as their objective a wide range of services to the broadest possible segment of the community, it is not surprising that expenditures have increased. At the same time, attempts to deal with hospital financing through prospective rate setting are subject to many theoretical and practical difficulties. Some have argued that with economic incentives as strong as they are for hospitals to elaborate their services under the current arrangement, some more comprehensive set of incentives that tie together the interests of underwriters, physicians, and hospitals is the most feasible and desirable approach to containing health service costs. In the absence of very fundamental changes in the health services system, the relationship between hospitals and governmental and voluntary insurers will continue to be of considerable importance.

HOSPITAL AND NON-GOVERNMENTAL INSURANCE RELATIONSHIPS

As will be discussed further below, voluntary health insurance underwriters have been very successful in enrolling a high proportion of employed persons and their dependents, with in-depth coverage of expensive episodes, and in competing in an insurance market characterized by very sophisticated group coverage buyers or their brokers. Voluntary third parties have assumed the social responsibility of improving access to care by removing financial barriers for much of the population and by spreading the risk of high family health expenditures.

At the same time, commercial carriers and non-profit prepayment plans such as Blue Cross have not played a major role in controlling the rise in hospital costs.

No control function was originally intended by either the commercial carriers or Blue Cross, however, and under current arrangements little control is likely to exist in the absence of regulatory intervention. This situation is the result of the current relationships between underwriters and providers, existing incentives, and the historical development of these relationships.

There are two fundamental approaches to voluntary underwriting: indemnification and service benefits. Indemnification is the approach employed by commercial insurance companies for health insurance as well as a wide range of casualty coverages. With the indemnity approach, a contractual relationship is established between the company and the insured under which the insured agrees to pay a premium and the company, for its part, agrees to pay the insured a cash benefit in the event of a loss. For example, the insured may receive a certain dollar amount for each day of hospitalization as a result of an accident or covered illness, plus an additional amount equal to the charges for various ancillary services used during the stay in the hospital, up to some limit.

The service benefit approach, on the other hand, guarantees the insured individual, usually referred to as a subscriber or a member, services when needed in return for the premium, rather than a cash amount. For example, under a Blue Cross service benefit agreement the subscriber would be assured needed hospital services in the event of an accident or covered illness.

Under indemnity arrangements, the only contractual relationship is between the insurance company and the insured. With service benefits the underwriter must have some way of arranging for the delivery of services in order to fulfill its contractual obligation to the subscriber. Thus, the third party with a service benefit must either contract for services or provide services directly. In the case of Blue Cross plans, the third party has agreements with member hospitals, usually including all community general hospitals in its service area. The hospitals agree to care for Blue Cross enrollees, accepting reimbursement as payment in full with the exception of co-payments and exclusions, while the Blue Cross plan agrees to reimburse the hospital on an agreed-upon basis. Another example of a service benefit would be that provided by a Health Maintenance Organization which may own and operate its own hospital, may have a close affiliation with a community hospital, or may engage in contractual relationships with several hospitals.

The commercial underwriter's liability is limited to the dollar amounts agreed to in the indemnity arrangement, and the patient is responsible for any additional amounts charged by the hospital. For these reasons and the absence of a contractual relationship between the insurance company and the institution, there is no reason to expect cost control behavior by insurance companies. Blue Cross plans might be in a better position to influence hospital costs and several voluntary efforts have been undertaken. However, in many parts of the country there is a balance of power between Blue Cross plans and the hospitals since the Blue Cross plan must have hospital members to offer a service benefit, while the hospitals enjoy favorable reimbursement arrangements with Blue Cross. Although the relationship is weaker today than it once was, hospitals and Blue Cross plans in many areas view themselves as closely allied. At the same time, Blue Cross plans must compete in the insurance market and therefore feel the impact of hospital cost increases very directly in establishing premiums for the following year. In many states, insurance commissioners have put pressure on Blue Cross at the time premium increases are up for approval, but in most cases these efforts have had little long-term impact.

Another approach to the relationship between hospitals and third parties is to consider the market objectives of the third parties themselves. A common objective is the maximization of enrollments or market share. This would be particularly true of non-profit third parties such as Blue Cross. As hospital costs increase, the utility of having third party coverage to protect against such costs also increases. Thus, rising hospital costs enable the third party to pursue its objective of increased enrollments and comprehensiveness of coverage, while at the same time supporting hospitals in their pursuit of greater quantity and quality of services. Thus, by financing hospital cost increases, Blue Cross increases the "potential negative impact on the consumers' wealth positions and thereby expands enrollments and coverage" (11). Also, to the degree that governmental programs such as Medicare reimburse hospitals for less than their full costs, these costs are likely to be passed on in the form of higher charges or reimbursement to those not covered by the governmental programs. The same insurance effect then results since the increased cost of hospitalization encourages additional insurance coverage because the expected loss to the prospective hospital patient is increased. These and other factors have been responsible for dramatic increases in insurance coverage for health services.

HEALTH INSURANCE COVERAGE IN THE UNITED STATES

In this section health care financing is considered from the consumer's perspective. What are the options available in terms of third party insurance coverage either from private underwriters or government programs, how do they market or otherwise make coverage available, and what kinds of benefit structures are typical?

DEVELOPMENT OF HEALTH INSURANCE COVERAGE

Third party coverage for health care costs is a phenomenon largely of the last 40 years in this country. In 1940, for example, less than 10% of the population had coverage for inpatient care, and a negligible portion had coverage for any other type of health service. By 1977, almost four out of every five Americans under the age of 65 had private health insurance for inpatient services of both hospitals and physicians, more than 60% had some type of coverage for out-of-hospital physician visits, and the proportion with coverage for dental care was approaching one out of four (Table 10–5) (12).

Virtually the entire population age 65 and over is covered under Medicare, with hospital benefits (Part A) that protect 98% and medical benefits covering 97% of the elderly. Further, more than three out of five persons over 65 have some form of private supplementary coverage, in addition to Medicare, for hospital services. An estimated 11% of the population under age 65 received benefits from the Medicaid program during 1976, and an additional 1% were covered under that portion of the Medicare program designed for the disabled under age 65. In contrast, census estimates (13) and a national survey supported by foundation sources (14) indicate that 12 to 13% of the U.S. population under age 65 have no insurance coverage at all.

In the early years of this century, it was not generally believed by those in the insurance industry that health care, particularly for illnesses, as distinct from accidents, was an insurable risk. To indemnify against a loss, the event causing the loss would ordinarily be expected to be clearly definable, undesirable from the point of view of the insured, and unpredictable on an individual basis but predictable, in the actuarial sense, for a group of individuals or for the entire population. Until the emergence of the twentieth century hospital (Chapter 5), care for illness did not fit this definition. Although there were numerous experiments in the first quarter of this century to spread the risk of financial loss due to illness, there were no large scale efforts.

During the late 1920s, a very comprehensive study of various facets of health care organization and financing under the aegis of the Committee on the Costs of Medical Care (15) demonstrated the degree to which a relatively small fraction of the population in any given year bore a substantial fraction of the costs of medical care. The hospital had emerged as the most appropriate setting for the treatment of serious illness for all socioeconomic classes, but had also resulted in substantial increases in health costs per episode of illness.

Rising health costs and the financial impact on families of the Great Depression led to the specter of potential debt for families with a member requiring hospitalization, and very real financial difficulties for community general hospitals. These hospitals were increasingly dependent upon income generated from charges to private patients. The combination of a definable event such as medical or surgical inpatient treatment, the recognition of the need to spread financial risk across the community, and the need of institutions for a more reliable source of revenue led to hospital prepayment which ultimately became the Blue Cross system. Blue Cross plans grew relatively slowly during the 1930s although they were widely recognized as an important social movement.

The two objectives of providing a stronger financial base for community hospitals and spreading the risk of economic loss from hospitalization were both viewed as socially worthy objectives. Also, the service benefit relationship between the third party and the hospital was markedly different from customary commercial indemnity insurance. As a result of these factors, special enabling legislation was passed in many states to encourage the development of Blue Cross on a nonprofit, tax-free basis, with exemption from the usual requirements of commercial insurance underwriters. Blue Shield plans, organized by the medical profession, also were developing during this period. However, the paid-in-full service benefit arrangement never took hold for physicians' coverage, with the exception of plans on the

TABLE 10–5. Estimates of Net Number of Different Persons Under Private Health Insurance Plans and Percent of Population Covered, by Age and Specified Type of Care, as of December 31, 1976

Type of Service	All Ages		Under Age 65		Aged 65 and Over	
	Number (in thousands)	Percent of Civilian Population*	Number (in thousands)	Percent of Civilian Population†	Number (in thousands)	Percent of Civilian Population‡
Hospital care	168,448	79.3	154,205	81.3	14,243	62.7
Physicians' services						
Surgical services	164,986	77.7	152,498	80.4	12,488	55.0
In-hospital visits	160,750	75.7	151,034	79.6	9,716	42.8
X-ray and laboratory examinations	156,717	73.8	148,293	78.2	8,424	37.1
Office & home visits	127,735	60.1	121,234	63.9	6,501	28.6
Dental care	34,477	16.2	33,840	17.8	637	2.8
Prescribed drugs (out-of-hospital)	149,276	70.3	144,335	76.1	4,941	21.8
Private-duty nursing	145,927	68.7	140,996	74.3	4,931	21.7
Visiting-nurse service	141,561	66.7	136,099	71.8	5,462	24.1
Nursing-home care	70,146	33.0	65,686	34.6	4,460	19.6

*Based on Bureau of Census estimate of 212,376,000 as of 1/1/76.
†Based on Bureau of Census estimate of 189,674,000 as of 1/1/76.
‡Based on Bureau of Census estimate of 22,702,000 as of 1/1/76.

Source: Mueller MS: Private health insurance in 1975: coverage, enrollment, and financial experience. *Social Security Bulletin* 40(6):3–21, 1977, p.5.

West Coast which were established to protect physicians, and their patients, from "contract practice," under which a particular physician or physician group would serve as the exclusive provider for an employer's workers to the exclusion of other physicians in the community.

During the 1940s and early 1950s major growth occurred in both hospital coverage and inpatient medical-surgical coverage. And during this period, the original social objectives of the Blue Cross system were undermined by the more conventional practices of commercial insurers.

Blue Cross plans originally spread the risk of loss across all segments of their communities. This was accomplished by establishing a premium which was essentially the same regardless of the potential subscriber's degree of risk. The premium rate was the same whether an individual or group of individuals was young and healthy or older and at greater risk. This approach was in sharp contrast to underwriting practices traditionally used by commercial carriers who attempt to estimate the claims that will be experienced by a group and establish a premium rate accordingly. The common rate approach, used originally by Blue Cross, is referred to as community rating and the commercial insurance approach is experience rating.

As Blue Cross began to develop coverage for employee groups, and as this form of fringe benefit became increasingly popular during the 1940s, commercial insurance companies were able to penetrate the market by selectively offering equal or improved benefits for lower premiums by selling to groups that were of below average risk. To the degree that more favorable groups obtained coverage from commercial underwriters, the remaining market was at greater risk and therefore the Blue Cross premium would necessarily be higher. As a consequence, Blue Cross plans eventually abandoned community rating, except in the case of small employers and individual coverage, and began to compete with commercial underwriters using experience rating. One consequence of this natural evolution of market forces was that neither Blue Cross and Blue Shield plans, nor commercial underwriters, were able to provide coverage in an economical fashion to two very important high-risk segments of the population: the aged, who were at high risk and had left the labor force, and the poor, who tended to be at higher risk and were typically not members of stable employee groups. This situation led to the passage of two federal programs, Medicare and Medicaid.

The competition for new enrollees between the prepayment plans (Blue Cross/Blue Shield) and commercial underwriters was particularly vigorous during the 1940s and 1950s. A major impetus for the rapid growth of voluntary health insurance was its increasing popularity as a fringe benefit, with at least partial contributions by the employer. During World War II and the wage and price control years that followed, health insurance was recognized as a negotiable item under collective bargaining agreements and, furthermore, one which was exempt from controls. Thus, both industry and labor found it an attractive component of employee compensation.

Over the years, through collective bargaining or simply competition in the labor market, health insurance plans have changed in two respects. First, an increasing number of benefits have been added to plans, while existing benefits have been improved in the sense that the plan pays for a higher proportion of expenses incurred. Second, an increasing proportion of all employers pay part or all of the premium for their employees and, concomitantly, an increasing proportion of all premiums are paid for by employers. For example, of the almost 500 group health insurance plans for groups of 100 or more employees which took effect during the first three months of 1977, all but 6% were paid for entirely by the employers (39%) or involved contributions by both the employee and the employer (55%). It is estimated that over 70% of all premium expenses for group insurance are paid for by employers.

In addition to group insurance available through Blue Cross/Blue Shield and commerical insurance companies, there is also coverage in the form of individual health insurance policies. These policies vary widely in the quality of the coverage and tend to be costly to administer. And since the individual who purchases a health insurance policy is not receiving coverage as a member of a group constituted for a purpose other than acquiring health insurance (employee group) which may be of lower than average risk, the claims experience for individual policy holders is usually less favorable. That is, an individual unable to obtain insurance through a group related to employment status or some other non-health related status such as being a student, would be more likely to apply for insurance if he or she anticipated illness. The same phenomenon may occur in the process of employment but then the effect would be swamped or "averaged out" by the large numbers of people in an employed group.

VOLUNTARY HEALTH INSURANCE PLAN ADMINISTRATION

Health insurance premiums vary tremendously, in large part because of the wide variation in benefit structure and in the composition of groups that buy the insurance. In addition, however, operating expenses (and profits) range from a relatively low proportion of the total premium to as much as half or more of the premium. Table 10–6 shows the operating expense experienced by different categories of underwriters, and for commercial insurance companies by type of policy, for the years 1970–1976. These percentages have not changed appreciably in recent years.

The operating expense of Blue Cross, nationally, and of the independent plans have consistently been the lowest. By far the highest operating expense is associated with individual policies marketed by commercial insurance companies. While Blue Cross and the independent plans have much lower than average operating expenses, the reasons are somewhat different. What these organizations have in common is that they offer service benefits and therefore, as discussed earlier, necessarily have a contractual relationship with providers. Thus, the administrative expense associated with reimbursement is in many instances lower. For example, cost reimbursement under Blue Cross is administratively easier than reimbursing on the basis of itemized bills for a multitude of different providers. Similarly, independent plans have well-established payment mechanisms developed for member providers, some of which may be as straightforward to administer as paying annual salaries.

TABLE 10–6. Operating Expense as a Proportion of Premium Income, 1970–1976

Type of Plan	Operating Expense as Percent of Premium Income by Year						
	1970	1971	1972	1973	1974	1975	1976
Total	14.0	13.9	14.2	14.0	14.1	13.1	12.8
Blue Cross-Blue Shield,* total	7.2	6.9	6.9	7.0	7.4	7.4	6.9
Blue Cross	5.6	5.2	5.2	5.2	5.4	5.5	5.2
Blue Shield	11.0	11.0	11.3	11.5	11.8	11.5	10.9
Insurance companies, total	20.4	21.2	21.5	21.2	21.0	18.8	18.9
Group policies	12.8	12.7	13.4	13.0	13.0	12.7	13.3
Individual policies	46.6	47.1	47.0	47.0	47.0	46.1	46.8
Independent plans, total	7.7	7.5	7.0	7.0	7.4	7.5	6.3
Community	7.2	6.7	6.9	6.8	7.1	6.6	6.6
Employer-employee-union	7.7	7.8	6.0	5.7	5.9	6.7	6.1

*Data are adjusted for duplication.

Sources: Mueller MS: Private health insurance in 1975: coverage, enrollment, and financial experience. *Social Security Bulletin* 40(6):3-21, 1977, p. 18; and Carroll MS: Private health insurance plans in 1976: an evaluation. *Social Security Bulletin* 41(9):3-16, 1978, p. 14.

Another important factor, however, involves the size of the average claim. It is less expensive to administer a smaller number of large claims, as for hospital coverage, than a larger number of small claims, as for fee-for-service physician coverage. Thus, Blue Cross, which primarily covers hospital services, has the lowest operating expense while the independent plans, which tend to be more comprehensive in their coverage, have somewhat higher expenses as a proportion of premium.

The group policies of insurance companies tend to have higher administrative costs than Blue Cross, Blue Shield, or the independent plans because they are heterogeneous, organizationally have a wider range of providers to pay, do not have established relationships with those providers, and offer more complex and often more limited coverage. The individual policies sold by commercial insurance companies have operating expenses, and profit, that average 47 cents for every dollar of premium collected.

In addition to the administrative costs associated with indemnity coverage, commercial insurance companies have much higher selling and administration expenses, including the cost of premium collections. In the group situation, health insurance is offered through an employer, thus enabling the underwriter to reach a relatively large number of subscribers through a single or master contract. In contrast, individual policies must be sold on a one-to-one basis. Further, the premiums for group policies are usually collected by the union or employer and paid to the insurance company in a lump sum. In contrast, insurance companies must collect directly for the premiums on individual policies. Finally, keeping track of eligible insureds is complicated in the individual policy case and is the responsibility of the underwriter. By comparison, in the case of group policies, the employer advises the underwriter, typically each month, of additions and deletions with respect to eligibility.

BENEFIT STRUCTURE OF HEALTH INSURANCE PLANS

Plans may range from very limited individual coverage, such as indemnity of $40 per day for hospitalization as a result of an accident, to very comprehensive coverage such as paid-in-full service benefits for all inpatient and outpatient services with few exclusions or limitations. The development of health insurance began with the identification of hospitalization as a definable and insurable risk. Medical-surgical benefits were the next to develop; these benefits usually included coverage for inpatient physician services, and most notably surgeons' fees.

During the latter 1950s, major medical insurance began to develop quite rapidly. This coverage paid for a wide range of medical services including hospital care, both inpatient and outpatient physician services, drugs, appliances, ambulance services, and so forth. Major medical insurance, however, included a deductible and coinsurance as well as an upper limit. The deductible is an amount to be paid by the insured before coverage takes effect. Coinsurance refers to a portion of the total expense that is expected to be borne by the insured. At present a common major medical policy would have a deductible of between $100 and $150, 20% coinsurance, and a maximum of anywhere from $100,000 to $250,000.

Basic hospital and medical-surgical coverage is often complemented by a major medical policy. Such a major medical policy superimposed on a base plan would generally have a much lower or possibly no deductible. Thus, the combination of plans would lead to payment in full for hospital confinements and physicians' services in the hospital, perhaps up to some limit under the basic plan, fairly substantial coverage for care in the hospital beyond such limits, and partial coverage for other medical services not included in the base plan.

Another approach which has become increasingly prevalent in recent years is a comprehensive coverage which directly combines the base and major medical plans. Under this benefit structure, most services are paid at 80 to 90% of reasonable charges after a fairly low deductible, such as $50 to $100 per year. Comprehensive plans often pay 100% after an out-of-pocket expense limit, such as $200 or $300 per year, has been reached by the insured. Certain types of benefits, such as psychiatric or dental coverages, may be subject to additional deductibles, coinsurance, or limits. For example, the psychiatric benefit may limit outpatient visits to the subscriber to a specified number of visits per year, or to a dollar ceiling such as $1,000. At the same time, there may be a coinsurance of 50%. Similarly, dental care may be paid-in-full for preventive services up to two visits per year but have a 50% coinsurance feature for restorative care, and no provision for orthodontics.

310 Resources for Health Services

The important point is that there are virtually an infinite variety of benefit packages. As noted earlier, the trend in recent years has been toward fuller coverage of traditional hospital and physician services, as well as the addition of new benefits. New benefits tend to be initiated with relatively conservative provisions including coinsurance and limits. As experience accumulates, these benefits may then be broadened or deepened. A summary measure of the depth of coverage for various types of care is reflected in Table 10–7 which presents the proportion of consumer expenditures paid for through private insurance since 1950.

In 1950, only 12% of such expenditures were financed through private insurance. Almost all of the insurance payments were devoted to inpatient hospital and physician services. Over the years the proportion of all consumer expenditures met by insurance has increased almost four-fold to 46.3% in 1976. Eighty-six percent of consumer expenditures for hospital care were paid for through private insurance in 1976, while 46% of physician services and 18% of outpatient dental care were paid for through insurance. Outpatient prescribed drugs and all other types of care are still largely paid for out-of-pocket by consumers.

In 1976, Blue Cross/Blue Shield plans accounted for 41% of gross enrollments for the most basic insurance, hospital coverage. These were largely enrollments under group policies. This type of policy underwritten by commercial insurance companies accounted for another 42% of all enrollments with individual policies underwritten by insurance companies yielding an additional 13%. The remaining 4% of enrollments for hospital insurance was accounted for by independent prepaid group practice plans, individual practice associations, and union plans. As their

TABLE 10–7. Proportion of Consumer Expenditures Met by Health Insurance 1950–1976

Year	Total	Hospital Care	Physicians' Services	Prescribed Drugs	Dental Care (out-of-hospital)	Other Types of Care
1950	12.2	37.1	12.0	NA*	NA	NA
1960	27.8	64.7	30.0	NA	NA	NA
1965	32.6	71.2	32.8	NA	NA	NA
1966	32.3	69.0	33.9	NA	NA	NA
1967	33.5	73.3	35.9	NA	NA	NA
1968	36.6	76.9	40.7	NA	NA	NA
1969	36.3	74.3	41.1	NA	NA	NA
1970	38.5	77.9	43.8	4.5	5.3	5.2
1971	39.8	82.5	43.9	5.5	6.3	4.6
1972	39.9	77.6	45.7	5.4	7.3	6.0
1973	39.9	75.9	46.1	6.0	8.6	6.8
1974	42.9	77.8	50.7	6.2	11.5	9.8
1975	45.0	86.8	46.8	6.9	13.9	8.3
1976	46.3	85.8	45.9	8.1	18.4	9.6

*NA—not available.

Source: Carroll MS: Private health insurance plans in 1976: an evaluation. *Social Security Bulletin* 41(9):3-16, 1978, p. 14.

name implies, independent plans tend to be locally oriented, but some represent large systems, as for example the Kaiser-Permanente medical care system.

HEALTH MAINTENANCE ORGANIZATIONS

In the early 1970s an umbrella label, the Health Maintenance Organization (HMO), was coined to characterize independent plans that offered service benefits for an enrolled population, covering hospital, physician, and related ancillary services. These plans offer service benefits which implies the requirement that both the source of hospital care and physician services be provided directly or on a contractual basis through the HMO.

The Health Maintenance Organization has received considerable attention since federal legislation was passed in 1973 intending to promote this type of financing and organization through planning and operational grants and loans. About 200 such organizations exist in the United States at various stages of development with quite diverse characteristics. The federal legislation included complex and very demanding requirements for these organizations if they were to become eligible for federal funding and mandatory inclusion in dual choice health insurance offerings by employers. Under dual choice the employer must offer to the employee more than one health insurance plan. Organizational aspects of HMOs are discussed in Chapter 4 and insurance considerations are presented here.

The ideals of community rating and very comprehensive services, characteristics of some of the more successful earlier prepaid group practices or HMOs, put the newer developing organizations at a considerable disadvantage in the marketplace. More recent amendments have made their promotion more feasible. At the same time, some states have passed legislation intended to protect developing HMOs and in particular to encourage their further development by requiring that employers include an HMO option in their fringe benefit offerings. What is it about the HMO that is so appealing from the public policy point of view?

Perhaps the major factor is that the HMO combines the insurance or underwriting function with the responsibility for delivering a broad range of health services. Thus, the underwriter (HMO) has to compete in the insurance market to be included as a benefit option for employees as the preferred employee choice among the alternatives, such as commercial insurance or Blue Cross/Blue Shield coverage. In addition, the plan must offer services that are professionally satisfactory and acceptable to patients. Thus, a central organization, the plan, has a strong incentive to offer services efficiently and in as cost effective a manner as possible so as to contain premium increases and expand benefits, both of which would attract enrollees in the dual choice situation. The HMO, then, has been an important model for encouraging natural regulation of the health care market through the usual forces of competition.

The better established Health Maninentenance Organizations, and particularly prepaid group practice plans, have been operating successfully in various areas, largely on the West Coast and in New York City and Washington, D.C., since the 1940s. The development of these plans has been steady in their local geographic areas, and some, such as Kaiser-Permanente, have expanded into new geographic areas over the decades.

These prepaid group practice plans have been characterized by far more comprehensive benefits than the typical health insurance program. Comprehensive HMO coverage, including hospital and physician services for both the subscriber and dependents typically without a deductible or coinsurance, has been a major attraction. The premium to cover this comprehensive benefit package has generally been higher than the premium associated with competing traditional health insurance programs. The total costs to the subscriber or member, however, must be considered in terms of premium payments combined with out-of-pocket expenses. On average, prepaid group practice is considerably less expensive, for the same benefit package, than traditional underwriting using independent fee-for-service physicians and community hospitals.

A drawback to prepaid group practice enrollment is the required use of plan physicians, who themselves are grouped into area medical centers. Thus, an enrollee must find a physician within the group practice with whom family members are satisfied, and must have reasonable geographic access to health services if this type of HMO is to be attractive. The slow but steady growth of prepaid group practice over the recent decades indicates that for many people the protection afforded by more comprehensive coverage at relatively less expense offsets limited choice of physician and lessened geographic availability.

Recent developments in financing health services, however, raise some serious questions about the attractiveness of prepaid group practice in the future. As was noted earlier, there is a tendency for a larger proportion of the premium, and often the entire premium, to be paid by employers and a tendency toward more comprehensive benefits to be offered by commercial insurance companies and Blue Cross/Blue Shield plans. These changes would appear to reduce the competitive advantage of prepaid group practice, since the latter arrangement still has inherent in it the organizational and geographic limitations, but is at a lesser advantage in terms of coverage and risk-sharing.

Employers and other purchasers of third party coverage, such as government, would benefit from the lower premium costs, given equal benefit structures, of prepaid group practice. But in the dual choice situation, it is the subscriber or employee who makes the decision as to which plan to use. The issue then becomes one of who will benefit from the savings that accrue by selection of a prepaid group practice in contrast to a traditional insurance program.

An alternative form of HMO to the prepaid group practice is the individual practice association (IPA) in which contractual arrangements exist between the plan and individual physicians and multiple medical groups, who are at some financial risk in the event that the costs of services exceed premium income, but practice in their offices, widely dispersed throughout the community. The IPA arrangement incorporates a broader range of physicians more geographically accessible to an enrolled population, and thus may offset the drawbacks to prepaid group practice mentioned above. The plan can also utilize physicians already in practice and hospitals already operating in the community, rather than invest the substantial capital required to start a group practice, particularly one that ultimately operates its own hospital. Further, physicians can be reimbursed on a prorated fee-for-service basis, a method close to that to which they are already accustomed.

Yet another approach is the primary care network plan. This system takes advantage of the gatekeeper role of the primary care physician by developing a contractual relationship with primary care physicians in the community, either on a fee-for-service or capitation basis, to deliver their own services. These physicians then have the responsibility for handling referrals of enrollees to specialists and to hospitals and of approving the charges for such care. Under this arrangement, reimbursement is withheld for care rendered by a specialist or in the hospital unless the patient was referred by the primary care physician. Ease of selection of a primary care physician depends, of course, upon the participating proportion and geographical dispersion of the primary care practitioners in the community.

A drawback of the individual practice association and network is that the plan or HMO has much less influence over the organization and method of physician practice than under the prepaid group arrangement. Such plans are more dependent upon the incentives built into the reimbursement agreement with physicians and sometimes hospitals. In contrast, the prepaid group can select physicians with practice styles consistent with the plan's operation, can organize facilities so as to encourage out-of-hospital management of illness, and can achieve the efficiencies inherent in combined ambulatory and inpatient delivery organizations.

To date, much of the experience with IPAs or primary care networks has been in settings in which they are competing with more traditional prepaid group practice, as well as with commercial insurance companies and Blue Cross-Blue Shield. Indeed, as noted in Chapter 4, in some instances IPAs have been developed by physicians to meet the competitive threat of prepaid group practices moving into their area. Under these circumstances, it is difficult to judge how much influence specific economic incentives have on physician behavior in the sense of putting physicians at risk through reimbursement schemes, and how much of the savings that seem evident under the IPA arrangement are because of broader physician motivation and peer control.

MAJOR GOVERNMENTALLY-FINANCED PROGRAMS

As noted earlier, the development of private health insurance in this country, and particularly the evolution of experience rating of premiums under both commercial insurance plans and Blue Cross/Blue Shield, left two major segments of the population without access to adequate coverage. The first group, the elderly, tend to be out of the labor force and therefore not eligible for group coverage, experience a substantial drop in income and typically a deteriorating wealth position, and are at increasing risk of major illness and therefore financial loss. The poor, on the other hand, are also at greater risk of illness and, in addition, are often either unemployed, or find themselves in occupations with irregular employment patterns or with low wages and poor fringe benefits.

These issues were especially evident during the 1950s and 1960s when voluntary health insurance was covering an increasingly expanding percentage of the population. Arguments against major federal programs to deal with these two groups could be persuasively opposed on the grounds that the voluntary system could do the job. Consequently, two titles were added to the Social Security Act in 1965. The first, Title XVIII, was the Medicare program for those age 65 and older; and the second was Title XIX, the Medicaid program, which substantially expanded the financial assistance provided to states and counties to pay for medical services for the poor.

Hospital insurance is provided to the elderly, and more recently to the permanently and totally disabled, beginning in the thirteenth month of Social Security disability, as well as to victims of end-stage renal disease, through Part A of Medicare. Part A also offers coverage in extended care facilities for post-hospital convalescence and home health services. Part B of Medicare, supplementary medical insurance, resembles major medical insurance for other than hospital services. Part B includes physician services, both inpatient and outpatient, ancillary services, and a wide range of other related medical services.

Part A is available without cost to the enrollee for virtually the entire elderly population and 98% of eligibles are covered. This hospital coverage includes a deductible that is roughly equivalent to the cost of one day of care in the hospital. This amount increases from time to time and in 1978 was $160. Coverage is provided for 90 days of hospital care for each illness episode with a copayment for the last 30 of these days ($40 per day for 1978), and 100 days of coverage per illness episode for extended care, with a copayment ($20 per day in 1978) for the last 80 days. Additional coverage for hospital days is available in the form of a "lifetime reserve" each day of which has a copayment associated with it. The lifetime reserve of 60 hospital days may be applied to any episode of care up to the reserve limit.

Part B of Medicare also includes a deductible, but on an annual basis. In 1978, this deductible was $60. A coinsurance of 20% of the reasonable charge is also applied. Often, the beneficiary must also make up the difference between "reasonable" and actual physician charges. Although it varies by region, overall approximately 50% of claims payments are accepted by physicians as payment-in-full (assignment). There are further limitations for mental and nervous conditions. A very high proportion of the elderly population (97%) are covered in Part B in addition to Part A. Unlike Part A, Part B is available on a voluntary basis with the requirement that the elderly person pay a monthly premium which is intended to be half the actual rate, based on loss experience. The other half is to be financed by the Health Care Financing Administration (which in reality finances more than two-thirds of the premium). The portion of the premium charged to the individual in 1978 was $8.70 per month.

The effects of deductibles, coinsurance, limitations in coverage, such as for psychiatric benefits, and service exclusions, such as routine dental and vision care, hearing aids, and particularly custodial skilled nursing home services, result in a Medicare program for the elderly that covers somewhat less than half of consumer expenditures for health services for this group of the population. Thus, the inadequacies are similar to those of private health insurance, with the important exception that the governmental programs provide coverage to a very high risk segment of the population that would ordinarily not be eligible for coverage under the voluntary system.

Medicare Part A is financed almost entirely by a portion, slightly over 1%, of the Social Security payroll tax through contributions by employees and employers. These funds are deposited in a separate trust fund. Premiums paid directly by a relatively small number of individuals who have not been participants in the Social Security or Railroad Retirement systems also contribute to the trust fund. Another trust fund receives monies from the voluntary premium payments of enrollees under Part B and premium payments from Medicaid on behalf of welfare recipients. The Part B trust fund also receives general revenues to make up the remainder of the funds required. Because of the rising costs of medical care, the amounts paid into the Medicare system from all sources have been substantially increased over the years.

Payments from these trust funds for both the administration of claims processing and reimbursement of providers is through fiscal intermediaries, who are voluntary underwriters, largely Blue Cross, Blue Shield, and commercial carriers, rather than directly by the government. As the program was developing in the late 1960s, the use of existing underwriters that had established administrative systems and relationships with both consumers and providers offered many advantages. More recently, the use of fiscal intermediaries has had the further advantage of requiring responsiveness to changes in federal policy under threat of changes in designation of fiscal intermediaries, a process that could not be used if administration were directly by the federal government. A major disadvantage of using fiscal intermediaries for claims processing and provider relations is the inevitable variation in practices that develop over time across the country; even with Blue Cross, the federal program is using scores of local plans, although they are tied together through a national association.

The Medicaid program for low income families is quite different in concept from the Medicare program. The Medicaid program developed out of the welfare system, which was originally local in both its administration and financing. During the Great Depression, local and state funds for welfare were quickly exhausted and the need for federal assistance became evident. The system that developed was one of federal matching funds to the states in support of welfare payments to various categories of the poor. Over the years, new categories were added, such as the totally and permanently disabled. An obvious need of the poor was assistance in paying for medical expenses. There developed a mechanism, "vendor payments," which simply meant that medical care provided to welfare recipients would be reimbursed by the county or state welfare authorities. Matching grants to the states from the federal government to partially offset the states' cost for vendor payments was formalized and expanded in the early 1960s. Medicaid built upon this welfare oriented system of federal grants to the states by matching state expenditures.

As originally envisioned, Medicaid included matching funds to states which met a set of requirements or standards including payment for five basic services, inpatient and outpatient hospital care, physician services, laboratory and x-ray services, and nursing home care, and reimbursed providers on a basis consistent with federally established Medicare policies including retrospective cost reimbursement for hospitals and fee-for-service payments to physicians. Thus states were obliged to reimburse hospitals on a reasonable cost basis, for example. These services had to be financed by the states for categorical welfare recipients such as families with dependent children, the elderly, the blind, and the totally and permanently disabled.

The original 1965 Medicaid law mandated certain minimum standards within the states in order for the states to receive matching funds, the amount of the match, ranging from 50 to 83%, being inversely related to the relative affluence of the residents of the state. States were also permitted to offer a much wider range of services than the minimum requirement, with partial federal reimbursement. Further, the states were permitted to establish their own income cut-off levels for determining eligibility. It was originally envisioned that by 1975, all states would be obliged to offer a full range of services to all residents in the state falling below a state-determined income level, without regard to whether or not they were categorical welfare recipients.

The cost to the federal government of the Medicaid program in its first year of operation and in subsequent years was substantially higher than had originally been forecast. Some states set income levels that were quite high by the standards then prevailing and offered a wide range of services. In the following years, amendments to the Medicaid law passed by the Congress reduced the freedom of the states to set high income cut-off levels, removed the requirements for expansion of services and eligibility originally envisioned, and tightened standards along a number of dimensions.

At the same time, state Medicaid budgets were stretched to the breaking point as a result of the rapid increase in costs of care due to the development and use of new services, upgraded services such as in nursing homes, and other factors. The original objective of eliminating "second-class" medical care for the poor was gradually eroded, in part because of the financial constraints that were placed on the programs, but also because of the great difficulty state governments had administering such a complex third-party payment program.

There was, and continues to be, considerable hostility toward state Medicaid programs by providers, but at the same time this source of funding remains crucial for the poor and dominant in certain sectors such as long-term care. Because Medicaid is not a program fully financed and administered by the federal government, there is tremendous variation between states with respect to benefits, eligibility, and administration. As a result, a truly national plan for health services has been seriously debated by federal policymakers.

PUBLIC POLICY ISSUES

It is evident from the preceding description of health services financing that a number of pressing issues are facing our society in this area. In this concluding section are summarized the more important issues, and consideration is given to general outlines of various proposed solutions, including strategies along the rather fundamental continuum that underlies the current debate: ranging from substantial government underwriting and direct regulation to a competitive market approach.

The major issues fall in the general categories of equity, effectiveness, and economy. With respect to equity, there are problems of risk-sharing across the population and income redistribution. The primary concerns in the effectiveness category are access to primary care and future technological development. The broad issue of economy encompasses concerns about total health services costs, cost effectiveness, and the visibility of expenditures.

Spreading the risk of a family's experiencing substantial expense due to medical care was a very early and very compelling force in the development of voluntary health insurance. Further, the inability of private health insurance to effectively cover the high risk associated with the elderly and the poor led to the passage of Medicare and Medicaid legislation. It was widely believed after the passage of these two programs that the problem of risk-sharing in our society had been largely resolved with voluntary insurance providing adequate protection to the majority of the population (generally those employed), and governmental programs (Medicare, Medicaid, and other programs designed for specific segments of the population) providing protection for the remainder.

Ironically, the reduction in the effective price of services at the time of delivery attributable to third-party coverage, coupled with cost reimbursement, have led to an elaboration of technological medical care to the point where even with health insurance coverage the population currently runs the risk of catastrophic loss. So-called "half way" technologies, or those which are very expensive relative to the measurable benefits that accrue to the patient because they do not definitively deal with the medical problem, seem to have further aggravated the problem of adequate risk-sharing through third party coverage. Further, even with the federal and voluntary programs now in effect, there is still a segment of the population, as noted earlier in the chapter, which falls between the eligibility cracks. A potential solution to these problems would be federally legislated universal entitlement with a mechanism to insure that every resident has access to some form of third-party coverage in practice as well as in theory. Universal entitlement might be coupled with a program of catastrophic health insurance coverage that is federally underwritten, or alternatively federally mandated but underwritten on a voluntary or mixed governmental and voluntary basis.

Another facet of the equity issue is the effect of redistribution of income as a result of policies followed in the financing of health services. There are three basic sources of revenue that have been described in this chapter: out-of-pocket payment for health services, premium payments by employers or employees, and tax revenues (primarily federal Social Security contributions and income taxes). The passage of a national health insurance plan, and its implementation, will result in changes in the relative money costs of health care to families at various income levels. The various proposals that have been put forth over the years differ substantially in their impact on families, with the regressive or progressive nature of a particular plan related not only to the use of a payroll tax versus the income tax (or general revenues), but also to the nature of mandated employer/employee paid premiums when this is part of the proposal, and the design of the benefit structure (yielding varying out-of-pocket burdens). It should be sufficient to note here that with expenditures for health services accounting for almost one-tenth of the Gross National Product, and assuming universal entitlement, the redistributive effects of any national health plan will be given serious consideration.

The broad issue of effectiveness includes the impact of third party coverage and reimbursement policies on the nature of the services that are encouraged or discouraged. Under the present system, the breadth and depth of coverage for inpatient care, coupled with cost reimbursement, has resulted in an increasing proportion of all health care expenditures being devoted to hospital care. It is interesting to note that in those parts of the country, particularly the West Coast, where third party coverage of out-of-hospital services and favorable reimbursement arrangements for physicians' care developed very early (in some cases prior to the establishment of Blue Cross) there is a markedly lower proportion of expenditures for hospital care, and a lower rate of growth in per capita hospital costs.

Third party coverage is an important factor in the issue of access to primary care. Beyond this, however, there is evidence to suggest that in large organized systems with enrolled populations, such as prepaid group practice, there appears to be a shift in resources from expensive and elaborate inpatient care to greater amounts of primary care, particularly for enrollees who are younger and healthier. In most parts of the country, however, the pattern is one of little or no coverage of preventive services and relatively poor coverage of routine ambulatory care generally.

At the other extreme, it is common to find substantial coverage for high-cost diagnostic and therapeutic technologies. Further, the apparent popularity of federally underwritten universal catastrophic coverage to address the problem of risk sharing, cited earlier in this section, would further encourage this disparity. Major efforts are only just getting underway to deal with the question of technology assessment in a manner that would give some guidance as to the effectiveness of various clinical strategies and therefore the merits of providing third party coverage in greater or lesser depth for particular types of services (as discussed in Chapter 8).

Under the general rubric of economy, an important factor is the cost-effectiveness of medical care. The present financing system removes much of the incentive for consideration of cost-effectiveness at the doctor-patient encounter level, as well as at the broader community or regional level. On the other hand, it is becoming clear that increases in total costs which exceed the growth rate of the economy as a whole are stirring the interest of a rather broad political coalition involving not only organized labor but industry as well. At the same time, the public has not been as conscious of rising personal health expenditures since ever-expanding third party coverage has kept out-of-pocket costs at a fairly stable level measured on a constant dollar basis. In other words, and as noted earlier in this chapter, costs have not been very visible to the consumer in comparison to the obvious increases in complexity, quality, and the amenity level of most health services. With respect to the latter, the public has rather high expectations which generally seem to be met.

Discussions of national health insurance up to the period of the late 1960s were almost exclusively concerned with improving risk-sharing across the community and providing better and more equitable access to care. In the last 10 years, however, at least equal if not greater attention has been directed toward the potential for cost containment and the correction of many of the market defects described in this chapter. As the debate has progressed, some have argued that it would be inflationary to implement a national health plan without first having firmly established a strong regulatory strategy designed to constrain both entry of capital into the health field and increases in hospital expenditures and, more generally, to promote cost effectiveness in the delivery of care. Others have argued that the only way to effectively implement such regulation is to incorporate it into a comprehensive national health insurance plan which both concentrates the dollars flowing into the system (through the federal government in order to provide more force to the regulatory effort) and makes the costs of the system more visible by such concentration.

More recently, the fundamental policy differences that have emerged address the relative merits of heavy regulation of the health care industry to contain costs, perhaps coupled with national health insurance, versus a restructuring of the system so as to rely on competition between voluntary health plans to provide a self-correcting market. Such plans would include both underwriting and delivery of care as exemplified by the HMO.

In reality, there is currently substantial regulation of the industry, as discussed in Chapters 5, 11, and 12, and no plausible system has been proposed that does not require a continuation of governmental regulation of some aspects of the field, including the framework within which market competition would take place. Similarly, even proposals that rely heavily on direct governmental financing and/or regulation must recognize that the forces of competition in the market will be at work, undoubtedly distorting the intended outcomes of any regulatory strategy.

To conclude this chapter, some of the problems with governmental under-writing and direct regulation on the one hand, and with the competitive market approach on the other are described. A good summary of the key weaknesses of the governmental approach is presented by Enthoven (16). In describing the weaknesses of the extreme case of a government monopoly on health insurance and therefore direct involvement of the government in regulation of the delivery system, Enthoven points out that: 1) Government differs from private enterprise in that it responds to well-focused producer interests whereas competitive markets respond to broad consumer interests, thus weighing decisions in the direction of the former rather than the latter interests; 2) Political decisions tend to be made on the basis of doing no direct harm but paying much less attention to indirect shortcomings. Because of this, government regulated systems are designed rigidly with bureaucrats having very limited discretion; 3) "When every dollar in the system is a federal dollar, what every dollar is spent on becomes a federal case" (17); 4) Government tends to encourage uniformity, which often means a bargained compromise that is satisfactory to no one; 5) If government were involved in direct provision of care it would face the weakness that it generally does a poor job of delivering direct services to individuals; 6) The government is not a cost-effective purchaser. This is partially a result of limitations on governmental employees in exercising their judgment; and 7) Government is disinclined to take chances and is intolerant of individuals' mistakes. This makes innovations within a governmental system difficult.

The alternate strategy would be to provide enough regulation to structure competitive markets in which comprehensive systems would be competing against one another (e.g., HMOs), and individuals would be responsible for enough of the premium payment as to encourage prudent selection among competing plans. To deal with some of the difficulties that have been described throughout this chapter, the regulatory framework for a competitive market model would need to include at least requirements regarding: 1) the information provided consumers; 2) open enrollment and premium rationing; and 3) minimum benefit packages. In addition, subsidies could be provided to assist those with lower incomes. This might be accomplished through vouchers to be used only for the purchase of health insurance. The remainder of the population might be provided partial payment for health insurance premiums either through tax credits or mandated employer payments, but would bear some substantial cost of the premium so as to encourage shopping for the most economical plan, given the family's quality preferences. It would be important to let premiums and/or health plan benefits vary so that the advantages of more efficient plans would accrue to the individuals making the choice within the market.

The principal difficulties with the market competition approach to improving upon the current financing of health services are two-fold: uncertainties with respect to provider response, and the degree to which there would be substantial competition (as opposed to a tendency toward ever-increasing industry norms for standards of operation and professional practice). Up to this point, providers have quite understandably been generally satisfied with the financial arrangements for health services. Certain organized comprehensive systems of care such as prepaid group practice have developed and grown in selected geographic areas, although the growth has not been as impressive as many would have liked. It has been argued that prepaid group practices are substantially more efficient than the rest of the medical care market because they must be in order to finance the more comprehensive benefits that are attractive to those who choose this approach to coverage and care. If competing systems offered equally comprehensive care but at higher premium levels, one could imagine the prepaid group practice or other HMO type system having little incentive to do other than ease the pressures toward efficiency allowing premiums to approach but not quite equal those of its competitors.

With respect to the impact of professional standards, even existing HMOs find it difficult to encourage the practice of substantially different styles of medicine than are found generally in the society. In a less highly organized system such as the individual practice association group norms would be weaker and greater reliance would have to be placed on financial incentives to providers. However, as was noted in an earlier section, it is not clear to what degree moderating financial incentives can offset the drive for more scientific, technological, and expensive patterns of diagnosis and treatment.

The coming years portend continued debate of the many issues raised in this chapter, and broader recognition of some of the underlying problems. The solutions to a number of the issues are incompatible, and all are politically sensitive. If it were otherwise, the country would probably have already come to grips with them, and would have adopted a coherent national policy on the financing of health services. These financing issues are among the central uncertainties in the continuing evolution of approaches to health planning and regulation as discussed in detail in the following chapters.

REFERENCES

1. Gibson RM, Fisher CR: National health expenditures, *Health Care Financing Review,* (Summer, 1979): 1-36.
2. Birnbaum H: *The Cost of Catastrophic Illness.* Lexington, MA, Lexington Books, 1978, pp. 1,2.
3. *Ibid,* p. 3.
4. Gibson RM, Mueller MS: National health expenditures, fiscal year 1976. *Social Security Bulletin* 40(4):3–22, 1977.
5. Scitovsky A, McCall N: *Changes in the Costs of Treatment of Selected Illnesses: 1951–1964–1971.* Research Digest Series, National Center for Health Statistics, U.S. Department of Health, Education, and Welfare, 1976.
6. Gibson, Fisher: National health expenditures, fiscal year 1977. *Social Security Bulletin* 41(7):3-620, 1978.
7. Somers AR: The high cost of health care for the elderly: diagnosis, prognosis, and some suggestions for therapy. *Journal of Health Politics, Policy and Law* 3(2):163–180, 1978.

8. *Ibid*, p. 163.

9. *Ibid*, p. 170.

10. Gibson, Fisher: National health expenditures, fiscal year 1977. *op cit.*, p. 9.

11. Jacobs P, Bauerschmidt AD, Furst RW: Hospital cost inflation and health insurance: a complex market model. *Inquiry* 15:217–224, 1978.

12. Mueller MS: Private health insurance in 1975: coverage, enrollment, and financial experience. *Social Security Bulletin* 40(6)3–21, 1977, p. 5.

13. *Ibid*, p. 5.

14. Robert Wood Johnson Foundation: *America's Health Care System: A Comprehensive Portrait. Robert Wood Johnson Foundation Special Report, No. 1.* Princeton, NJ, 1978.

15. Richardson WC: Group payment since the CCMC: policy implications of the ignored and the unforeseen. Mimeo. University of Washington, Seattle, WA, 1978.

16. Enthoven, AC: Consumer-choice health plan (Part One): Inflation and inequity in health care today--Alternatives for cost control and an analysis of proposals for National Health Insurance. *New England Journal of Medicine* **298**:650–658, 1978.

17. *Ibid.*, p. 655.

Part Five
Assessing
and Regulating
System Performance

CHAPTER 11

Health Services Planning and Regulation

Thomas W. Bice

In the post-World War II era, modern nations of all political and economic colorations have turned increasingly to planning and regulation to guide economic and social development (1). Expanding conceptions of the welfare state, imperatives of technological complexity and change, and unwanted consequences of industrialization and urbanization have given rise to new forms of collective rationality and control that extend over enlarging segments of economic and social life (2). Nowhere is this trend more evident than in modern nations' health services industries. While the basic forms of their organization and financing vary considerably among countries, all are being subjected to direction by mixtures of the market and of state planning and regulation (3).

This chapter reviews these trends as they have materialized in the United States. The discussion begins by defining planning and regulation and laying out the rationales underlying their use as social and economic instruments. Following this, historical sketches of major milestones in the development of planning and regulation aimed at improving the health industry's performance are discussed. In the concluding section, lessons and issues drawn from this nation's experiences with planning and regulation are tied together and speculation about where the United States appears to be heading and alternative future worlds is presented.

PLANNING AND REGULATION

DEFINITIONS

Rational action by collectivities involves four fundamental steps: 1) delineation of problems and objectives; 2) formulation and valuation of alternative means of attaining objectives; 3) implementation of chosen means; and 4) evaluation of program processes and impacts (4, 5). When performed by individuals, these steps constitute rational behavior, and when performed by groups, the entire process is ordinarily considered planning. This chapter makes a somewhat arbitrary distinction between the steps involving decision-making about problems, objectives, means, and program effectiveness, which are referred to as planning, and the implementation stage, which in most instances involves regulation.

Accordingly, planning is viewed as an essentially symbolic process, the results of which are statements of alternative ends and means, and choices among them. Regulation, by contrast, refers to a diverse set of means by which individuals or institutions are either induced or compelled to behave in specified ways.

RATIONALES FOR PLANNING AND REGULATION

The needs for planning and regulation arise from several features of modern industrialized nations, among them the increasing complexity and interdependence of relationships among specialized institutions; the expansion of the concept of the general welfare; and a variety of circumstances referred to as "market failures."

Modern industrialized nations are characteristically comprised of highly specialized institutions which, to accomplish their objectives, must coordinate activities. In countries whose political and economic institutions are based on the principles of political pluralism and free enterprise, the vast majority of such coordination is accomplished through market mechanisms, contractual agreements and, within the limits set by anti-trust laws, by private associations. Such arrangements minimize the need for government-sponsored planning when society collectively has no particular interest in what is produced and consumed and when other assumptions of the market are met.

Since no society is totally indifferent to the living conditions of its members or to the types of goods and services that are produced and consumed, government is charged with the functions and powers to protect persons' rights and to promote the general welfare (6). These functions and powers grow in proportion to the numbers and varieties of rights, entitlements, and other claims that citizens can legitimately make upon government. Faced with increasing claims, government has two broad alternatives: to provide goods and services directly or to induce or compel private actors to provide them (7). Socialist countries are inclined toward the former solution, and capitalist nations favor the latter. In either case, the amount and extensiveness of government-sponsored planning and control expand.

Another impetus for planning and regulation is a variety of "market failures." The presumption that market mechanisms will achieve a socially optimal allocation of goods and services rests on several assumptions that are untenable in particular situations, including the following:

1. that individuals know what they want and are able to make informed choices among alternative products;
2. that an individual's consumption decisions affect only himself or herself;
3. that people can select from products offered by a large number of independent suppliers; and

4. that suppliers bear the full costs of producing their products.

The first two assumptions pertain to consumers' abilities to make informed choices and to the consequences of their decisions for others. Instances of departures from these conditions abound in highly industrialized and urbanized nations, where consumers have only limited knowledge about many of the products they consume and where opportunities for "neighborhood effects" multiply. The lack of consumers' knowledge about pharmaceutical products, for instance, combine with the potential risks of learning by experimentation to lead government to plan and regulate the production and the distribution of drugs; and the harmful and bothersome pollutants emitted by automobiles lead government to require drivers to equip their vehicles with emission control devices.

The second pair of assumptions deals with the characteristics of a market's structure and so-called externalities of production. The former assumes that industries are comprised of large numbers of competitive suppliers who freely enter and leave markets and who independently decide what to produce and the prices they will charge for their products. The several circumstances that violate these assumptions call for planning and regulation. In situations where it is economically efficient for particular goods or services to be supplied by a single producer (e.g., natural monopolies), government applies public utility regulation to protect the public against monopolistic practices. In others, high costs of entry and other barriers limit the numbers of suppliers, or collusive decision-making among suppliers limits the ranges of products and prices available to consumers. Finally, as in the case of the polluting driver, government intervention is evoked by producers who externalize to the public such costs as those associated with environmental pollution.

The combination of these conditions within the health services industry makes it particularly subject to government planning and regulation (8). The composition of the industry and the nature of the demands made upon it cause it to be one of the more complex sectors of the economy, and trends of the past few decades have greatly increased the need for coordination. Advancements in medical knowledge and technology have created high degrees of specialization and segmentation within the medical profession and vast increases in the numbers and varieties of ancillary medical personnel and services. Concomitantly, the types and relative prevalences of health problems have changed from a preponderance of acute and infectious diseases to chronic, emotional, and social problems that require long-term management by other helping professionals and agencies as well as by traditional health care providers. Yet, the prevailing modes of organization and financing within the industry continue to reflect their roots in earlier periods and discourage voluntary coordination of the various levels and varieties of services that might better meet the needs of patients. Because the industry is dominated by private entrepreneurs, each being reimbursed independently for services provided, few incentives exist to encourage coordination and change. The industry is thus prone to continue oversupplying the highly sophisticated and expensive services of medical specialists and acute care hospitals, and undersupplying less technologically complex primary medical care and life support services.

The intimate relationships between health services and modern nations' notions of the general welfare also invite planning and regulation. Because health care is prominent among the necessities of life, all nations have established means to assure their citizens access to health services. In the United States this has prompted the federal and state governments to provide subsidies to consumers and suppliers of health services and to those who train health care personnel and conduct research, and to directly provide services to particular population groups. Because health services are cloaked in the public interest and because governments are paying growing shares of their costs, public pressure is brought to bear on governments to assure that services are equitably and efficiently allocated. Increasingly, those pressures are being manifested in more government-sponsored planning and regulation.

Finally, virtually all of the market failures that evoke planning and regulation apply to the health services industry. Given the complexity of medical knowledge and technology, few people are equipped to select among alternative modalities of treatment. Hence, patients essentially abdicate to physicians responsibilities for choosing the combinations of goods and services they consume. Even if consumers were able to make such decisions, extensive insurance coverage renders them virtually indifferent to the relative prices of alternative modes of treatment. On the suppliers' side, the industry is dominated by professions that limit entry into their ranks and discourage competitive pricing, and by hospitals that enjoy the status of non-profit community institutions. Neither physicians nor the hospitals bear the full costs of producing their services. In the case of physicians, they are typically free to employ the facilities and personnel of hospitals in the treatment of their patients without regard for the costs imposed on the hospitals. In turn, the now common practice of reimbursing hospitals retrospectively on the basis of their costs allows hospitals to pass these costs on to the insurers and, through them, to the public. In consequence, neither physicians nor hospitals would be expected to economize voluntarily.

Many of the features of the health services industry that invite planning and regulation were visible nearly a half century ago. Others have developed only rather recently. Despite changing circumstances, however, the appeals for comprehensive planning and greater coordination voiced in the opening decades of this century are strikingly similar to those heard today.

ORIGINS AND DEVELOPMENT OF HEALTH SERVICES PLANNING

Health services planning began in the United States in the 1930s as voluntary efforts and subsequently developed primarily under the auspices of the federal and state governments. Since the beginning of the federal government's involvement in the 1940s, the objectives, scope, and organization of planning have been largely determined by federal policy as expressed in five programs: The Hill-Burton Program, The Hospital Survey and Construction Act of 1946 (P.L. 79-725); The Regional Medical Programs, The Heart Disease, Cancer, and Stroke Act of 1965

(P.L. 89-239); The Comprehensive Health Planning Program, The Partnership for Health Act of 1967 (P.L. 90-174); The Experimental Health Services Delivery Program; and The National Health Planning and Resources Development Act of 1974. The provisions of the programs and the experiences of the processes they established are milestones in the transformation of health planning from its origins in elite-dominated, categorical planning to the present participatory, comprehensive planning, and from planning in the absence of regulation to the partial joining of these functions (9).

ORIGINS OF HEALTH PLANNING

Health services planning emerged in the United States in the 1930s, joining two elements that continue to shape the organization and objectives of planning. One established the organizational foundations of health planning in local voluntaristic groups. The other developed the idea of a regionalized health services system that remains to this day the ideal to which comprehensive health planning is directed.

Prior to the 1940s, health planning was limited to localized efforts aimed primarily at coordinating activities of municipal public health and welfare departments and hospitals. The attention of the health and welfare councils established to accomplish these ends focused on problems of providing services for the indigent rather than on fundamental reforms of the health services industry (10). The first organized attempt to deal specifically with such matters was initiated in the 1930s in New York City with the founding of the Hospital Council of Greater New York (11). The economic depression had produced severe overcrowding of municipal facilities that provided free services and depleted patient censuses in the voluntary hospitals. These and other conditions were documented in an extensive survey of hospitals, leading the group of prominent citizens that sponsored the study to recommend the establishment of a permanent planning body. A few other cities followed New York's example, urged by philanthropists interested in seeing that their contributions to hospitals were being wisely used (12).

Supported largely by philanthropic donations, these early planning agencies functioned outside the ambit of government. Their governing boards typically were comprised of influential citizens who oversaw the activities of their small staffs. Initially, planning concentrated almost exclusively on estimating the numbers of hospital beds needed in communities.

The concept of health services planning achieved national prominence in the early 1930s with the publication of findings and recommendations of the prestigious Commitee on the Costs of Medical Care. The Committee had been established in 1927 following a national conference on health care attended by leading physicians, social scientists, public health practitioners, and the lay public (13). With funds provided by several philanthropic foundations, the Committee undertook extensive studies of the use, organization, and financing of health services that culminated in 28 published reports and numerous staff papers. Among the Committee's principal conclusions was a recommendation calling for the establishment of local and state agencies for the purposes of conducting research and devising plans for coordinating health services. Further, the Committee presented a plan for organizing health services institutions and personnel in accordance with the principles of regionalization detailed in the Dawson Report issued 12 years earlier in the United Kingdom (14).

The notion of regionalization outlined in the Dawson Report and in the recommendations of the Committee on the Costs of Medical Care envisioned a division of functions among hospitals, clinics, and medical personnel based on vertically integrated levels of specialization and intensity of services. Choices of sites of care and the placement of patients would be dictated by the levels of services required. The beginnings of such arrangements were already recognizable in Sweden and Denmark by the opening of this century, and the idea has been adopted as a guiding principle for health planning in the United Kingdom and elsewhere.

The rationales offered for health services planning in the 1930s and early 1940s combined several notions that appealed to deeply rooted social values. As practiced in New York City and later in Rochester (New York), Detroit, and Pittsburgh, planning was a voluntary endeavor in which leading citizens and health care providers applied the tools of business management to attain greater efficiency and improved health care. Moreover, the concept of regionalization embodied ultimate designs of rationality and offered possibilities for resolving the then pressing problem of providing health services to the nation's small towns and rural areas.

THE HILL-BURTON PROGRAM

The Second World War and its aftermath placed health services planning on the public agenda as the Great Depression had done the decade before. Concerns about the educational and physical fitness of the population raised by findings from examinations of military inductees led to a Senate inquiry into the adequacy of the nation's health services and their bearing upon the health of the population. Pursuant to its charge, the Subcommittee on Wartime Health and Education conducted hearings at which the then Surgeon General of the United States Public Health Service proposed establishing planning agencies throughout the country to guide the development of "coordinated hospital systems" (15). His testimony and subsequent discussions with members of the Subcommittee clearly evidenced the influence of the Dawson Report and, although the label attached to his proposal referred specifically to "coordinated hospitals," the plan itself extended to virtually all aspects of contemporary comprehensive health planning.

Following the War the conditions of hospitals prompted the federal government to establish the nation's first major health services planning and construction subsidy program. Having suffered two decades of neglect imposed first by the Depression and then by the War, the country's stock of hospital facilities was obsolete and unevenly distributed; and wartime migrations of people from rural areas to cities, rapid population growth, and rising construction costs strained the private sector's ability to make needed improvements. In response, the Congress enacted the Hospital Survey and Construction Act of 1946, discussed in Chapter 5, a two-part law that provided funds for states to:

1. inventory their existing hospitals, to survey the need for construction of hospitals, and to develop programs for construction of such public and other non-profit hospitals as will, in conjunction with existing facilities, afford the necessary physical facilities for furnishing adequate hospitals, clinics, and similar services to all people; and

2. construct public and other non-profit hospitals in accordance with such programs (16).

The avowed purpose of the program was to eliminate shortages of hospitals, particularly in the nation's rural and economically depressed regions. This objective was incorporated in the formula devised to allocate funds among the states and, within the states, in the fixed bed-to-population ratios used to identify underserved areas. Over its more than twenty years of operation, the program was successful in distributing construction funds to hospitals and, as the shortage of hospital beds diminished, the act was repeatedly amended to extend its benefits to hospital modernization and replacement, and later to neighborhood health centers and emergency rooms. Additionally, the thought that increasing the numbers of hospitals in rural areas would entice physicians to locate in them appears in retrospect to have had at least some validity (17).

The record of Hill-Burton in planning and inducing coordination among hospitals is less favorable, however. The program was administered in each state by an agency of state government assisted by an advisory Hospital Planning Council typically comprised of hospital administrators and representatives of trade associations and local government agencies. These councils reviewed applications for grants and provided other assistance. In view of their members' ties to the industry, one would not have expected them to be vigorous proponents of major changes, and, even if they had been so, Hill-Burton agencies faced other problems that limited their ability to plan and coordinate. Initially, they were provided few resources with which to plan. Consequently, their decisions on whether to award grants to particular applicant hospitals were often made without the benefit of well-formulated guidelines (18). Furthermore, agencies' purviews encompassed only a minority of the nation's hospitals, and their authorities to enforce compliance with plans were strictly circumscribed. An applicant whose request for assistance was denied was free to engage in construction projects using funds from other sources, and those who were either ineligible for subsidies or chose not to apply for them were outside the agency's control altogether.

Despite these limitations, the program provided states with at least some experience in planning hospital facilities and in dealing with the difficult problems of defining and estimating populations' needs for hospital beds. The replacement of the bed-to-population formula by a more sensitive indicator of need represented an important advancement in the techniques of planning, and the grants for research and demonstration programs authorized in 1964 stimulated investigation into a variety of issues pertaining to the structure and dynamics of hospitals.

By the early 1970s, however, history had reversed itself: the problem of shortages of hospital beds had been eclipsed by concerns about their oversupply.

Hence, Hill-Burton's *raison d'etre* evaporated, as had its focal role of planning with the establishment of the Regional Medical Programs and Comprehensive Health Planning Program in the mid-1960s. In 1974, the Hill-Burton authority was allowed to expire, and its few remaining functions were incorporated in the National Health Planning and Resources Development Act.

REGIONAL MEDICAL PROGRAMS

Among the enduring problems of the American health services industry has been the variance in the quality of health services rendered in the nation's medical research and teaching centers versus that provided by community-based practitioners. Once licensed upon completion of their training, physicians find it difficult and have few incentives to stay abreast of new discoveries and improved techniques. Medical schools, in turn, have had little contact with community-based providers. Throughout this century the lacuna has widened, as specialization has accelerated the growth of medical knowledge (19).

To remedy this situation, Congress enacted in 1965 an amendment to the Public Health Service Act intended, among other purposes, "to encourage and assist in the establishment of regional cooperative arrangements among medical schools, research institutions, and hospitals, for research and training (including continuing education) and related demonstrations of patient care" (20). The law was an outgrowth of a report by the President's Commission on Heart Disease, Cancer, and Stroke, which had been empanelled to make recommendations regarding the control and treatment of these three dreaded diseases (21). Upon completion of its task, the Commission envisioned the establishment of regional centers through which advanced technology would be channeled to communities from research and training institutions, and where services would be delivered and community-based physicians informed of new techniques through continuing education.

The amendment, however, authorized considerably less than the Commission had recommended. The program was essentially stripped of its services providing authorities and, thereby, was transformed primarily into a grants-in-aid program (22). Powerful interest groups, particularly the American Medical Association, opposed the federal government's sponsoring centers that would compete with local practitioners in the practice of medicine. Hence, the compromises required to attain passage led to a program that was to coordinate services without interfering with existing patterns of health services delivery.

The Regional Medical Programs Act was implemented by Regional Advisory Groups (RAGs) constituted in 56 regions. Comprised of representatives of medical schools, teaching hospitals, state and local health departments, private practitioners, and the general public, RAGs were charged with devising plans and authorizing expenditures of federal grant monies for innovative programs. Thus, the Regional Medical Programs were to enhance coordination and integration of health services through a voluntary, pluralistic mechanism that decentralized decision-making directly from the federal government to the 56 RAGs, which were dominated by the interests of providers, particularly by those of the medical schools and teaching hospitals. Although most of the regions embodied portions of various states, state governments were given no role in the program's implementation or funding.

As the substance of Regional Medical Programs was left within broad limits to local determination, considerable variation occurred in both their structures and activities. In consequence, as Glaser notes (23), it became increasingly difficult over time to characterize the program's national purposes (24). The RAGs stimulated federally-funded demonstrations of a variety of innovations, including continuing education for physicians and training for ancillary personnel. However, no overlapping plans appeared in any of the 56 regions. When other local planning agencies began to be established pursuant to the Partnership for Health Amendments of 1967, the Regional Medical Programs' stated goals shifted from concern with specific diseases to the promotion of comprehensive health services. Federal monies were then made available through the Programs for several types of system-oriented demonstrations, prominent among them efforts to develop and improve emergency medical services (25). In Glaser's words, "the Regional Medical Programs became an effort to obtain federal money for worthy projects rather than a disciplined system for framing and implementing plans" (26).

Because the Regional Medical Programs Act was popular among the nation's medical schools and teaching hospitals, it was able to withstand the Nixon Administration's attempts to abolish it. However, in 1974 the program was swept with Hill-Burton and other planning efforts under the umbrella National Health Planning and Resources Development Act, and shortly thereafter the Regional Medical Programs became extinct.

THE COMPREHENSIVE HEALTH PLANNING PROGRAM

Although the federal government had attempted to promote planning and coordination of health services through Hill-Burton and the Regional Medical Programs, it had done so following categorical approaches. Hill-Burton dealt only with construction of and planning for facilities; the Regional Medical Programs ostensibly concentrated, at least at the outset, on particular diseases. No agency had responsibility for overall, comprehensive health planning. Only one year after enactment of the Regional Medical Programs' legislation, Congress moved to fill this void. The instrument was to be a network of voluntary comprehensive health planning agencies with mandates to develop long-range, statewide, and local plans for environmental as well as personal health services.

As with the Regional Medical Programs, Comprehensive Health Planning legislation was preceded by a report of a national commission that called for more sweeping roles and authorities than were ultimately incorporated in the authorizing statute (27). "Planning" was defined as an " action process" in which councils would not only devise blueprints, but also would take steps to implement their plans. Based on careful and extensive study of health service needs and through exercise of their pluralistic influence, councils were to effect major and permanent changes in health services delivery (29).

However, legislation authorizing the program, like the Regional Medical Programs before it, specified that planning was to be accomplished without interfering with the prevailing patterns of medical practice. This constraint and the absence of any regulatory authority over health services institutions left Comprehensive Health Planning agencies created under the act devoid of official powers to pursue "active planning" as defined by the National Commission. In effect, these agencies were given the mandate to develop plans but were prevented from implementing them.

Comprehensive Health Planning (CHP) was organized in two layers. Each participating state established a statewide—CHP(a)—agency to oversee planning throughout the state. At the local level, areawide—CHP(b)—agencies were responsible for planning within designated regions. Plans developed by these so-called "b" agencies were to be reviewed by the umbrella "a" agency and incorporated in its statewide plan.

Unlike the Regional Medical Programs, Comprehensive Health Planning was structured as a cooperative effort among the federal and state governments and local areas rather than as a direct federal to local decentralization. Moreover, the Partnership for Health Amendments reflected the policy of encouraging maximum feasible participation that was incorporated in much of the social legislation of the 1960s. CHP(a) agencies were to be advised by councils comprised of not less than 51% consumer members. Similarly, CHP(b) agencies were to be voluntary corporations with equivalently constituted boards. To preserve local autonomy, CHP agencies were funded by formula grants in which federal monies were to be augmented by contributions from state and local shares, which were divided about evenly (30).

It is generally agreed that CHP agencies were unable to accomplish all of their intended aims. Although empirical data on improvements in health levels, health care costs, and the like attributable to CHP planning are virtually nonexistent (31), observations accumulated since 1967 on the organization and process of planning in various sites suggest that CHP was structurally, fiscally, and politically unable to bring about the kinds of changes that are required to significantly affect major trends in the costs, quality, and accessibility of health services (32). Few statewide or areawide agencies were able to develop long-range plans; most lacked the resources to gather information to develop them, and few had the power to enforce compliance with their recommendations. As a result, CHP agencies existed on the fringes of the major forces that shape the nation's health services industry. They attempted to plan in a turbulent and recalcitrant environment, while the power to act remained in the hands of institutions and associations that comprised their memberships and provided local funds.

During the late 1960s and early 1970s, CHP agencies began to acquire advisory roles in federal and state regulatory processes. In keeping with its New Federalism policy, the Nixon Administration delegated to CHP agencies the function of reviewing and commenting on requests for federal Public Health Service grants by institutions within their jurisdictions. Also, several states assigned advisory roles to CHP agencies in their implementation of certificate-of-need controls (33). However, for the most part, CHP agencies continued to practice "consensus planning," lacking the "teeth" to move forcefully to the implementation stage. Moreover, by the early 1970s, it had become apparent to officials in the Nixon Administration that federal agencies engaged in planning had become as confused as the health services industry itself. On that point, the then Secretary of the Department of Health, Education, and Welfare remarked that:

> . . . six years ago, the federal government attempted to systematize and bolster planning efforts by creating and funding state and local comprehensive health agencies (sic). Today, all states and territories have comprehensive health planning agencies. And more than 170 local and areawide agencies now serve about 70 percent of the nation's population.
>
> But from their inception, these agencies have been underfunded and understaffed. Even more pertinent, they haven't had any real authority to coordinate planning. They have served principally as advisory groups and, while some can claim successes here and there, for the most part, their advice has been ignored.
>
> Thus we see a planning system in which, as with its operational counterpart, interrelationships among functions are very poorly thought out—if any real thought has even been given to the possibility of interrelationships—and which is thus hopelessly confusing and sometime duplicative and overlapping.
>
> It is, again, a "non-system" incapable of either rationally identifying shortfalls or gaps in performance or of rationally addressing needs (34).

Dedicated to the elimination of programs that "don't work" and to streamlining the federal bureaucracy (35), the Nixon Administration had sought to combine the Regional Medical Programs and the Comprehensive Health Planning Program under a single authority. Its proposal, submitted to the Congress as the "National Health Care Improvement Act of 1970," had failed, leaving these programs intact as separate entities. The consolidation was ultimately accomplished with the enactment of the National Health Planning and Resources Development Act of 1974, when Comprehensive Health Planning gave way to a more vigorous form of planning linked to regulatory controls.

THE EXPERIMENTAL HEALTH SERVICES DELIVERY PROGRAM

The federally sponsored health services planning programs described to this point shared an important feature: the principal impetus behind each was the federal government's recognition of deficiencies *within* the health services industry. By the late 1960s, however, other elements were becoming visible as sources of concern to the federal government, namely, the so-called "bureaucracy problem" (36) and rapidly escalating health care costs stemming from the Medicare and Medicaid programs. Hence, several problems within the health services industry were increasingly being attributed to the federal government's involvement. Such recognitions gave rise to yet another planning effort, the Experimental Health Services Delivery System (EHSDS) program.

The EHSDS program grew out of attempts to reorganize the internal affairs of the federal bureaucracy and its dealings with local communities. Beginning with the Johnson Administration's War on Poverty in the early 1960s and continuing throughout the decade, Congress enacted a landslide of health legislation that vastly increased the federal government's administrative responsibilities (37). Characteristically, programs bypassed the states, going directly to "targeted" areas in which local groups dealt directly with federal agencies (38, 39). A variety of demonstration authorities had established health centers for the impoverished—first under the Office of Economic Opportunity and later others under the Partnership for Health Programs—migrant workers' health centers, maternal and infant care centers, mental health centers, and Model Cities health clinics. All were supported with federal funds administered by newly created or expanded federal agencies (40).

Several of these agencies were brought together in 1968 under the administration of the newly created Health Services and Mental Health Administration (HSMHA). Established as part of a general reorganization of the health activities of the Department of Health, Education, and Welfare (41), HSMHA's nine agencies and Fiscal Year 1970 budget of $1,300,000,000 made it one of the three largest federal organizations concerned exclusively with health and health services (42, 43, 44).

Impressive as the scope of activities subsumed under HSMHA was, the creation of the agency by no means solved all the problems of disorganization among the federal government's health programs. Most of the government's health effort, as measured by budgets, remained with other agencies, (e.g., Medicare and Medicaid), and each of HSMHA's programs operated under Congressional authorizations that defined at least in general terms how their appropriations were to be allocated. HSMHA was not an integrated agency with a set of well-ordered priorities or abilities to combine budgets and personnel of its member programs. It was, rather, a confederation of programs, each with its own purposes, procedures, constituencies, and interests (45).

The need for transforming HSMHA's disparate functions and programs into a coherent whole gave impetus to ideas that ultimately led to the EHSDS program. A solution that emerged was the notion of "conjoint funding": HSMHA programs were to increase their efficiency by working together and, more importantly, by pooling their resources and delegating allocative decisions to local groups.

Within HSMHA, the National Center for Health Services Research and Development (NCHSR&D) was designated as the "lead agency" to develop the EHSDS program. NCHSR&D was a newly established agency whose principal mission was to provide grants and contracts for research into and development of health services (44). The agency came to view EHSDS as the ultimate embodiment of rationality and as a mechanism for bringing together various innovations being developed and tested under its grants and contracts (45). In selected states and communities, systemwide planning based on research and development was to combine with the rational allocation of funds by local management agencies, that is, EHSDS corporations. These funds were to be channelled from various federal agencies directly to the management corporations, thus eliminating federal agencies' direct administrative involvement in determining the uses of federal monies in local communities.

To accomplish these aims, in 1971 NCHSR&D established twelve EHSDS corporations scattered throughout the United States, and six others were added the following year. Like Comprehensive Health Planning "b" agencies, EHSDS corporations were voluntary, nonprofit corporations. Unlike the "b" agencies, however, boards of EHSDS corporations were mandated to include representatives of four interests groups (the "4 P's")—public, providers, payers (i.e., insurance companies and government agencies), and politicians—in proportions such that no group consituted a majority.

While EHSDS members could also participate on Comprehensive Health Planning and Regional Medical Program boards, the EHSDS corporations were to remain corporately distinct from these and other agencies. NCHSR&D developed a triangular model of the division of labor among Regional Medical Programs, Comprehensive Health Planning, and EHSDS bodies. Regional Medical Programs were seen as instruments of providers to develop and test innovations in the delivery of health services. Comprehensive Health Planning agencies would, in turn, incorporate these ideas in their long-range plans and communicate to the Regional Medical Programs the issues that planners deemed important for research and development. EHSDS bodies would then incorporate these priorities in their shorter term investment decisions. In sum NCHSR&D envisioned a network of cooperative and mutually facilitating exchanges among the three planning and coordinating bodies.

As the EHSDS experiment proceeded, none of the prerequisites required for its full implementation materialized. Each EHSDS site was given two years to charter a conforming corporate body and to conduct community surveys and other studies with which to establish priorities. Meanwhile, NCHSR&D and HSMHA endeavored to conjoin funds of HSMHA and other federal agencies and to deliver these to EHSDS corporations. No such conjoining occurred, however. As might have been expected, other HSMHA agencies resisted NCHSR&D's urgings to delegate funding decisions to EHSDS bodies and declined even to give EHSDS communities priority claims upon their funds. In consequence, the principal functions of the EHSDS corporations were vitiated, and their activities became increasingly indistinguishable locally from those of Comprehensive Health Planning and Regional Medical Programs. Instead of mutual cooperation and coordination, conflict and duplication characterized the triangle of agencies. On this point, in 1974 the Acting Associate Director for Health Resources Planning of the Bureau of Health Resources Development observed that the EHSDS experiment demonstrated that communities will accept federal funds when they are offered and will engage in conflict when competing programs are established (48).

While the EHSDS experiment failed to attain its principal objectives, it introduced a new element into the evolving debate about health planning that had reemerged in the early 1970s, and it contributed valuable experience to the body of planning methods. The experiment's focus on implementation and systemwide management of conjoined federal funds—although none were forthcoming—was in marked contrast to the long-range perspectives of Comprehensive Health Planning and the narrower, categorical interests of the Regional Medical Programs. Also, EHSDS' emphasis upon linking decisions to thorough empirical research on communities' health services needs and utilization and their flows of health services monies was notably different from the paucity of such information in most Comprehensive Health Planning agencies. Indeed, the vision of regional health authorities not unlike those in the United Kingdom that underlay the EHSDS ideology anticipated by several years contemporary debate about the roles of current planning agencies in gathering and analyzing data and in implementing regulatory controls.

The experiment never gained the support of officials in the Nixon Administration, who in 1973 ordered its orderly termination. Lacking explicit legislative authorization, the EHSDS program thus died within the bureaucracy, causing little comment. With Hill-Burton and the two other sides of the planning/innovation-management triangle, EHSDS corporations closed their doors shortly after the enactment of P.L. 93-641.

THE NATIONAL HEALTH PLANNING AND RESOURCES DEVELOPMENT ACT OF 1974

The National Health Planning and Resources Development Act of 1974 (P.L. 93-641) is currently the nation's principal health planning legislation. It embodies several features that attempt to deal with inadequacies of its predecessors and, as experience accumulates, the programs that it has established will undoubtedly evolve into still newer forms.

As Klarman has observed, P.L. 93-641 mandates several improvements of the planning structure and process (49). The law preserves the two-tiered state and regional structure of Comprehensive Health Planning and reinforces the policy of participatory planning, adding two new layers. Health Systems Agencies (HSAs) are at the base of the structure as were the "b" agencies before. These HSAs are constituted as nonprofit corporations or government agencies with boards comprised of representatives of the "4 Ps"—public, providers, payers and politicians—the majorities of whom are consumer representatives. HSAs are charged with fulfilling a variety of functions whose objectives and means are detailed in the statute. An HSA's principal mission is to develop plans for its Health Services Area and to communicate these plans to counterpart agencies higher in the structure, specifically to the State Health Planning and Development Agency (SHPDA), which is analogous to the previous "a" agency, and to the intermediate State Health Coordinating Committee (SHCC). The latter is a new element mandated by P.L. 93-641 that serves as an advisory body to the SHPDA, and is constituted in part by representatives of regional HSAs and in part by persons appointed by the state's governor. Finally, the law establishes a National Health Planning Council at the federal level charged with advising the Secretary of the Department of Health, Education, and Welfare on the national health planning goals and standards that he is directed to formulate and disseminate.

The statute also explicitly defines the expected products of each layer of this structure and the means to be employed in arriving at them. Most important in this respect is the requirement that each agency generate not only long-range comprehensive plans (e.g., Health Systems Plans, State Health Plans, and State Health Facilities Plans) but formulate as well shorter-range plans for implementing components of the longer-range plans (e.g., Annual Implementation Plans). All plans are supposed to be based on current quantitative information about populations' health services needs and about the accessibility, availability, costs, and quality of health services.

The basic program is funded on a formula basis entirely with federal revenues, with allowances for additional federal matching of contributions by state and local governments and other permissible donors. The latter excludes named groups and organizations whose contributions might be construed as constituting conflicts of interest (e.g., individual hospitals).

Finally, the program places planning and regulatory functions within a single structure. Each participating state is required to enact a certificate-of-need law that conforms with federal guidelines and to establish within its SPHDA means of determining which proposals from designated health care institutions for capital investments and changes in service will be certified as conforming with needs documented in the state's health plans. Failing that, the agency is to deny the request and enforce its decision. Similarly, grants to hospitals and other health care institutions provided for by Title XVI of the act are to be in conformance with needs documented in separate facilities plans. In each of these processes, the SHPDA is to heed advice from the SHCC and from the HSA, which conducts prior reviews of proposals emanating from its jurisdiction.

Because P.L. 93-641, as originally written, was extremely explicit as to both ends and means and placed a great deal of authority in the Office of the Secretary of the Department of Health, Education, and Welfare, the program has occasioned considerable debate and resistance at each stage of its implementation. Several state governors who found portions of their states being joined in HSAs with portions of other states challenged the Department's designations of Health Services Areas. Some entered with the American Medical Association and other parties into suits alleging that the law's certificate-of-need provisions violate constitutional guarantees of states' rights by coercing (through the threat of terminating particular federal health subsidies) states to enact such regulatory programs. Still others challenged the compositional requirements of HSAs and SHCCs, and the issuance of the first set of planning guidelines detailing quantitative criteria for hospital beds and other health services per population (50) evoked a veritable flood of dissenting comments.

To date, the courts have consistently ruled in favor of P.L. 93-641 in cases based on fundamental constitutional issues and on the Secretary's authority to implement the law's various features (51). Other legal matters are certain to arise, however. For instance, the antitrust implications of planning agencies' both serving as parties to regulatory decisions and assisting particular health care institutions in the formulation of plans have yet to be considered in detail. Meanwhile, the planning and regulatory system created by P.L. 93-641 is evolving throughout the nation, undoubtedly at varying paces and in somewhat different directions among the states and localities (52). While speculation abounds as to whether P.L. 93-641 is on balance desirable or undesirable, little is known about its benefits and costs. These are difficult matters to measure for broad-aimed, multiple-objective planning programs (53), and the difficulty is compounded by the rush of regulatory fervor that swept through the federal and several state governments in the early 1970s.

ORIGINS AND DEVELOPMENT OF HEALTH SERVICES REGULATION

It was noted at the outset of this chapter that regulation subsumes a variety of instruments by which government induces or compels persons to engage in (or refrain from) behaviors that promote (or are injurious to) some aspect of the public interest or general welfare. The objectives pursued through regulation embrace a large and growing set of socially desirable ends, including directing the development of entire industries and sectors of the economy, and protecting individuals from a host of hazards accompanying modern life (54, 55). The means available to government to pursue such ends are nearly limitless, ranging from subsidies provided either indirectly through tax policies or directly through cash transfers to direct command and control mechanisms enforced by varieties of legal and economic sanctions (56). Further, the types of agencies involved in the implementation of regulatory programs defy simple enumeration. All branches of government—legislative, executive, and judicial—are directly implicated (57), and in many instances basically private bodies are enlisted into governments' regulatory efforts (58).

In view of this complexity, one cannot hope to comprehend either the entirety of regulation within the United States or even its totality within a single sector of the nation's economy (59). Accordingly, the discussion that follows is selective and highlights the general features of, and trends in, regulation rather than attempting to comprehensively plunge into the details of the highly fluid and uncertain regulatory environment surrounding the health services industry.

Specifically, the origins and development of three types of regulation that rather recently have been imposed upon the health services industry are examined: 1) capital expenditures and services (CES) controls, 2) utilization review as practiced by the Professional Standards Review Organizations (PRSROs), and 3) prospective rate setting applied to hospitals and nursing homes. Each of these programs is intended, *inter alia,* to contain health care cost inflation, and each contributes an ingredient to a whole that approximates public utility regulation as applied in other industries (60). Before proceeding to these particular forms of regulation, the principal types of regulation are briefly described and illustrated to alert the reader to the proportions of the discussion's selectivity.

TYPES OF REGULATION

In the interest of simplicity, Figure 11–1 is presented to roughly categorize and illustrate types of regulatory instruments that are operative in the health services industry. The four fundamental instruments in the rows of the figure are:

1. subsidies
2. entry controls
3. rate or price setting, and
4. quality controls (61).

Objects of Regulation

	Individuals	Institutions

Subsidies	Supply
	   Training grants
	
	Demand
	   Medicare / Medicaid
	   Tax exemptions
		Supply
		   Construction grants, loans,
		   loan guarantees
		   Tax exemptions
		Demand
		   Tax exemptions to
		   employers

Entry Restrictions	Personnel licensure	Facilities licensure Capital expenditures controls

Rate
Controls
	Fee schedules under
	   Medicaid & the Economic
	   Stabilization Program
		Rate setting commissions
		   Medicare and Medicaid
		   reimbursement limits

Quality Controls	Professional Standards Review Organization	Certification for Medicare and Medicaid

Regulatory Instruments

Figure 11–1. A typology of regulatory instruments and examples from the health services industry.

The columns classify objects of regulation as natural and corporate persons.

Subsidies are generally the oldest and most widespread means employed by governments to regulate the supplies of, and demand for, health services. These take many forms. On the supply side, governments have conferred tax exempt status upon voluntary, nonprofit hospitals and nursing homes and have provided them with direct grants, loans, and loan guarantees for construction, renovation, and modernization. Likewise, governments support the training of health services professionals and the conduct of health-related research and development and have made available construction subsidies to institutions that engage in training and research. On the demand side, tax credits offered to employees and employers defray the costs of health insurance and, above specified limits, individuals' health care expenditures are exempted from the personal income tax. Governments also act as third parties for the aged under Medicare, for the impoverished under Medicaid, and increasingly for persons receiving treatment for chronic, catastrophic diseases (e.g., end stage renal disease).

Ordinarily, subsidy programs are accompanied by administrative regulations that define eligibility criteria, specify the legitimate uses of subsidies and, increasingly, define terms of trade. Examples of the latter are provisions of the Hill-Burton program requiring hospitals to provide specified volumes of "free care" in return for government grants, and sections of personnel training legislation that establish for medical schools target mixes of types of physicians to be educated and for trainees "forgiveness clauses." Furthermore, it should be noted that the principal of the nonexistence of free lunches applies to all subsidy programs and, under current fiscal constraints, increasingly so. That is, eligibility requirements and definitions of scopes of goods and services covered by subsidy programs often entail for both givers and receivers considerable administrative costs in the forms of paperwork and "red tape" (61).

Entry controls apply to producers. They generally seek to limit persons' abilities to offer particular goods or services to those who have satisfied at least minimal tests of competence or character or to those whose products are needed in their communities. In the case of health personnel and facilities, these controls take the familiar forms of licensure and certification. More pertinent to the discussion below, capital expenditures and services controls are applied to health care institutions to assure the public that offerings of health services are balanced with communities' needs.

Rate or price setting authorities are usually assumed by governments as a *quid pro quo* for protection afforded producers in markets that are subject to mandated entry restrictions or in industries where government is the dominant (i.e., monopsonistic) purchaser of their outputs. The former rationale is applied most purely in so-called natural monopolistic markets such as those found in the production and distribution of electrical power and local telephone services. In these and similar situations, where a sole producer is optimally efficient, governments protect monopolies from competition by restricting entry and, in turn, protect the public from the monopolies by controlling their rates and the quality of their products. The latter rationale—that of the government monopsony—appears to underlie the imposition of price controls in the health services industry, even where governments are not the principal purchasers of its services. In the inpatient sector of the industry, such controls are universally applied by states to nursing homes, and various combinations of voluntary and state-mandated rate setting efforts are imposed on hospitals in about a dozen states.

The category of "quality controls" subsumes various regulatory mechanisms aimed at reducing adverse risks and other socially undesirable practices associated with the product or consumption of goods and services. This class is frequently labelled "social regulation," as opposed to "economic regulation," which embraces the other types of controls described above (62, 63). Especially prominent among the group of social regulations are efforts to eliminate hazards in workplaces, environmental pollution, and other so-called external costs of production, and to assure the safety and efficacy of consumer goods and services. These controls differ from entry restrictions, some of which attempt to assure quality, in that they apply to all designated suppliers whether or not they exist in markets with entry controls. In the health services industry, for instance, hospitals, like all other firms, must comply with construction and fire codes, fair employment rules, and environmental pollution standards. Further, the Food and Drug Administration's reviews of the safety of drug products and PSROs' scrutiny of physicians practices are intended, respectively, to assure consumers that the drugs they ingest and the medical services they receive are at least not injurious to their health or proffered fraudulently.

Having summarily dispensed with a great deal of the regulatory apparatus that affects portions of the health services industry, the focus can turn to features of the structure and financing of hospital services that have prompted the imposition of entry restrictions and "quality" and price controls.

THE BASES OF CONTROLS ON HOSPITALS

Hospitals are the principal targets of regulatory programs, as discussed in Chapter 5, aimed at controlling health care cost inflation (64). This may be due to the hospital industry's large and growing share of the nation's health care expenditures. It accounts for about 40% of the total and has been increasing annually at a rate of approximately 15%. It may also reflect tradition and political forces. As discussed previously, hospitals have been the major focus of the health planning movement from its inception. Since the regulatory movement now afoot builds on that tradition, it follows that controls on hospitals would be the first to appear. It is also the case, as noted in Chapter 5, that hospitals have historically been a less potent political force than physicians and, therefore, are correspondingly more vulnerable to government intervention. Alternatively, if one takes the view that regulatory controls—particularly entry restrictions—are sought by industries to thwart competition, it might be argued that physicians' greater power was exercised earlier in this century in the establishment of their cartel and that hospitals have only recently been able to accomplish this feat (65). Regardless of one's conception of the origins of regulation, the fact remains that the newest forms of regulation concentrate on hospitals.

The principal problem that has stimulated regulation of hospitals is cost inflation attributable to inefficiencies in the industry. Basically, two related types of argument are advanced: 1) that hospitals "overinvest" in sophisticated and expensive services and 2) that such services are "overutilized" by the population (66). The overinvestment and overutilization, in turn, result in "unnecessary" expenditures for health services that contribute wastefully to cost inflation.

Recalling the earlier comments on the structure and financing of the health services industry, several features of the market for inpatient hospital services appear to warrant regulation. Specifically, assuming consumer ignorance, four features combine to justify regulation: 1) the nonprofit status of most hospitals; 2) their relationships with community-based physicians; 3) the so-called "Roemer Law" (more generally the availability effect); and 4) insurance.

The hospital industry is dominated by multi-product, nonprofit firms whose investment and output decisions are amalgams of interests of their communities, lay boards of trustees, management, and medical staffs. Because hospitals must be responsive to the demands of these various constituencies, their investment decisions reflect considerations other than profit maximization. Among the various objectives attributed to hospitals by economists are prestige and status (67), the quality and quantity of services produced (68), and social welfare (69). While all such specifications are conceived as being subject to the constraint that revenues must cover costs, all imply that nonprofit hospitals' investment and output decisions do not conform to the model of a pure profit-maximizer.

Related to these observations is the argument that hospitals' investment and output decisions are strongly influenced by physicians' preferences (70, 71). Because physicians select both the hospitals into which their patients are admitted and the mixes of services patients receive, they exert pressures on hospitals to provide the types and amounts of facilities, services, and support personnel that they desire. These pressures join with competition among hospitals for prestige to encourage investment in expansion and, more importantly, in upgrading styles of care (72). Moreover, the role of the physician as both an advocate for the patient and an entrepreneur invites conflicts of interest that apparently are frequently resolved in favor of the entrepreneurial segment (73). As physicians' incomes are enhanced by their use of hospital services, whose costs are paid by insurance, one would expect them to give little attention to hospital cost inflation (74).

The availability effect observed in the hospital industry protects the hospital from losses due to investment in facilities and services for which demand is low (75). In effect, this phenomenon implies that the availability of health services stimulates their use. Hence, within limits, hospitals can expand capacity and services with the assurance that additional beds will be filled, and services will be used.

Insurance for hospital services affects hospital investment in two ways. First, the typically more extensive coverage of inpatient services versus those rendered in ambulatory care settings shifts patients into hospitals, where, due to low deductibles and co-insurance rates, patients pay out-of-pocket only a small portion of their charges. Patients are therefore relatively indifferent to costs incurred at the time of treatment. Second, retrospective cost-based reimbursement schemes protect hospitals from losses that might otherwise occur from poor investment decisions. Together, the assurances of high cash flows due to the availability effect and insurance and the guaranteed retroactive payment of costs (including debt service) place hospitals in favored positions in the capital market (76, 77). This, in turn, facilitates more investment. The three types of regulation discussed next are intended to rectify the consequences of these structural and financial characteristics.

CAPITAL EXPENDITURES AND SERVICE CONTROLS

Capital expenditures and services (CES) controls attempt to eliminate unnecessary investment in expansion of capacity and to halt offerings of new services that are deemed to duplicate existing ones (78–83). To the extent that this occurs, needless expenditures for health services will be averted by preventing initial outlays for construction, renovation, and new equipment and avoiding future operating costs. Proponents of CES regulation point to two indicators of unnecessary expenditures: excess capacity and inappropriate utilization. Excess capacity, as evidenced by empty hospital beds and idle equipment and services, is taken to be an obvious sign of overinvestment and a portion of their fixed costs as an indication of unnecessary expenditures. Also, expenditures for inpatient services are considered unnecessarily high in instances where patients' problems are viewed as amenable to treatment in less expensive ambulatory care settings and, for patients who require hospitalization, where less expensive combinations of diagnostic and therapeutic services could be substituted for more costly ones (84).

These controls, which are currently in force in all but one state, are mandated by state certificate-of-need (CON) laws and the federally sponsored Section 1122 program (85). Both attempt to attain equilibria between supplies of and needs for services by requiring hospitals' plans for major capital investments and offerings of new services to be certified by regulatory agencies as needed in their communities (76). State CON statutes typically levy legal sanctions against institutions that either fail to seek certificates or proceed with their plans after certificates have been denied. The Section 1122 program employs only financial sanctions: institutions that implement plans that have not received prior authorization are denied reimbursement for costs associated with their investments (e.g., interest payments) by the Medicare, Medicaid, and Maternal and Infant Care programs. As provisions of P.L. 93-641 require states to adopt CON laws by 1980 in order to qualify for various grants-in-aid from the U.S. Public Health Service, it is likely that this more stringent form of CES regulation will soon blanket the nation.

CES programs are administered by agencies created by the National Health Planning and Resources Development Act of 1974. The review process is initiated when a hospital submits a proposal for a major capital investment or a significant change in its services to its local Health Systems Agency (HSA). This body makes a determination as to the need for the proposed project and transmits its recommendation to the State Health Coordinating Committee (SHCC) and the State Health Planning and Development Agency (SHPDA). Based on its review and the recommendations from the HSA and SHCC, the SHPDA decides whether to issue or deny a certificate (87, 88).

As these controls have been in force for only a relatively short time, little is known about their effects on health care cost inflation. What little is known is from research based on the period before 1973, when about half the states had CON programs. In general, assessments of the impacts of this form of regulation on hospitals' investment behavior suggest that it had no discernible influence on overall investment before 1973 (89). One study found, however, that CON controls may have caused shifts in investment from growth-related investment to purchasing new equipment and modernizing facilities. The control over expansion of capacity was thus offset by increased investment in other types of projects, and the net result of these patterns was to negate any overall savings in per capita expenditures for inpatient hospital care (90, 91). Although findings from assessments of hospitals' purchases of particular types of sophisticated equipment are inconsistent, taken together they provide no strong evidence that CON regulation had a significant influence on such decisions. In sum, early experience with this form of regulation suggests that it is ineffective as a cost-control device.

PROFESSIONAL STANDARDS REVIEW ORGANIZATIONS

The soaring costs of Medicare and Medicaid prompted the Congress to enact in 1972 sweeping reforms in these programs' reimbursement procedures. Among the amendments attached to the Social Security Act by P.L. 92-603 were provisions establishing Professional Standards Review Organizations (PSROs), discussed also in Chapter 12. These organizations were

> to promote the effective, efficient, and economical delivery of health care services of proper quality for which payment may be made (in whole or in part) under this Act and in recognition of the interests of patients, the public, practitioners, and providers in improved health care services, it is the purpose of this part to assure, through the application of suitable

procedures of professional standards review, that the Social Security Act will conform to appropriate professional standards for the provision of health care (92).

The clear intent of the statute was to curtail overutilization and excessive costs of inpatient hospital services by subjecting physicians' admitting and treatment decisions to reviews by colleagues. To accomplish this, PSROs comprised of local physicians were created throughout the nation. These bodies were to establish standards of medical care for categories of health problems, develop profiles of individual physicians' practices, and monitor the inpatient services they provide or order for beneficiaries of the Medicare, Medicaid, and Maternal and Infant Care programs (93). Failing this test, the federal government withholds payment to the offending physician for the unnecessary services and levies more severe financial penalties on repeating and fraudulent offenders.

At the federal level, a National PSRO Council was empanelled, *inter alia,* to review local PSROs' standards and to advise the Secretary of Health, Education, and Welfare on the program's structure and operation.

From its inception the PSRO program has been beset by controversy. During the legislative process, the American Medical Association mounted a ferocious, albeit belated and unsuccessful campaign to defeat the bill. While the Association endorsed the bill's delegations of responsibilities and authorities to its members, it was appalled by what it regarded as an unwarranted and ominous gambit that allowed the federal government to intrude directly in individual physicians' practices. Associations representing other health professions viewed the program as a government endorsement of the dominance of physicians, and spokesmen for consumers' interests saw it as a sellout akin to appointing the fox to guard the henhouse (94). Moreover, as the program has developed, its principal mission has become clouded. Physicians are inclined to view it primarily as aimed at improving the quality of health services, while advocates of PSRO in the Congress and federal bureaucracy see it as a cost-containment effort (95).

However one conceives PSRO's objectives, evidence assembled to date indicates that, as of 1976, the program had no profound impacts on the use of inpatient hospital services or their costs and produced no measureable improvements in the quality of care (96). While some savings have been identified in some areas of the nation and for selected types of expenditures (97, 98), the current informed opinion is that, like CES regulation, PSRO has not materially lowered hospital cost inflation.

PROSPECTIVE RATE SETTING

By the late 1960s, the brunt of health care cost inflation from the Medicaid program was being felt in state legislatures. Among the several factors identified as causing the problem was the prevailing mode of paying hospitals for their services. The reimbursement scheme for the Medicare and Medicaid programs had initially been modeled after the Blue Cross procedure of retroactively paying hospitals their costs plus a fixed percentage (99). As noted earlier, this approach to financing in combination with other features of the hospital industry reinforced its tendencies toward inefficiency (100).

To remedy this, in the early 1970s several states established rate setting programs by which hospitals' budgets are set prospectively (101). Although the several programs currently in operation employ various means to establish budgets, all are based on the assumption that the strategy will impel hospitals toward more cost-conscious behavior and greater overall efficiency (102, 103). In effect, hospitals receive funds at the outset of a budget period to cover subsequent costs. Those whose actual costs are lower than the budgeted amount may retain the net revenues; those who overspend must cover costs with monies from other sources.

By 1978, some form of prospective rate setting was in force in at least portions of 28 states (104). About half of these programs are voluntary efforts involving Blue Cross plans and/or bodies established by state hospital associations. In six other states rate setting is mandated by state laws that are implemented by commissions (105). Given the current fiscal and political climate, it is reasonable to assume that rate setting may be widely adopted in the near future. The Health Care Financing Administration of the U.S. Department of Health, Education, and Welfare is promoting rate setting through grants-in-aid to states that establish experimental programs (106), and the Carter Administration has adopted the idea as a central feature in its legislative proposals for a national strategy to contain the costs of health services (107).

On the basis of existing evidence, it appears that rate setting has not had a major impact on cost inflation (108, 109). However, this evidence is difficult to interpret because rate setting programs—with the exception of the Indiana effort (110)—have appeared rather late in the regulatory movement and function alongside other controls. Also, the almost exclusive attention given by evaluation studies to *per diem* rates as the outcome of interest leads to ambiguous results (111). As Dowling has observed, hospitals probably respond differently to different types of rate setting strategies, and they may pursue many of several options to lower *per diem* rates (112). Some of these would be considered desirable (e.g., effecting greater efficiency within departments); others would be perverse (e.g., selecting only low-cost, high profit patients). As Salkever notes, a more informative test of a regulatory program's impact on health care costs would be its consequences for a population's total per capita expenditures for all health services (113). To date, studies show that prospective rate setting has only a minor dampening influence on *per diem* costs, and it remains to be determined how this affects health care costs more generally.

AN ASSESSMENT OF PLANNING AND REGULATION

The comprehensive health planning and regulatory movements began in this nation in an era in which philanthropic and, later, government subsidies sought to develop health care resources and to assure their equitable and efficient deployment. Over the years, the nation took sometimes halting but always compassionate steps toward the fulfillment of deeply rooted political and social values by expanding government's role as the guarantor of an elusive right to health care. It did so, however, in the characteristically American fashion of "muddling through," attempting to enlarge government's functions without at the same time extending its authorities. Gradually, but inevitably, the country reached an impasse that is visible today as the rush to regulation to contain the costs of our beneficence. While our society has not abandoned the values that spawned the planning movement nearly a half century ago, their economic meanings are painfully in view and perhaps on a collision course with the growing mood of fiscal conservatism.

Equally apparent is the antagonism between this nation's devotion to free enterprise as the bedrock of its economy and the widespread reliance on increasingly stringent regulatory controls (114). The federal government first embraced this political-economic instrument to protect free enterprise from the abuses of monopolies (115, 116). The government continues to employ controls for that purpose, but increasingly they are imposed to remedy the untoward consequences of modern existence and, in health care, to rectify behaviors of an industry that has enjoyed a half century of virtually unfettered subsidies. Regulation has as yet not effected its intended goals in the health services industry, and the regulatory movement is now evoking its dialectic in the form of a "deregulation" movement.

Faced with pervasive and significant strains, people voice extreme and all-encompassing proposals for their resolution. Such abound in the debate about health services planning and regulation. One view holds that planning and regulation have been ineffective because we have pursued the strategy only half-heartedly with fragmented responsibilities and partial authorities. The solution from this perspective lies in the welding of fragments and extending the resulting superstructure more broadly over and more deeply into the health services industry (117). At the opposite pole is the belief that planning and regulation are inherently clumsy—in Lindblom's words, "thumbs without fingers" (118)—and that they should therefore be abandoned in favor of other incentives that would unleash latent market forces (119, 120).

Given the incrementalist nature of policy formation in modern democracies, their abhorrence of great leaps, and the seeming vastness of uncharted details of market-oriented schemes, our society appears to prefer to continue on the current regulatory path. If that is so, much remains to be done to perfect our instruments. Presently, the nation lacks the intellectual capacity and the political will that are required to effectively manage the health services industry by collective decision making. These laments are voiced as regards each of the types of regulation described in this chapter. Health planning and regulation via capital expenditures and services controls assume that need for health services can be defined and measured (121). Regulation by Professional Standards Review Organizations assumes that effective standards can be established and applied to the immense variety and complexity of problems brought to the health services industry (122). Prospective rate setting assumes the equally plentiful and complex alternatives open to managers of hospitals can be comprehended and monitored (123). While progress on all these fronts has been impressive, one cannot fail to realize that it barely stays in sight of the inventiveness which changes the industry and discovers ways to accomplish strongly held objectives. The regularity with which governments enact regulatory statutes, however, attests to the vitality of our desire to regulate.

Perhaps the regulatory route upon which the nation has embarked has stimulated innovativeness within the industry and a willingness to entertain alternatives that a decade ago would have been unthinkable. If so, the unanticipated consequences of our present course may outweigh its temporary costs. Exciting and innovative proposals for invigorating market forces are appearing, and private institutions and associations are devising new organizational forms and strategies. To be sure, much of the current activity in the formation of independent practice associations, voluntary cost containment programs, and the like is motivated by threats of more draconian regulation and the uncertainty they engender. However, motives are less important than actions.

Planning and regulation will not disappear, for they are essential activities in modern societies. Were the industry, with the assistance of community-oriented and competent planning, to reform itself, much of the acrimonious, uncertain, and litigious atmosphere surrounding the health services industry could be diminished. Planning and regulation could then be directed to the humane and creative purposes to which they owe their origins.

REFERENCES

1. Lindblom CE: *Politics and Markets: The World's Political-Economic Systems.* New York, Basic Books, 1977.
2. Weidenbaum ML: *Business, Government, and the Public.* Englewood Cliffs, Prentice-Hall, 1977.
3. Blanpain J, Delesie L, Nys H: *National Health Insurance and Health Resources: The European Experience.* Cambridge, Massachusetts, Harvard University Press, 1978.
4. Dahl RA, Lindblom CE: *Politics, Economics, and Welfare.* New York, Harper, 1953.
5. Bice TW, Eichhorn RL: Evaluation of Public Health Programs. In Guttentag M and Struening EL, editors: *Handbook of Evaluation Research,* Volume II, Beverly Hills, California, Sage, 1975, pp. 605–620.
6. Okun AM: *Equality and Efficiency: The Big Tradeoff.* Washington, D.C., The Brookings Institution, 1975.
7. Accuracy requires more subtlety than is possible in this introduction. See: Lindblom CE: *Politics and Markets: The World's Political-Economic Systems.* pp. 3–116.
8. Fuchs VR: Health Care and the United States Economic System—An Essay in Abnormal Physiology. In McKinlay JB, editor: *Economic Aspects of Health Care.* New York, Prodist 1973, pp. 57–94.
9. Bice TW, Kerwin C: Governance of Regional Health Systems. In Saward EW, editor: *The Regionalization of Personal Health Services,* New York, Prodist, 1976, pp. 61–105.
10. Palmiere D: Community Health Planning. In Corey L, Saltman SE, Epstein MF, editors: *Medicine in a Changing Society,* St. Louis, C. V. Mosby, 1972, pp. 59–82.
11. Klarman HE: Planning for Facilities. In Ginzberg E, editor: *Regionalization and Health Policy,* Washington, D.C., U.S. Government Printing Office, 1977, pp. 25–36.
12. Thompson P: Voluntary Regional Planning. In Ginzberg E, editor: *Regionalization and Health Policy.* Washington, D.C., U.S. Government Printing Office, pp. 123–128.
13. Pearson DA: The Concept of Regionalized Personal Health Services in the United States, 1920–1975. In Saward EW, editor: *The Regionalization of Personal Health Services.* New York, Prodist, 1976, pp. 10–14.
14. *Ibid.*, pp. 5–10.

15. *Ibid.*, pp. 14–19.
16. Cited from May JJ: *Health Planning: Its Past and Potential.* Chicago, Center for Health Administration Studies, Perspectives No. A5, University of Chicago, 1967, p. 25.
17. Lave JR, Lave LB: *The Hospital Construction Act: An Evaluation of the Hill-Burton Program, 1948–1973.* Washington, D.C., American Enterprise Institute for Public Policy Research, 1974, pp. 41–43.
18. Gottlieb SR: A Brief History of Health Planning in the United States. In Havighurst CC, editor: *Regulating Health Facilities Construction.* Washington, D.C. American Enterprise Institute for Public Policy Research, 1974, pp. 7–26.
19. Stevens R: *American Medicine and the Public Interest.* New Haven, Yale University Press, 1971.
20. Cited from Hilleboe HE, Barkhuus A: Health planning in the United States: some categorical and general approaches. *International Journal of Health Services* 1:137, 1971.
21. President's Commission on Heart Disease, Cancer and Stroke: *A National Program to Conquer Heart Disease, Cancer and Stroke.* Volume I, Washington, D.C., U.S. Government Printing Office, 1964.
22. For a comparison of the Commission's recommendations and the actual provisions of the amendment, see: Pollack J: Health services and the role of medical school, *Milbank Memorial Fund Quarterly* 46:151–152, Part 2, 1968.
23. Glaser WA: Experiences in Health Planning in the United States. (mimeo) Paper prepared for the Conference on Health Planning in the United States: Past Experiences and Future Imperatives, New York, Columbia University, June, 1973.
24. Bodenheimer TS: Regional medical programs: no road to regionalization. *Medical Care Review* 26:1125–1166, 1969.
25. Regional Medical Programs Service: *Selected Vignettes on Activities of Regional Medical Programs,* Washington, D.C., Health Services and Mental Health Administration, U.S. Department of Health, Education, and Welfare, 1971.
26. Glaser WA: Experiences in Health Planning in the United States, *op. cit.*, p. 16.
27. National Commission on Community Health Services: *Health Is A Community Affair.* Cambridge, Massachusetts, Harvard University Press, 1966.
28. *Ibid.*, p. 131.
29. *Ibid.*, pp. 167–183.
30. Comptroller General of the United States: *Comprehensive Health Planning As Carried Out by State and Areawide Agencies in Three States.* Washington, D.C., U.S. General Accounting Office, Congress of the United States, April, 1974, p. 8.
31. May's studies are a notable exception. See May JJ: *Health Planning: Its Past and Potential. op. cit.*, pp. 25–36.
32. Havighurst CC: Regulation of health facilities and services by 'certificate of need.' *Virginia Law Review* 59:1143–1232, October, 1973.
33. These and other regulatory controls are discussed below.
34. Richardson EL: Address before the Institute of Medicine. Washington, D.C., National Academy of Sciences, May 10, 1972.
35. Iglehart JK, Lilley III W, Clark TB: New federalism report/HEW department advances sweeping proposal to overhaul its programs. *National Journal* Jan. 6:1–10, 1973.
36. Wilson JQ: The bureaucracy problem. *The Public Interest* 3–9, Winter, 1967.
37. United States Congress, Senate Committee on Government Operations, Subcommittee on Executive Reorganization and Government Research: *Federal Role in Health: Report Pursuant to S. Res. 390. 91st Congress,* 2nd Session, S. Report 91–801, 1970.
38. Sundquist JL, Davis DW: *Making Federalism Work.* Washington, D.C., The Brookings Institution, 1969.
39. Liebman L: Social intervention in a democracy. *The Public Interest* 14–29, Winter, 1974.

40. Stevens R: *American Medicine and the Public Interest. op. cit.*, pp. 496–527.

41. United States Congress, House of Representatives: *Hearings Before the Subcommittee on Department of Labor and Health, Education, and Welfare and Related Agencies of the Committee on Appropriations,* 91st Congress, 1st Session, 1969, pp. 426–431.

42. English JT: Mission of the Health Services and Mental Health Administration. *Public Health Reports* 85:95–99, 1970.

43. All of the planning programs discussed in this chapter were within HSMHA.

44. The Health Services and Mental Administration was abolished in 1973, and its agencies were divided between the present Health Services Administration and Health Resources Administration.

45. For a more complete enumeration of such programs, see: U.S. Congress, Senate Committee on Government Operations, Subcommittee on Executive Reorganization and Government Research: *Federal Role in Health: Report Pursuant to S. Res. 390. op. cit..*

46. The National Center for Health Services Research and Development is now the National Center for Health Services Research. For a description of this agency's history and current functions, see: The Institute of Medicine: *Health Services Research.* Washington, D.C., Institute of Medicine, National Academy of Sciences, 1979, Chapter 5.

47. Sanazaro PJ: Federal Health Services Research and R and D Under the Auspices of the National Center for Health Services Research and Development. In Flook EE, Sanazaro PJ, editors: *Health Services Research and R and D in Perspective.* Ann Arbor, Health Administration Press, 1973, pp. 150–183.

48. Rubel EJ: Testimony before the U.S. Congress, House of Representatives, Committee on Interstate and Foreign Commerce, Subcommittee on Public Health and Environment. *Hearings on the National Health Policy and Health Resources Development Bill and Related Bills,* 93rd Congress, 2nd Session, March 15; April 30; May 1, 6–9 and 14, 1974, p. 408.

49. Klarman HE: Health planning: progress, prespects, and issues. *Milbank Memorial Fund Quarterly/Health and Society* 56:78–112, Winter 1978.

50. Public Health Service, U.S. Department of Health, Education, and Welfare: National guidelines for health planning. *Federal Register* 43:13,040–13,050, March 28, 1978.

51. Glantz LH: Legal Aspects of health facilities regulation. In Hyman HH, editor: *Health Regulation: Certificate of Need and Section 1122.* Germantown, Maryland, Aspen, Aspen Systems Corporation 1977, pp. 75–104.

52. Buntz CA, Macaluso TF, Azarow JA: Federal influence on state health policy. *Journal of Health Politics, Policy and Law* 3:71–86, 1978.

53. Bice TW, Eichhorn RL: Evaluation of Public Health Programs, *op. cit.* pp. 617–618.

54. Stone A: Planning, Public Policy and Capitalism. In Lowi TJ, Stone A, editors: *Nationalizing Government: Public Policies in America.* Beverly Hills, California, Sage Publications, 1978, pp. 427–442.

55. Weidenbaum ML: *Business, Government, and the Public.* pp. 24–91.

56. Stone A: Planning, Public Policy and Capitalism. pp. 433–439.

57. Woll P: *American Bureaucracy, 2nd Edition.* New York, W.W. Norton, 1977.

58. Truman DB: *The Governmental Process: Political Interests and Public Opinion, 2nd Edition.* New York, Alfred A. Knopf, 1971.

59. For a personalized attempt to do so for a single state's health services regulatory structure, see: D.M. Kinzer, *Health Controls Out of Control: Warnings to the Nation from Massachusetts.* Chicago, Illinois, Teach'Em, Inc., 1977.

60. Stigler GJ: The theory of economic regulation. *The Bell Journal of Economics and Management Science* 2:3–21, 1971.

61. Weidenbaum ML: The Costs of Government Regulation of Business. A study prepared for the use of the Subcommittee on Economic Growth and Stabilization of

the Joint Economic Committee, Congress of the United States, Washington, D.C., U.S. Government Printing Office, 1978.

62. Green M, Nader R: Economic regulation vs. competition: Uncle Sam the monopoly man. *Yale Law Journal* 82:871–889, 1973.

63. Weidenbaum ML: *Business, Government, and the Public. op. cit.*, pp. 11–23.

64. Zubkoff M, editor: *Health: A Victim or Cause of Inflation.* New York, Prodist, 1976.

65. Havighurst CC: Regulation of health facilities by 'certificate of need.' *op. cit.*, pp. 1148–1151.

66. Throughout this section terms are used such as "need," "overinvest," "unnecessary costs," and the like recognizing that these are elusive concepts. For a critique of the practice of basing health planning on notions of need, see: Klarman HE: Planning for Facilities. *op. cit.* For a more general critique of the language of health planners, see: Kessel R: Commentary on the Papers. In Havighurst CC, editor: *Regulating Health Facilities Construction. op. cit.*, pp. 33–35. Also Posner RA: Certificates of Need for Health Care Facilities: A Dissenting View. In Havighurst CC, editor: *Regulating Health Facilities Construction. op. cit.*, pp. 113–118.

67. Lee ML: A conspicuous production theory of hospital behavior. *Southern Economic Journal* 38:45–58, 1971.

68. Newhouse JP: Toward a theory of nonprofit institutions: an economic model of a hospital. *American Economic Review* 60:64–74, 1970.

69. Feldstein PJ: *An Empirical Investigation of the Marginal Cost of Hospital Services.* Chicago, Illinois, Graduate Program in Hospital Administration, University of Chicago, 1961. For a review of economics literature on hospitals' objective functions, see: Berki SE: *Hospital Economics.* Lexington, Massachusetts, Lexington Books, 1972, pp. 19–30.

70. Fuchs VR: *Who Shall Live: Health Economics and Social Choice.* New York, Basic Books, 1974.

71. Redisch MA: Physician Involvement in Hospital Decision Making. In Zubkoff M, Raskin IE, Hanft RS, editors: *Hospital Cost Containment,* New York, Prodist, 1978.

72. Feldstein MS: Hospital cost inflation: a study of nonprofit price dynamics. *American Economic Review* 60:853–872, December 1970. Pauly MV, Redisch M: The not-for-profit hospital as a physicians' cooperative. *American Economic Review* 63:87–99, 1973.

73. Monsma Jr. GN: Marginal Revenue and the Demand for Physicians' Services. In Klarman HE, editor: *Empirical Studies in Health Economics.* Baltimore, Maryland, The Johns Hopkins University Press, 1970, pp. 145–160.

74. Pauly MV, Redisch M: The not-for-profit hospital as a physicians' cooperative. *American Economic Review,* 63:87–99.

75. Feldstein MS: Hospital cost inflation: a study of nonprofit price dynamics. **op. cit.**, pp. 871–872.

76. Clapp DC, Spector AB: A Study of the American Capital Market and Its Relationship to the Capital Needs of the Health Care Field. In MacLeod GK, Perlman M, editors: *Health Care Capital: Competition and Control.* Cambridge, Massachusetts, Ballinger Publishing Company, 1978, pp. 275–304.

77. Kelling Jr. RS, Williams PC: The Projected Response of the Capital Markets to Health Facilities Expenditures. *Ibid.*, pp. 319–348.

78. Curran WJ: A National Survey and Analysis of State Certificate-of-Need Laws for Health Facilities. In Havighurst CC, editor: *Regulating Health Facilities Construction.* op. cit., pp. 85–112.

79. Lewin L and Associates, Inc.: *Nationwide Survey of State Health Regulations.* Washington, D.C., Social Security Administration, 1974.

80. Macro Systems, Inc.: *The Certificate of Need Experience: An Early Assessment.* Silver Springs, Maryland, Macro Systems, Inc., 1974.

81. O'Donoghue P, and Policy Center, Inc.: *Evidence About the Effects of Health Care Regulation*. Denver, Colorado, Spectrum Research, Inc., 1974.

82. Salkever DS, Bice TW: *Hospital Certificate of Need Controls: Impact on Investment, Costs, and Use*. Washington, D.C., American Enterprise Institute for Public Policy Research, 1979.

83. Urban Systems Research and Engineering and Policy Analysis, Inc.: *Certificate of Need Programs: A Review, Analysis, and Annotated Bibliography*. Washington, D.C., U.S. Government Printing Office, November 1978.

84. McClure W: *Reducing Excess Hospital Capacity*. Washington, D.C., U.S. Department of Commerce, National Technical Information Service, 1976.

85. Hyman HH, editor: Health Regulation: *Certificate of Need and Section 1122*. op. cit.

86. Curran WJ: A National Survey and Analysis of State Certificate-of-Need Laws for Health facilities. p. 85.

87. Of course, the process rarely proceeds so simply. See: Kinzer DM: *Health Controls Out of Control: Warning to the Nation from Massachusetts*. op. cit. Also Lewin and Associates, Inc.: *Evaluation of the Efficiency and Effectiveness of the Section 1122 Review Process, Part I*. Washington, D.C., U.S. Department of Commerce, National Technical Information Services, 1975.

88. Public Health Service, U.S. Department of Health, Education, and Welfare: Health Planning: Capital expenditure review, certificate of need and review of new institutional health services. *Federal Register* 42:4,002–4,032, 1977.

89. Urban Systems Research and Engineering and Policy Analysis, Inc.: *Certificate of Need Programs: A Review, Analysis, and Annotated Bibliography*. pp. 1–37.

90. Salkever DS, Bice TW: The impact of certificate-of-need controls on hospital investment. *Milbank Memorial Fund Quarterly/Health and Society* 54:185–214, 1976.

91. Salkever DS, Bice TW: *Hospital Certificate of Need Controls: Impact on Investment, Costs, and Use*. pp. 53–73.

92. 42 United States Code 1301, Sec. 1151.

93. Blumstein JF: The role of PSROs in hospital cost containment. In Zubkoff M, Raskin IE, Hanft RS, editors: *Hospital Cost Containment*, **op. cit.** pp. 461–488.

94. Bellin LE: PSRO: quality control? or gimmickry? *Medical Care* 12:1012–1018, 1974.

95. Havighurst CC, Blumstein JF: Coping with quality/cost tradeoffs in medical care: the role of PSROs. *Northwestern Law Review* 70:6–68, 1975.

96. Office of Planning, Evaluation and Legislation, Health Services Administration, U.S. Department of Health, Education, and Welfare: *Professional Standards Review Organizations: Program Evaluation, Volume I*. Washington, D.C., U.S. Department of Health, Education, and Welfare, 1978.

97. *Ibid.* pp. 22–29.

98. Brook RH, Williams KN, Rolph JE: *Controlling the Use and Cost of Medical Services: The New Mexico Experimental Medical Care Review Organization–A Four-Year Case Study*. Santa Monica, California, The Rand Corporation, November 1978.

99. The plus portion of this formula was subsequently deleted. For a detailed analysis of the original Medicare reimbursement procedures, see: Somers HM, Somers AR: *Medicare and the Hospitals: Issues and Prospects*. Washington, D.C., The Brookings Institution, 1967, pp. 154–196.

100. Klarman HE: The Financing of Health Care. In Knowles JH: The responsibility of the individual. *Daedalus* **106**:215–246, Winter 1977.

101. Actually, the first major effort of this type was begun in 1960 in Indiana as a cooperative voluntary program sponsored by Indiana Blue Cross and the Indiana Hospital Association. See: O'Donoghue P: *Controlling Hospital Costs: The Revealing Case of Indiana*. Denver, Colorado, Policy Center, Inc., 1978.

102. Bauer KG: Hospital Rate Setting—This Way to Salvation? In Zubkoff M, Raskin IE, Hanft RS, editors: *Hospital Cost Containment.* pp. 324–369,

103. Salkever DS: Measuring the Impact of Rate-Setting: An Overview of Recent Econometric Research. In *Hospital Sector Inflation.* Lexington, Massachusetts, Lexington Books, in press, Chapter 4, pp. 1–15.

104. Editorial: State rate controls: documentation of the bureaucracy's imperfect plan. *Federation of American Hospitals Review,* pp. 11–13, December 1978.

105. *Ibid.,* pp. 12–13.

106. Hellinger FJ: An Empirical Analysis of Several Prospective Reimbursement Systems. In Zubkoff M, Raskin IE, Hanft RS, editors: *Hospital Cost Containment.* pp. 370–400.

107. Dunn WL, Lefkowitz B: The Hospital Cost Containment Act of 1977: An Analysis of the Administration's Proposal. In Zubkoff M, Raskin IE, Hanft RS, editors: *Hospital Cost Containment.* op. cit., pp.166–216.

108. Hellinger FJ: An Empirical Analysis of Several Prospective Reimbursement Systems. op. cit., pp. 372–393.

109. For an extensive and thorough review of recent studies, see: Salkever DS: An Overview of Recent Econometric Research, *op. cit.*

110. The Indiana program appears to have been successful in containing hospital costs. See: O'Donoghue P: *Controlling Hospital Costs: The Revealing Case of Indiana. op. cit.*

111. Salkever DS: An Overview of Recent Econometric Research. op. cit., pp. 1–6.

112. Dowling WL: Prospective reimbursement of hospitals. *Inquiry* 11:163–180, 1974.

113. Salkever DS: An Overview of Recent Econometric Research. op. cit., p. 5.

114. Schultze CL; *The Public Use of Private Interest.* Washington, D.C., The Brookings Institution, 1977.

115. Hofstadter R: *The Age of Reform.* New York, Vintage Books, 1960.

116. Lowi TJ: *The End of Liberalism: Ideology, Policy, and the Crisis of Public Authority.* New York, W.W. Norton, 1969.

117. For broad outlines of extensive regulatory strategies, see: Blum HL: *Expanding Health Care Horizons: From a General Systems Concept of Health to a National Health Policy,* Oakland, California, Third Party Associates, 1976, pp. 161–196. Also, Joe T, Needleman J, Lewin LS: Health Care Capital Financing: Regulation, the Market, and Public Policy. In McLeod GK, Perlman M, editors: *Health Care Capital: Competition and Control.* op. cit., pp. 63–80. Also, Krause EA: *Power and Illness: The Political Sociology of Health and Medical Care.* New York, Elsevier, 1977, pp. 324–350.

118. Lindblom CE: Politics and Markets: *The World's Political-Economic Systems. op. cit.,* pp. 65–75.

119. Enthoven A: Consumer choice health plan. Parts I and II. *New England Journal of Medicine* 298:650–658, 709–730, 1978.

120. McClure W: The medical care system under national health insurance: four models. *Journal of Health Politics, Policy and Law,* pp. 22–68, Spring 1976.

121. Klarman HE: Health planning: progress, prospects, and issues. *op. cit.*

122. Brook RH: *Quality of Care Assessment: A Comparison of Five Methods of Peer Review.* Washington, D.C., Bureau of Health Services Research, U.S. Department of Health, Education, and Welfare, 1973.

123. Bauer KG: Hospital Rate Setting—This Way to Salvation? *op. cit.,* p. 328

CHAPTER 12

Evaluation of Health Services and Quality of Care

James P. LoGerfo

Robert H. Brook

This chapter concerns the evaluation of health services and the assessment and assurance of the quality of medical care. The assessment of the quality of care is inextricably intertwined with societal, professional, and patient expectations concerning the role of health care in society. Quality—the degree of excellence or conformation to standards—cannot be assessed without a clear understanding about the expected standards of excellence. This is true at both the programmatic level and at the level of the individual patient and physician interaction. Unfortunately, many of society's expectations concerning health and medical care have not been explicitly delineated and one is left with the dilemma reflected in the title of a recent book, *Doing Better and Feeling Worse: Health Care in the U.S.* (1). The title reflects that changes in medical care or its results, such as better access to care for disadvantaged populations and increased life expectancy, have been accompanied by criticism of the quality and efficiency of health care.

The purpose of this chapter is to present an overview of the issues, methods, and applications relevant to assessing the quality of health and medical care. The first part of the chapter is directed toward exploring aspects of program evaluation as they relate to the health system. The remainder of the chapter addresses issues relevant to assessing and assuring the quality of care at the individual patient and physician level. System level evaluation is discussed with respect to three topics: generic issues of program evaluation; the relationship between health and medical care; and the importance of evaluating the quality of care provided to populations. The section on quality of care assessment addresses the following topics: sources and selection of data on provider performance; generic issues of measurement of quality including reliability of data, sensitivity, specificity, and reliability of judgments concerning quality of care; specific methods of measuring quality of care and each method's strengths and limitations; and the implications for quality assessment of imperfect knowledge concerning the true effectiveness of many medical services. Illustrative studies of quality of care are also presented. Finally, mechanisms and programs for assuring the quality of care are reviewed. While the chapter addresses most of the issues in the above areas, it is not an exhaustive review and the reader may wish to consult other reviews and bibliographies on assessment and assurance of the quality of medical care (2–5).

GENERIC ISSUES OF PROGRAM EVALUATION OF HEALTH SERVICES

In its broadest sense, medical care can be viewed as one of several activities that have a major emphasis on the promotion, restoration, or maintenance of health. In order to maximize health, society will need to make many complex decisions and tradeoffs that could be made better if critical evaluations of health services are performed. Assessment of the quality of medical care is only one aspect of health services evaluation and the broader issues of evaluations must be discussed before quality of care is considered.

Evaluation of health services can assume numerous forms. In all instances, however, the objective is to assess some aspects of health care critically weighing the pluses and minuses and providing some insight and direction for the development of policy and administrative actions. Although health services in this country are too fragmented to be viewed as a single program organized in response to health needs, the assessment of selected components of health services can proceed using the framework established for health program evaluation. In this context a program is any organized effort to provide services. The components evaluated may range from the effectiveness of specific clinics providing ambulatory care to the clinical efficacy of medical procedures. Taken together, all of the evaluation activities conducted will help answer critical questions about the future direction of health care; and when their results are integrated into a "systems approach" as discussed in Chapter 3, hopefully will lead to more effective delivery of health services.

Two issues of health program evaluation that are particularly important concern the motivation for performing evaluations, and the specification of program goals and objectives.

REASONS FOR EVALUATION

There is a myriad of reasons given in response to the question "Why evaluate a program?", and the reasons differ depending on one's perspective (6). From the viewpoint of consumer groups the reasons might include the ability to answer the following questions: 1) Are the benefits of health care adequate and can they be improved? 2) Are the dollars spent on health care being used efficiently? 3) What is the value of planned changes in health services programs? and 4) How can community participation in major health and social programs be increased?

Providers may be interested in evaluating programs to: 1) identify deficiencies or weaknesses as a basis for planning future actions; 2) demonstrate the effectiveness in order to justify expenditures for the programs; 3) gain support for expansion of various aspects of a program (personnel, facilities, equipment); and 4) determine the costs of the program.

Individual administrators within a program might have other motivations such as bringing favorable attention to the program or increasing the administrator's status as a means of gaining support for greater program control. In many instances, evaluation will be required by funding agencies who want to know what they are paying for, or how efficient the program is, or because they seek to demonstrate the value of the program in a political context.

This list is not exhaustive, but rather serves to illustrate that any evaluation of a program intervention is designed to meet the needs of certain constituencies, possibly to the exclusion of the needs of other groups. The assessment of the quality of care, especially, is multidimensional, and the assessment of only a few aspects of care will probably not yield a composite picture of the overall effectiveness or efficiency of a health care program necessary to meet the needs of all constituencies. For example, in assigning a value to the costs of a health service, a third party might be primarily interested in direct costs of care while the consumer of the service may also be interested in time and convenience costs.

SPECIFICATION OF OBJECTIVES

A fundamental tenet of program evaluation is that there be clearly defined objectives. It is also important to order the objectives, the "measurable" results of any program or intervention, by the establishment of priorities. Higher order health program objectives might include improvement in health status as measured by life expectancy or number of days lost from work or other usual activity; intermediate order objectives might be how well the services that are needed to achieve the higher order objectives are provided. The lowest order objectives might reflect the operating characteristics of the program such as the opening of an office or the hiring of specific kinds of personnel. The ordering of objectives in the evaluation of a health program might appear as in Figure 12–1. The "impact variables" are those that measure the outcome or effect of the program or services such as longer lifespan or reduced illness or morbidity as measured by the number of days of disability. The "bridging variables" measure the intermediate objectives of the health program such as the provision of "good" quality care based on technical criteria or the satisfaction of patients with the care received. The "operational variables" at the lowest level of objectives are concerned with the specific details of the program such as hiring qualified staff.

At the programmatic level, the ordering of variables should reflect a causal chain of objectives with clearly understood relationships among the different levels.

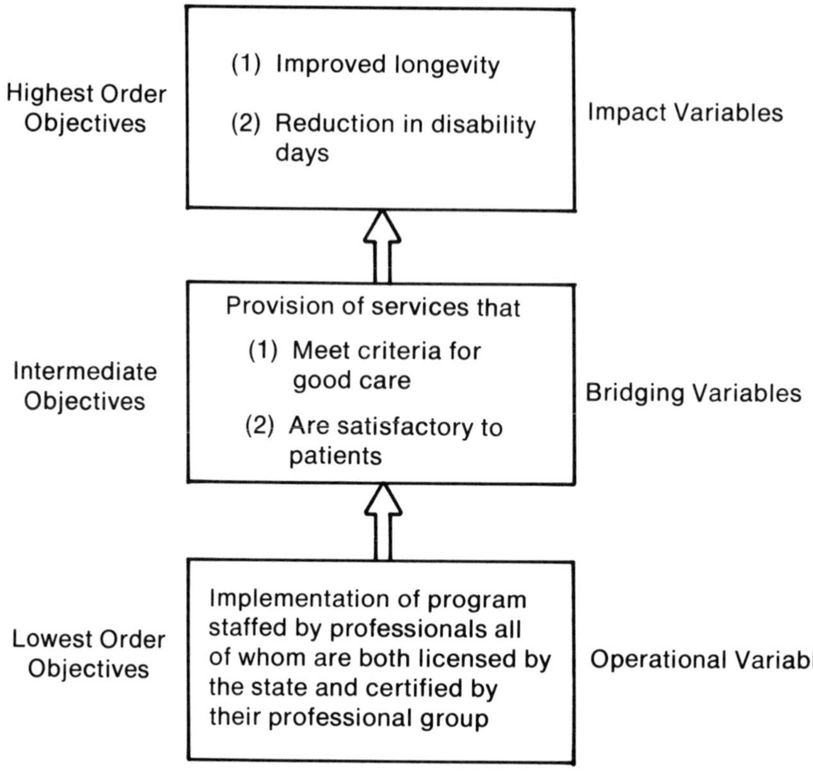

Highest Order
Objectives

(1) Improved longevity

(2) Reduction in disability
days

Impact Variables

⇧

Intermediate
Objectives

Provision of services that

(1) Meet criteria for
good care

(2) Are satisfactory to
patients

Bridging Variables

⇧

Lowest Order
Objectives

Implementation of program
staffed by professionals all
of whom are both licensed by
the state and certified by
their professional group

Operational Variables

Figure 12–1. Illustrative objectives for evaluating a health services program.

Efforts designed to measure the highest-order objectives are termed summative evaluations, and those at the lowest-order formative evaluations.

While these concepts might seem simplistic and self-evident, inadequate attention has been directed to the specification of objectives for health services. Some of the failure in this area derives from the historical origins of the provision of personal health services in Western society in general, and the United States in particular. As discussed in Chapters 1 and 2, most health care historically resulted from individuals with perceived illnesses contacting other individuals who claimed to be able to define the causes of illness and to provide care. The "health services" were the collective sum of all such care. The resulting goals were implicit and as diverse as the individual patient's perceived needs and the individual provider's personal desires, both altruistic and selfish. No proof of efficacy was required by society. All that was necessary for the system to evolve was the patient's sense that the care was beneficial in some way—such as the alleviation of fear, the removal of pain, the increase in happiness from knowing someone (a provider) cares about them, the restoration of function, the validation of disease as an excuse from work or other usual activity, or the prolongation of life. Widespread use of health care came into vogue long before societies formally regulated its provision or expressed concern for assessing the quality of care that was provided.

In view of the historical foundation, it is not surprising that there have been few explicit objectives at the societal level that would be used as a basis for evaluating health care. Of the implicit goals noted above, the improvement in health might be the most universally accepted first-order objective. If so, an ideal health care system that provided a specified level of resources would optimize health status in a manner most consonant with the cultural and social mores of the society. If there were "good methods" for measuring health, the "quality" of the system could be measured by the extent to which the people's actual health compared to the expected level to be achieved for the level of resources that were expended on health care. In this scheme, the provision of services would be an intermediate objective with a known causal relationship to the higher-order (or ultimate) objective of improved health status. Unfortunately, the relationship between health care and the improvement of health is not well defined, a deficiency that has significant implications for the assessment of health care.

THE RELATIONSHIP BETWEEN HEALTH AND MEDICAL CARE

The improvement and maintenance of health are nearly universally accepted as objectives of medical care. These objectives would ideally be achieved by a sequence of events, represented in Figure 12–2 and discussed in more detail in Chapter 3. As has been known for over 20 centuries, however, many factors besides medical care have a profound effect on health. In addition, as reflected in various ancient codes of law dealing with the adverse outcomes of care, such as removing the hand of a surgeon for a "poor quality" operation, not all care is efficacious; that is, not all care contributes to a positive outcome. Indeed some care has the potential to be harmful, leading to iatrogenic illness caused by the care itself (e.g., infections after surgery). Accordingly, a more extensive model is presented in Figure 12–3.

The final outcome of care for any patient is a function of the likelihood that they actually need care, that a correct diagnosis is made, that the correct treatment is given, that the treatment is efficacious, and that the treatment was adhered to by the patient. The probability of all of these events occurring in a positive manner represents the positive contribution of medical care to health. Most of these probabilities are not precisely known. Even if the probabilities are known for specific medical care interventions, it is critical to recognize the contributions of the

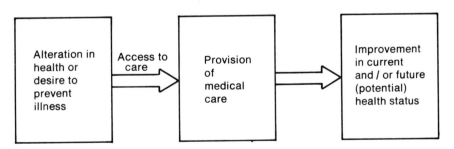

Figure 12–2. Idealized model of an episode of medical care.

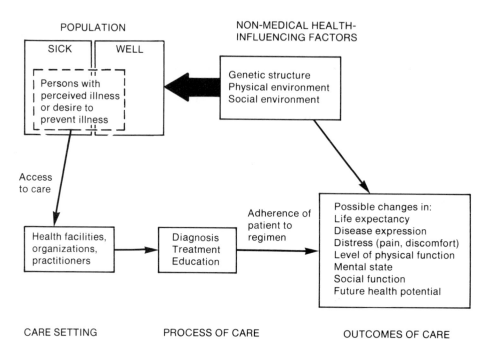

Figure 12–3. Model of a single episode of medical care.

nonmedical factors (such as environment) to the production of health. This recognition is important because lack of an understanding of the multifactorial determinants of outcomes of disease processes can lead to major errors in evaluation of health services. For example, critics of the United States health care system often cite this country's higher infant death rate and lower life expectancy compared to selected European nations as evidence that the health care system in this country is inferior. Infant death rates, however, are influenced by demographic and social factors that are difficult to adjust for when performing these comparisons. Similarly, life expectancy is influenced by personal behavior such as smoking, drinking, and involvement in violence. Thus, criticism of a health care system based on mortality statistics is less a condemnation of the health care system than might be thought at first glance. This is not meant to imply that medical care has no influence on health as measured by mortality rates, but rather that the rates are imperfect measures for the evaluation of medical care. Accordingly, planners, policymakers, and providers should be cautious in the use of such global measures as the sole basis for criticizing a health care system or recommending changes in it. This argument also applies to other measures of health that are affected by nonmedical factors.

While the above discussion sounds a cautionary note about the use of broad measures of health in assessing medical care, it is also important to note that a focus on very narrow, professionally defined technical measures of health might also cause a distortion if they are used as the sole basis of evaluation. For example, triumphs in the treatment of congenital heart disease by surgery, and the prevention of strokes through the treatment of high blood pressure are often cited as unequivocal examples of effective medical care. Even in these two areas of "undisputed" efficacy, however, there could be harmful effects if, for instance, people who do not have the disease were erroneously labeled as having the disease.

The negative effect of medical care on the health of nondiseased individuals was demonstrated in a study of junior high school children in Seattle, Washington, who had notations in school records indicating the presence of a heart condition (7). On detailed examination of these 93 students, only 18 had evidence of heart disease; the other 75 were probably misdiagnosed. In the latter group, 30 were significantly restricted either psychologically or physically. The result was that screening for cardiac disease that is potentially curable by surgery may have produced more disability among those with "nondisease" than it cured in those with heart disease.

In another study, the effects of labeling were noted in a hypertensive screening program. Absenteeism significantly increased when persons were identified as hypertensive even though many had had documented, but unlabeled, elevated blood pressures prior to screening (8). If the program had used narrowly defined measures of program outcome, such as number of cases identified, this important effect would have been missed. These examples both illustrate the importance of knowing the effects of medical care on the health of populations and being careful to select appropriate measures to assess health programs.

USE OF POPULATION-BASED RATES FOR PROGRAM EVALUATION

A crucial, often neglected concern in evaluation, is the use of measures of assessment that are directed at the entire population at risk rather than simply the users of services. The latter approach commonly implies assessment of care only for patients definitively diagnosed as having a specific disease (case rate analysis). The importance of using population based rates (occurrence of diseases in populations) rather than case rates for program evaluation has always been accepted by epidemiologists accustomed to concern for "denominators." The point is vividly illustrated in assessing the effect of various organizations or programs on the disease appendicitis, an entity frequently included in evaluations of care.

In cases of appendicitis, the dilemma confronting physicians is a choice between operating on patients who have abdominal pain at a time when the signs and symptoms are such that some of the patients may have a less serious, nonsurgical illness mimicking appendicitis versus waiting until the signs and symptoms are more definite and clearly indicate that an inflamed appendix is the cause of the pain. Unfortunately, if one waits too long, the inflamed appendix might perforate in some people and produce peritonitis (a general inflammation and infection of the abdomen). In essence, the choice is between operating "too early" on some people with abdominal pain and removing some normal appendices versus operating "too late" and having a few patients with appendicitis progress to peritonitis. Recognition of this trade-off has led to acceptance of the fact that even the best surgeons will operate on some patients at a time when the diagnosis is not certain so as to decrease the number of perforations. This means that some people who have undergone surgery will be found to have a normal appendix. The optimum rate of such removals per 100 cases of true appendicitis has not been rigorously defined, but the implications of the tradeoff have been discussed in detail (9).

In view of the above considerations, the logical inference is that the evaluator could assess the results described in the operative and pathology reports to classify the proportion of a facility's cases that are either normal ("unnecessary"), or abnormal but not perforated (best result), or perforated—possibly reflecting unnecessary delay before surgery. The case rate for these outcomes has been used to judge the extent to which a hospital or provider organization acts to reduce unnecessary surgery without significantly increasing the risks of perforation. Interestingly, the natural course of appendicitis is such that not all abnormal appendixes will perforate; rather, some will improve without specific therapy or surgical intervention. The possible fates of patients who present to a physician with abdominal pain are represented in Figure 12–4. Surgical intervention is only beneficial to groups III and IV, in the former case to prevent perforation and in the latter to prevent continued leakage of bacteria into the abdomen by removing the source of the bacteria and providing drainage of any abscess that might be present. Note that in an absolute biological sense, all operations on patients in groups I and II are "unnecessary." In assessing performance of a provider, a crucial question is the extent to which physicians can differentiate between groups II and III. If they can, and if case rates are used, the

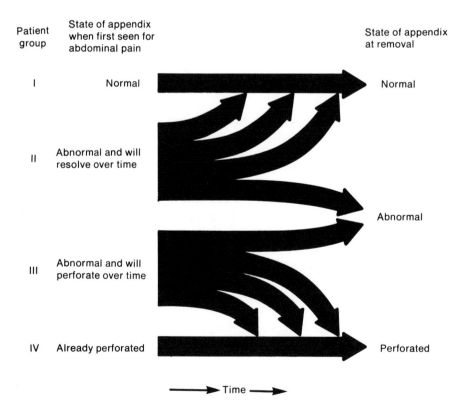

Figure 12–4. Changes in the state of the appendix in patients with abdominal pain.

relative sizes of those groups in any population will have a dramatic impact on the results of an assessment of care (Fig. 12–5).

Assume two different medical organizations provide care to biologically similar populations of 100,000 people each. The staff in organization A cannot distinguish patients with abdominal pain who have abnormal appendixes that are likely to perforate, either initially or after careful observation, from those patients whose abnormal appendixes are not likely to perforate. Thus, they admit all such patients to the hospital and operate on them. The physicians in organization B can make such distinctions and do not admit nor operate on patients in group II. In addition, they are able to distinguish correctly all patients with normal appendixes from those with abnormal ones and thus do not hospitalize or operate on anyone in group I. Analysis of operative case rates using only hospitalized patients would suggest that organization B is trading off lives (over 50% higher death rate) for efficiency. On a population basis, however, organization B has exactly the same number of deaths as organization A and in addition performed less than one-half as many operations. A practical demonstration of this problem in evaluating health care has been described (10).

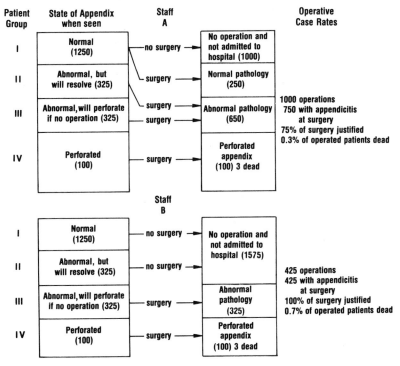

Figure 12–5. Hypothetical outcomes of care for two cohorts of 2,000 patients each with abdominal pain cared for under two different systems of care.

This illustration has implications for both quality assurance and cost-containment programs that are aimed at hospitals. For example, a hospital might respond to a cost-containment program by reducing admissions. An evaluation of the effect of that program on the quality of care may require a population-based assessment. Unfortunately, the identification of a hospital's denominator population is difficult and an evaluation of the impact of the cost-containment program on quality may be impossible.

COST-BENEFIT AND COST-EFFECTIVENESS ANALYSES

In addition to discussing the impact of a program on health, program evaluation implies that a value judgment can be made (i.e., are the results worth it?). Two techniques to aid in developing value judgments are cost-benefit analysis and cost-effectiveness analysis (11). In cost-benefit analysis, specific values (usually dollar values) are placed on all costs and all benefits of a health services program. If benefits are greater than costs, the program will be considered to have a net positive impact. While this system has great intuitive appeal, it has limited value in evaluation of health programs because of the problems inherent in placing a dollar value on life and on the relief of pain and suffering. Some of the methods proposed for establishing such values differentially favor higher socioeconomic groups over lower ones, men over women and working-age groups over the very young or very old.

Cost-effectiveness analysis is a subset of cost-benefit analysis, and is designed to provide an estimate of the costs incurred in achieving a given outcome. A cost-effectiveness analysis of a renal dialysis program might use the costs per additional year of life as the variable of interest. In addition, if programs happen to have similar outcomes such as the same number of additional years of life at age 40, they can be valued in rank order on the program cost variable without having to place a dollar value on an additional year of life for a 40 year old person.

SUMMARY OF GENERAL HEALTH PROGRAM EVALUATION ISSUES

This brief discussion of some of the more "global" topics related to evaluation of health services demonstrates the importance of asking critical questions about health care. These questions run the gamut from what effect does medical care have on health to how can services be provided most efficiently while assuring access to care. All of the preceding chapters have addressed such evaluative issues although they have not always been explicitly labeled as such. It is imperative that all groups involved in health care, including the consumer, raise questions of this kind. The importance of thinking in terms of populations rather than only in terms of those individuals who seek care has also been stressed, and solutions to health care problems require that this type of perspective be adopted.

QUALITY ASSESSMENT IN HEALTH CARE

The discussion below shifts from health care as a social benefit to the assessment of care at the level of the individual provider and patient. As noted in previous chapters, there are annually over one billion visits to physicians in the United States. While some care might be for trivial reasons, most of it has potential for either enhancing or harming the health of patients. It is essential, therefore, to use knowledge of the assessment and assurance of the quality of care to help achieve improved health. Most of the knowledge acquired thus far has been based on care given by physicians, but the general principles apply to care given by other health professionals, especially nurses (12, 13).

CHOICE OF WHOM TO STUDY

Just as in the case of program evaluation, the choice of what aspects of quality to assess and whether or not one should focus on selected providers will depend on the motivations for assessing care and on assumptions concerning the distribution of poor quality of care.

The potential units from which samples for study can be selected are numerous and selection of a sample will depend on the objectives of the effort. Samples may be physician-based; hospital or other facility-based; or can be based on the patient. A physician-based sample can be drawn by either sampling a few types of care given by all physicians who provide care for these conditions or by sampling care given for a large number of conditions by a few physicians. If poor care is assumed to be randomly distributed across physicians the former approach should be used. If poor quality is not randomly distributed, but is associated with physicians who have certain practice patterns, then physicians whose pattern of use of laboratory tests, drugs, or numbers of visits characterize them as "outliers" in comparison to their peers should be more intensively studied. Physician-based samples may not be appropriate if care is likely to be received from multiple providers for one illness episode. In this situation, the providers' competence must be assessed by choosing samples based on episodes of illness for selected conditions or by assessing all care given to selected patients (14).

Another sampling method is to select individuals randomly, regardless of whether they have been diagnosed as having certain conditions or have even seen a specific provider. This approach is particularly helpful in evaluating case-finding for an asymptomatic disease that might benefit from early treatment. It has been incorporated into a population-based quality assessment strategy known as the tracer method (7).

CHOICE OF WHAT TO STUDY

An important criterion for selecting what aspect of care to study is whether it is believed that this is an area of poor quality of care. This knowledge could be based on either studies performed elsewhere that suggest that a problem could exist or should be investigated, or based on local anecdotal evidence. Poor quality of care includes care that is currently provided but is known to be ineffective and potentially harmful (e.g., use of certain drugs), as well as care not being provided from which selected patients could benefit. These are referred to as errors of commission and omission, respectively. In addition, a topic might also be chosen because it represents a common medical problem for which large numbers of people are treated and there is a desire to routinely "check" to determine if the care given to this large group of people is of acceptable quality. Finally, a topic might be chosen because large sums of money are being expended on it and there is concern about unnecessary utilization and cost.

Topics for study can be classified as disease-oriented, treatment-oriented, or prevention-oriented. A disease-oriented study includes assessing those elements of diagnosis and treatment for a specified disease that are considered "good" practice (e.g., performing certain tests). Treatment-oriented studies focus on the provision of a certain procedure or drug (i.e., patterns of use of a specific drug or procedure). Prevention-oriented studies focus on case finding for asymptomatic conditions (e.g., community screening programs).

SOURCES OF DATA FOR QUALITY ASSESSMENT

Data sources that can be used to study the quality of care are numerous and include direct observation; video or audio recordings of patient-provider contacts; direct interviews and examinations of patients; review of medical records; review of insurance claims forms; and review of public documents such as pharmacy records; birth or death certificates.

MEASUREMENT ISSUES

After specifying the subject or sample frame, topic, and data source, there are measurement problems that must be considered (2). These include issues of validity, reliability, sensitivity, and specificity. In addition, quality of care assessment can be based on outcomes, processes, or structural aspects of care.

VALIDITY AND RELIABILITY

The validity of a measure is the extent to which a measure actually assesses what it purports to measure. For instance, the number of deaths due to cancer of the pancreas is not a valid measure of the quality of care because alteration in the level of quality of care will not affect this number. In general, the most valid measures of quality of medical care tend to be defined quite narrowly (e.g., the percentage of people with uncontrolled blood pressure).

Reliability reflects the extent to which the same result occurs from repeated application of a measure to the same subject. Reliability has been of considerable interest at two levels: the reliability of clinical observations by professionals and the reliability of the judgments of quality as assessed by certain methods. The reliability of a clinical observation can be determined by having the same observer repeat the same examination on the same subject (e.g., a repeat physical exam or a rereading of x-rays) to determine if the same results (e.g., normal versus abnormal, getting better versus getting worse, need for a treatment versus no need for treatment) are obtained. This is termed intra-observer reliability.

A second method involves having different observers review the same subject and comparisons of the results of the observations are made. This is termed inter-observer reliability and is similar to what occurs in second opinion surgery programs in which more than one surgeon determines whether surgery is indicated. The results of observer-reliability testing have generally demonstrated poor levels of reliability of clinician-based data and judgments (16). For example, substantial lack of reliability has been shown for such information as whether or not patients have a heart murmur, or a diagnosis of coronary artery disease or whether they should have a certain elective surgical procedure. The order of magnitude of such disagreements varies from 5 to 40% disagreement using conventional reliability tests. When more sophisticated (Kappa Statistic) tests are performed the results are even more disquieting. The advanced method adjusts for the expected distribution of agreement based on chance alone (16). The implications of these problems in the reliability of clinical observations have not been adequately explored and most methods of assessing quality assume that clinical observations are correct.

RELIABILITY OF SECONDARY DATA SOURCES

Assuming that clinical observations are reliable, the next level of concern is the recording of data and its incorporation into data systems useful for quality assessment purposes. This includes entry of data into the medical record by providers followed by abstracting or synthesis of that information by medical records personnel. Abstracts include discharge diagnoses listed on the cover or summary sheets of medical records, summary abstracts such as those prepared for the Commission on Professional and Hospital Activities, insurance claims forms, and hospital discharge summaries; these "abstracted" sources are termed "secondary" data. There have been very few studies of what bias occurs when the events occurring in a patient-provider encounter are recorded in the medical record. Studies have compared tape recordings of medical encounters to the extent to which the physician's notes of these encounters reflected the verbal content (17). Significant underrecording occurred and was most pronounced for information relating to patient education and number of pills prescribed. A study of patients undergoing tonsillectomy and/or adenoidectomy indicated that phrases in hospital records such as "frequent" and "numerous" episodes of tonsillitis were open to considerable variation in interpretation when compared to the actual disease experiences of the patients (18).

It is assumed that there is greater discordance between actual care provided and that recorded in office settings as compared to such discordance in inpatient settings. Indeed, one large study of office care for children documented numerous deficiencies in recording and found that over half the physicians felt their records did not adequately reflect the care they provided (19).

Finally, with respect to data reliability, there is concern over information that is routinely abstracted from medical records and recorded on magnetic computer tapes. Studies conducted by the Institute of Medicine of the National Academy of Sciences assessed the reliability of hospital discharge diagnostic data and showed major disagreements on such critical items of information as principal diagnosis (20). As a result, concern has been raised of the utility of using such data for many quality assessment programs. These studies do not negate the utility of such data systems for identifying possible areas for more intensive review at the individual case level. Reliable judgments of the quality of care at the individual level (either patient or physician) will require the use of the medical record, however, except for those few providers whose practice patterns are so deviant from the norm that problems such as those discussed above are inconsequential.

EVALUATING METHODS USED TO ASSESS QUALITY OF CARE

The sensitivity, specificity, and predictive value of methods of quality assessment have major implications for the efficiency of the quality of review procedures. To illustrate these concepts, assume the presence of an omniscient quality-assessor who knows whether or not people are sick, what happens to them, and what the relative contribution of medical care is to improving their illness. Such an assessor would provide a "gold standard" for true judgments against which other methods of assessing quality could be compared. If a new method of identifying cases of bad quality care were proposed, a comparison of the "new" and "true" methods would result in a distribution of cases into four categories (Fig. 12–6). The sensitivity of the new method represents the extent to which it identifies all truly bad cases of quality; in this case, sensitivity = $a/(a + c)$. Specificity reflects the extent to which cases that are classified as good by the test actually are good; specificity = $d/(b + d)$.

Results by "New" Method	Results by "True" Method	
	Bad care	Good care
Bad care	a	b
Good care	c	d

Figure 12–6. Testing a new method of assessing the quality of care.

At the operational level, methods that have high sensitivity and specificity are desirable. In general, increases in the sensitivity of a method achieved by loosening the criteria for bad versus good care, without changing the method itself, will tend to decrease the specificity of the method.

The concepts of positive predictive value or negative predictive value of a method are also of interest. In Figure 12–6 the new method attempts to identify bad care as indicated by a positive test result. The positive predictive value of the test is the probability that a positive result by the "new" method reflects a positive result by the "true" method; positive predictive value = $a/(a + b)$. The accurate reflection of a negative result yields negative predictive value = $d/(c + d)$.

Knowledge of these characteristics of a method for assessing quality of care helps one to use such methods. If the primary goal of an assessment of quality is to identify all episodes of bad care, then highest priority should be given to increasing the sensitivity of the quality assessment method used. If the primary goal is to lower the cost of identifying a case of bad care, then specificity or positive predictive value would be emphasized.

QUALITY ASSESSMENT METHODS

The preceding discussion sets the stage for presenting the categories of measures of quality that can be monitored. The selection and design criteria outlined above are generic and apply to all measures of the quality of care. Quality of care measures generally fall into one of three categories: 1) outcome measures that reflect the results or impact of care (e.g., changes in health status); 2) process measures that reflect what was done (e.g.,number and types of laboratory tests performed); and 3)structural measures that reflect the setting in which care is provided (e.g., licensure of personnel or facilities).

OUTCOME MEASURES OF QUALITY

Outcomes of care reflect the net changes that occur in health status as a result of health care and are appealing because of their face validity; their use in assessing care has been extensively reviewed elsewhere (21, 22). As discussed previously, many factors affect health and if outcomes are to be used as an indicator of the quality of care, they must be sensitive to different levels in the quality of the process or content of care; that is, outcomes should change when process changes.

The two major groups of outcome measures are general health-status indicators and disease-specific indicators. A general health-status measure is multidimensional and may include physical, emotional, and social aspects of health. The measures can be based on a person's own perception of his health or on independent assessments that do not rely on the patient's own perceptions (23–26). An example of a health-status measure that relies on self-reported perceptions and covers several dimensions of health is the Sickness Impact Profile (27). This profile is an index based on patients' responses to a series of statements such as: 1) I am going out less to visit people; 2) I do not walk at all; 3) I often act irritable toward my work associates, for example, snap at them, give sharp answers, criticize easily, 4) I am doing less of the regular daily work around the house than I usually do; and 5) I stop often when traveling because of health problems. Changes in these aspects of an individual's function can be produced by a variety of diseases.

General health status indicators have the advantage of reflecting changes in several dimensions of health that might not be detected by technically derived, disease-specific measures (e.g., changes in blood pressure levels). They have the disadvantage of possibly being too sensitive to nonmedical factors. For instance, in assessing outcomes of care for an operation to fuse a spine because of back pain, a general health-status instrument might detect deficiencies in work productivity and in the emotional state of the patient, but there are many factors besides the surgery that could affect a patient's productivity and propensity to depression.

Disease-specific outcome indicators include death rates due to a given disease, presence of symptoms known to occur with a disease, or behavioral disabilities commonly associated with a specified disease. For example, in patients with coronary artery disease assessments could be based on deaths from heart attacks on the number of people with symptomatic chest pain with exertion, or on the avoidance of specific work or social activities by patients with heart disease due to fears of incurring a heart attack.

Data on many outcome measures must be obtained directly from patients because such data may not be recorded in the medical record. To obtain reliable outcome information by either a self-administered or interviewer-administered questionnaire may be expensive and the cost may limit the usefulness of the outcome methods on a routine basis.

Outcome measures can be used in operational settings to assess quality of care. At the very least, adverse outcomes related to treatment can be monitored as indicators of suboptimal quality (e.g., many infections following surgery). Similarly, while five years may have to elapse before determining if survivors of a surgical procedure have better or worse than expected death rates, immediate (within a "short" time period) surgical mortality rates can be used as indicators of poor technical quality for such procedures as gastrectomies for patients with stomach cancer or replacement of heart valves in patients with rheumatic heart disease. Before passing judgment on such mortality rates, however, the severity of illness in the individual cases treated must be considered as was done in a recent study of the variation by hospitalization in surgical death rates (28). In this study, unadjusted death rates for various operations varied five-fold across study hospitals, but the differences were generally less than two-fold after adjustments for case-severity were made.

In addition to the use of treatment-related adverse outcome measures, quality of care can be reflected in intermediate outcomes that are known to relate to a final outcome that is a goal of care. For example, the treatment for high blood pressure seeks to avoid the future occurrence of stroke or heart failure by lowering blood pressure. Rather than waiting 10 to 14 years to determine if the incidence of stroke or heart failure has been altered by a treatment program, an intermediate outcome can be measured. In this case one could assess the extent to which blood pressure has been reduced to levels that are known to be associated with a lower long-term probability of stroke or heart failure.

The use of intermediate outcomes is inherent in the "staging" approach to assessing quality of ambulatory care (29). An example of the use of this technique derives from the fact that death rates from certain cancers are related to how advanced the cancer is at the time of detection, and many cancers should be detectable at an early stage if the quality of ambulatory care is high. The stage of a cancer is reflected in pathology, laboratory, and x-ray reports and presumably a "good quality" ambulatory care program would identify tumors at an early stage (i.e., the intermediate outcome) and improve long-term survival.

PROCESS MEASURES OF QUALITY

The process of care, as defined by Donabedian, refers to what is done to patients (30). DeGeyndt has elaborated this into the notion of the content of care (i.e., activities performed) and uses the word process to denote the sequence and coordination of these activities (31). A further refinement of the concept separates the "technical" aspects of care from the affective and interpersonal skills (how the patient was "treated") implied in the "art" of care (32).

The use of process measures has considerable attraction because they are operationally much easier to collect than outcome measures. Specifically, they are less time-dependent and less dependent on expensive patient followup studies because the medical record, despite its imperfections, does reflect certain processes of care reasonably well. Most of the process approaches to assessing care depend on the establishment of agreed-upon criteria for good care and applying these criteria to individual cases.

The most common process method is based on the development of a list of elements of good care and on whether or not these elements are documented in the medical record. Physicians frequently argue that they do not think in checklist fashion, or more perjoratively, in a "laundry list" format. Instead, they argue correctly that in making decisions they use a contingency-based format that considers case-severity, test results, and the presence or absence of certain signs and symptoms. Accordingly, simple checklists may not be an optimal or the most relevant means of assessing the process of care.

An approach to assessing the process of care that more closely mirrors clinical decision-making is the criteria-mapping approach (38). In this approach, criteria for good care can be met in a variety of ways depending on the presence or absence of certain signs, symptoms, laboratory tests, or more general reflections of case-severity. The criteria-mapping approach should be as sensitive in detecting poor care as the list, but should also be more specific. Additionally, it may afford the possibility of identifying excess use of certain tests or procedures that should be done only in very selected circumstances. A comparison of criteria that might be used by these two approaches is shown in Table 12–1.

While the assessment of the process of care is inherently attractive, several criticisms have been voiced about the use of process measures. The most common criticism is that outcomes should be of most concern and few studies have

TABLE 12–1. Comparison of Lists and Mapping Approaches for Assessing the Process of Care: Hypothetical Criteria for Diagnostic Tests in Patients with Newly Discovered Hypertension

Checklist Approach	Illustrative Criteria-Mapping Approach
Abdominal exam for bruits	Abdominal exam for bruits
Serum Potassium level	Serum Potassium level
Serum Bicarbonate level	Serum Bicarbonate level
Fasting glucose level	Fasting glucose level
Test of Catecholamine or VMA excretion for pheochromocytoma	Test for pheochromocytoma only if there is history of palpitations, or weight loss, or elevated fasting glucose, or orthostatic drop in blood pressures off treatment, or family history of this tumor.
Plasma Renin or Intravenous Pylogram to rule out renal artery stenosis	Test for renal artery stenosis only if there is one of the following: abdominal or flank bruit, serum potassium less than 3.6 meq/L or bicarbonate greater than 28 meq/L.

demonstrated a strong relationship between the process and outcome of care. While this contention is often correct, there are several biologic and methodologic reasons for the failure to establish a strong relationship between process and outcome in quality of care studies. The biologic explanation is that not all health care is necessarily efficacious. Accordingly, variations in the process of care will not alter outcomes. For example, radical mastectomy could be required as an element of good process for treating breast cancer. But this procedure is not clearly superior to a simple mastectomy, and no difference in outcomes may be measured for patients who had either "good" or "suboptimal" process. Lack of such discrimination, however, does not mean that neither approach is efficacious or that care is irrelevant; rather it simply means that different strategies of treating patients with breast cancer may not produce large enough differences in outcomes to be detectable in quality of care studies. Examples of process criteria for good care that have not been validated are numerous and extend to time honored exhortations such as requiring that all patients with sore throats should have a throat culture before antibiotic therapy is started (34).

There are also conceptual and methods deficiencies in those studies that demonstrate low (or even negative) correlations between process and outcome. The choice of the strategy used to assess the quality of the process of care is critical; a strategy that emphasizes diagnosis rather than treatment ignores those aspects of process that are most proximate to determining good outcome. For example, hypertension is a treatable condition and therapy for it is efficacious. In over 90% of treated cases, hypertension is *not* due to a readily identifiable etiology, yet it will respond to therapy. Process-oriented studies of the quality of care given to hypertensive patients frequently focus on the degree to which physicians establish the level of end-organ damage when a hypertensive patient is identified, and the extent to which a differential diagnostic strategy is pursued to identify those few patients with a specific etiology for their hypertension. A more critical factor in changing outcomes, however, is whether an antihypertensive drug is prescribed. For the vast majority of patients, an antihypertensive drug will have more importance in determining whether blood pressure is lowered than will performance of a laboratory test to detect rare causes of hypertension. Accordingly, unless much greater weight is attached to initiation of therapy than to ruling out a rare diagnosis, there will be very little positive correlation between process and outcome assessments of quality of care.

The use of criteria for good care that are process-oriented but are not of proven efficacy in operational quality assurance programs may result in the increased use of unnecessary tests and drugs without any improvement in outcome. Much of the concern about using a process-oriented approach can be alleviated if it is employed primarily to identify a lack of optimal process in cases with known poor outcomes, (e.g., use of antihypertensive drugs in patients with uncontrolled hypertension) or to discourage the use of practices that are known to be harmful (e.g., use of chloramphenicol in most of its applications in ambulatory care).

The lack of definitive studies of efficacy of some clinical strategies does not require that they be excluded from a quality of care study. Practicing physicians should not be expected to conduct basic research to demonstrate conclusively the efficacy of a procedure which the overwhelming professional opinion already holds is appropriate to use; that should be the role of academic research centers. This reiterates the fundamentals of good care developed 50 years ago by Lee and Jones (35):

> Good medical care is the kind of medicine practiced and taught by recognized leaders of the medical profession at a given time and period of social, cultural, and professional development in a community or population group . . .
>
> The concept of good medical care . . . is based upon certain "articles of faith" which can be briefly stated:
>
> 1) Good medical care is limited to the practice of rational medicine based on the medical sciences . . .
>
> 2) Good medical care emphasizes prevention . . .
>
> 3) Good medical care requires intelligent cooperation between the lay public and the practitioners of scientific medicine . . .
>
> 4) Good medical care treats the individual as a whole . . . Good practice requires that the patient be considered as a person, a member of a family living in a certain enviroment. All factors which concern his [her] health—mental and emotional, as well as physiological—must be weighed in diagnosis, prevention, and treatment. It is the sick or injured person and not merely the pathologic condition which must be treated . . .
>
> 5) Good medical care maintains a close and continuing personal relationship between physician and patient . . .
>
> 6) Good medical care is coordinated with social welfare, work . . . love

of [people] must be clarified by an understanding of [people] and must take note of his [her] social environment and economic needs . . .

7) Good medical care coordinates all types of medical services . . .

8) Good medical care implies application of all the necessary services of modern scientific medicine to the needs of all the people. Judged from the viewpoints of society as a whole, the qualitative aspects of medical care cannot be dissociated from the quantitative. No matter what the perfection of technique of one individual case, medicine does not fulfill its functions adequately until the same perfection is within reach of all individuals.

STRUCTURAL MEASURES OF QUALITY

Measures of the structure of care relate to the personnel and facilities used to provide services and the manner in which they are organized. Examples of structural measures of care are presented in Table 12–2.

From an administrative viewpoint, structural assessments are attractive because much of the information they require can be readily obtained from existing documents or a simple inspection of a facility. Assessments based solely on the structure of care assume that if the structure is optimal, then the appropriate processes will necessarily follow and outcomes will be maximized. The assumptions underlying many structural criteria, however, have not been validated. For example, consider the criterion of whether or not the physicians in a hospital are board-certified. Presumably physicians with longer training programs who become board-certified in their specialty will treat diseases related to that specialty better than noncertified physicians. Much medical training, however, is oriented toward teach-

TABLE 12–2. Examples of Structural Measure of Quality

Resource	Illustrative Criteria
Facility	Does it meet fire and safety codes? Is it clean?
Personnel	Are the physicians licensed? Are the physicians board certified? Is the ratio of registered nurses to practical nurses over 0.3? Is the nurse to patient ratio over 0.2?
Organization	Is there an organization structure with clearly defined responsibility? Is there a mechanism for peer review?

ing the process of care as best known at the time of training. Because the presumed "best" process of care 10 years ago may not now result in the best outcome, board-certified status may not be a powerful prediction of quality of care.

There is also some evidence that "better" qualified physicians do not necessarily perform at a substantially higher level, i.e., have higher process scores, than similarly trained physicians who are not board-certified. A large study in Hawaii showed that self-declared specialists tended to treat diseases related to their specialty better than nonspecialists, but it also found little difference in quality of care provided by physicians with formal board certification in a specialty versus those who were self-identified specialists, but not board-certified (14). This example is especially pertinent in view of recent trends stressing board certification as an indicator of quality in consumer's guides to choosing a physician and as a mechanism to control the number of "unnecessary" surgical procedures. The objective of making all physicians board-certified could increase the total costs of care for society substantially with only a marginal affect on the quality of the process of care and perhaps no positive effect on outcomes. Similar concerns can be raised with a large number of other structural criteria for good care including an increased interest in having only nurses with baccalaureate training be eligible for licensure as a registered nurse.

Do limitations of structural measures mean that they should not be included as an element of a quality assessment or assurance program? While reliance on structural criteria does not guarantee that good processes and outcomes will follow, some level of structure must be obtained in areas such as professional responsibility, peer review, and life safety if good processes are to occur. Good structure is a necessary but not sufficient correlate of good care.

EFFICIENCY AND QUALITY

Efficiency of care reflects how much care of a given quality is provided for a specified cost, and can be expressed as net outcomes achieved per unit of cost. With concern over the rising costs of health care in relation to the Gross National Product (Chapter 10), increasing attention has been directed toward inefficient use of resources as reflected by such terms as "inappropriate hospitalization," "unnecessary surgery," and "defensive medicine." A hypothesized relationship between costs and outcomes is presented in Figure 12–7. Initial investments in care produce rapid increases in positive outcomes (zone A). When only difficult and costly problems are left to be overcome, there is little, and eventually no increase in positive outcomes from further investments (zone B). Finally, a negative slope could even occur in one of two ways (zone C). First, direct application of increased medical care at very intensive levels might produce more iatrogenic injury than benefit. Second, costs of care could become so high that resources that might be used to produce health in areas of the economy other than medical care are diverted to medical care. Thus, auto safety devices may not be produced in favor of investments in medical care that produce less impact on health. Note, however, that Figure 12–7 is very simplistic. A more complex figure would have a series of curves that takes account of the multidimensional nature of the outcome of care,

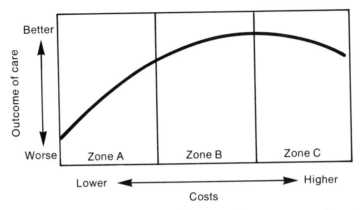

Figure 12-7. Hypothetical relationship between the outcomes and costs of care.

(e.g., disability days, symptom status, mortality) and would relate each of these outcomes to costs of care.

Because outcomes are multidimensional, even a simple disease process produces a family of efficiency curves rather than a single curve; the tradeoffs of favoring one efficiency curve over another must be understood. For example, two outcomes of interest in the management of high blood pressure might be work status and age-specific death rate. There is no question that investing more resources in the identification and adequate treatment of all hypertensives would reduce overall cardiovascular age-specific death rates. There may be, however, high rates of work loss in treated patients secondary to the psychological effects of being labeled hypertensive, or because of complications of therapy such as depression, or due to work loss to go see a physician. These latter effects will occur when treated patients are in their third or fourth decade of life while reduction in death rate might not occur until the fifth decade of life. The net effect might be substantially more disability days in a treated, as compared to an untreated, population in order to achieve a reduction in strokes and heart failure in later life. Many people who would never have had a stroke or heart failure are treated to prevent these events that will occur in some hypertensives. For those individuals who would never have developed a stroke or congestive failure, all of the treatment essentially had a negative effect with no clear benefit. Unfortunately, tradeoffs such as these are common in current medical practice and these tradeoffs will need to be considered in studies of the quality of care.

EFFICIENCY AND PROVIDER-PATIENT RELATIONSHIP

When efficiency is stressed, providers must play a larger role of social policeman vis-a-vis their role of patient advocate. This shift in emphasis has substantial implications for patient-provider relationships, especially under prepayment arrangements. For example, a physician may know that less than one in a hundred patients with adult onset seizures has a treatable form of brain tumor. The physician may also know that certain associated signs and symptoms make that possibility more or less likely. The physician cannot determine with absolute certainty, however, whether a given patient is, or is not, that one in a hundred. It is unethical for the physician to tell the patient that there is a 100% likelihood that the patient does not have a serious and treatable problem. How many tests and what expense should be incurred to determine if the patient is the rare case of that treatable disease? What should be the provider's response to a patient who says "Look Doc, I'm fully covered by insurance and I'd like you to order a computerized axial tomography scan for me because I just want to be sure?" These and similar questions have no simple answer and they pose major ethical dilemmas for professionals entrusted with the dual functions of advocate and policeman.

PATIENT SATISFACTION AND THE QUALITY OF CARE

Patient satisfaction is a measure than can reflect the outcome, process, and structure of care. Satisfaction has been viewed as a multidimensional concept involving the cost, convenience, technical and interpersonal aspects of care, and outcome of care (36, 37, 38). Satisfaction with care can be assessed for a specific illness episode, for a patient's own personal care, or for medical care in general. From a technical medical perspective, satisfaction is important because it is positively correlated with patient adherence to prescribed therapeutic regimens. It may positively affect subsequent care-seeking behavior, and probably has some impact on the propensity to file a malpractice claim.

At any point in time, using existing measures, the overwhelming majority (usually over 85%) of people are satisfied with their own health care. This is in marked contrast to claims to the contrary that occasionally appear in the mass media. The apparent high level of satisfaction may be because most patients finally find a provider who meets their needs after a long odyssey, or because existing measures of satisfaction are not sensitive to people's actual feelings, or to all components of satisfaction. However, despite the generally high rate of satisfaction with most aspects of personal medical care, there is room for improvement, especially in the area of satisfaction with the interpersonal aspects of care.

ACCESS TO CARE

Access to care has been discussed in earlier chapters and is an important element of quality assessment at the programmatic and social level. Access to care as a dimension of quality at the individual provider level is more difficult to conceptualize and measure. A provider who agrees to be a regular source of primary care for a "panel" (those patients who identify that provider as their regular source of care) should be responsible for assuring access to services for those patients. Poor access may be reflected in delayed care-seeking, absence of preventive care, and low levels of patient satisfaction. Whether equity of access for all members of society is a measure of quality at the individual provider level is an unresolved issue. This issue includes questions about the extent to which individual providers should be accountable for assuring access to care by working longer hours, treating more patients, working more efficiently, or encouraging or actively seeking out potential patients with limited access to care as reflected in the types of measures presented in Chapter 3.

A provider's patterns of practice can affect access to care quite markedly, and studies of physicians in group practices show marked variations in the number of patients per physician and number of visits per patient despite relatively similar populations of patients (39). In the absence of optimal visit schedules for acute and chronic illnesses by which such data could be judged, it is difficult to determine which physicians are practicing "better medicine" or are requiring too many or too few follow-up visits. Whether or not providers who treat patients obtain similar or different outcomes should lead to considerable concern about the relationships between efficiency, quality, and access to care.

ILLUSTRATIVE STUDIES OF THE QUALITY OF CARE

The quality of care assessment literature has expanded rapidly and selected major studies performed since 1950 are highlighted here for illustration purposes.

OUTCOME-ORIENTED STUDIES

Outcome-oriented studies have been based on death certificates, face-to-face and telephone interviews with patients, medical records, and secondarily abstracted medical records. Shapiro and associates studied the quality of care under two different organizational systems in New York by analyzing the perinatal mortality of infants born to low income women (40). Their findings indicated a lower death rate for those infants whose mothers were enrolled in a prepaid practice plan. The study highlights the importance of defining a denominator population and raises several issues concerning epidemiologic and statistical adjusting procedures when dealing with problems of selection bias in quality of care studies based on outcome measures.

Forrest and associates studied the outcome of surgical care in 17 hospitals by direct assessments of the status of patients during a 40 day post-operative interval (28). They found significant variations across hospitals with death rates that were nearly twice as high in the "worst" as compared to the "best" hospital in the sample. This study is important because it illustrates the need to adjust for case-severity. Forrest and associates also found that the use of data from a medical abstracting service as opposed to a direct assessment produced results with similar trends but not magnitudes. This means that with proper adjustments for such factors as case mix, hospitals with unusually adverse outcome rates can potentially be identified for further investigation by means of analysis of data collected by a medical abstracting service. Additionally, the study identified some organizational features of hospitals that might be associated with better care (41). For example, both stringent control over admission to membership on the surgical staff and the ratio of registered nurses to other nurses were positively related to better outcomes of care. Interestingly, teaching status, size of medical staff, and board certification of surgeons were not significantly correlated with quality of care. Because of the nature of the study, a causal relationship between these structural features and outcomes of care could not be inferred, but prospective studies using this information are clearly in order.

Kessner and associates conducted a population-based study of the quality of ambulatory care for children using the outcome oriented "tracer" methodology (42). They assessed outcomes for iron deficiency, ear infection, and vision correction. The study sample consisted of 1,436 families with 2,780 children aged 6 months to 11 years in Washington, D.C. Over 25% of the children aged six months to three years had anemia, 20% of them had ear disease, and nearly 25% aged 4 to 11 failed a vision screening test. After controlling for the social class of the patents, no significant correlation between the outcome and type of provider organization was found. Inappropriate or ineffective treatment was provided to a large proportion of children in the sample.

Schroeder and Donaldson applied the outcome-oriented method known as "health accounting" to a Health Maintenance Organization (43). This method was developed by Williamson and requires a consensus estimate of what outcomes are achievable with specific interventions. The extent to which the outcomes achieved deviate from expected outcomes is then determined. The outcome assessment can usually be performed by telephone survey or mailed questionnaire. Applied to the diagnoses of depression, high blood pressure, and "contraception," the method revealed major problems of underdiagnosis for all the conditions (44–74%) and unacceptable therapeutic outcomes for depression and high blood pressure. The operational difficulties for using this outcome-based method in ambulatory settings delivering care to large numbers of disadvantaged people were also emphasized.

Intermediate outcomes have been assessed from medical records in several studies. Gonnella and colleagues applied the "staging" approach to hospitalized patients as an outcome measure of the quality of their ambulatory medical care (29). They studied 5,000 patients admitted to hospitals in two cities in California. For 6 of the 18 conditions studied, they showed significant differences in the stages of disease severity present at time of hospitalization in patients from various population groups. Level of disease severity was generally worse in patients with government sponsorship other than Medicare.

PROCESS-ORIENTED STUDIES

Process-oriented studies can be conducted by direct observation of medical encounters, by review of medical records, and by review of insurance claims. Observational studies provide a wealth of information not otherwise obtainable, but suffer from high cost and potential alteration of behavior resulting from the presence of an observer. These problems notwithstanding, a few observational studies of process have been completed, the most noteworthy of which in the United States was a study of 88 general practitioners in North Carolina by Peterson and associates in 1953 (44). They developed a semistructured review protocol that included observable elements of history taking, physical diagnosis, use of laboratory services, preventive care and clinical record keeping. In addition to an index score based on these observations, the authors developed a five point qualitative ranking system. With the ranking system, 8% of the physicians were in rank 5 (essentially outstanding) and 18% in rank 1. The physicians in rank 1 had a very superficial, disorganized approach to clinical medicine. Overall, 39 of the 88 physicians were in rank 1 or 2. This study was of considerable importance because it demonstrated the feasibility of carrying out direct observations of practicing physicians in their offices and because it demonstrated major deficiencies in the level of care in office settings and thus established the need to assess the quality of care.

There have been numerous large scale process-oriented studies of hospital and ambulatory care utilizing medical records. In his pioneering work in Monroe County, New York, Lembcke identified numerous deficiencies in care given to patients undergoing hysterectomies (45). Similar findings were noted by Doyle in a study of over 6,000 hysterectomies in the Los Angeles area (46). More recently, major problems in surgery judged to be unnecessary by process criteria were noted in a population-based study of hysterectomies in Saskatchewan (47). Lest gynecologists feel singled out, McCarthy and Widmer have identified "potentially" unnecessary surgery in nearly one-third of patients recommended for a variety of elective procedures in a second surgical opinion program (48).

In one of the largest studies of the process of care, Payne and Lyons found numerous deficiencies in care provided to patients admitted to hospitals in Hawaii. This study was based on a random sample of all hospital patients in the state who had selected discharge diagnoses in the year 1968 (14). A group of practicing physicians established criteria for good care which were then applied to the hospital records. For each disease, a physician's performance index (PPI) was developed which represented the percentage of process criteria (e.g., performance of certain laboratory tests) for which evidence of compliance could be found in the medical records. Overall, they found a PPI of 0.71 for hospitalized patients. In a companion study of office-based care in 1970, they found an average PPI of only 0.40 (49). These studies are important demonstrations of the feasibility of carrying out large scale quality assessment efforts and have identified several organizational and structural features which tend to be associated with good care, even though the correlations were relatively low.

In addition to studies using direct observation or medical record review, the process of care has been studied through the use of claims forms. In tennessee, Ray and associates established criteria for the appropriate use of certain drugs and applied them to claims data (50). Their first analysis was concerned with chloramphenicol, a broad spectrum antibiotic that can cause death due to agranulocytosis (absence of white cells necessary to fight infection). The use of this drug has been recommended only for serious, well-defined infections for which there are no reasonable therapeutic alternatives. The analysis indicated that nearly 6% of all antibiotic prescriptions filled by pharmacies were for this drug and it was prescribed by 6% of the physicians participating in the Tennessee Medicaid program. About half of the prescriptions were for upper respiratory infections for which the drug is never indicated. Most of the remaining prescriptions were also inappropriate. This study is important because it documented the ability to indentify inappropriatte practice patterns by analysis of claims data. In a similar study, Brook and colleagues analyzed the use of injectable antibiotics in Medicaid patients in New Mexico and showed that claims data could indentify physicians whose practice patterns were both atypical and inappropriate (51). They further showed that practice patterns could be altered by the use of an ongoing monitoring system with feedback to physicians whose practice patterns were at variance with established and accepted standards.

QUALITY ASSURANCE IN MEDICAL CARE

The application of quality assessment methods to the "assurance" of acceptable care to patients is of considerable concern to providers. Quality assurance means those activities that are designed to partially guarantee that the care received meets some reasonable professional standards. In general, there are two major mechanisms that assure that care is of some minimal level of quality; these are either structure-oriented systems or systems that actively monitor the events and outcomes of the care actually provided.

STRUCTURE-ORIENTED APPROACHES TO QUALITY ASSURANCE:LICENSURE

The most pervasive, oldest, and most fundamental assurance mechanism is licensure. With rare, but highly publicized exception, licensure assures a patient that a physician or nurse has a specified level of educational achievement relevant to their profession. For physician licensure, states require graduation in good standing from a recognized medical school, passing of a state-required examination or the equivalent thereof (e.g., those offered by the National Board of Medical Examiners), no record of conviction for any major crime (such as a felony), and letters of recommendation from other licensed physicians. In addition, over 90% of the states require that the applicant has completed an accredited internship program. Persons not meeting these requirements are denied the right to practice their profession legally in a defined geographic area. In essence, the licensing mechanism sets a minimal floor on the quality of the resources available to provide care.

It is interesting to note that in professional licensure, the licensing body represents public interests, but the determination of whether certain schools are acceptable often lies (to a great extent) in the hands of nonpublic groups. In this instance, the determination of whether a given medical school is to be accredited is performed by a mixture of academic and professional organizations. This arrangement has raised certain questions as to whether an organization representing professional interests, such as the American Medical Association, should have any direct or indirect influence in determining whether certain training programs are accredited because potential conflict of interests might exist.

Licensure mechanisms are very general in relation to actual professional practice. For example, most physicians' licenses state only that they are physicians and surgeons and, in theory, they are allowed to perform any act in the scope of medical practice. Accordingly, they could attempt procedures they had not been specifically trained to do. For instance, substantial concern has been raised concerning the use of potentially toxic chemotherapeutic drugs in cancer patients by physicians not trained in this area. In view of such concern, the "general" nature of licensing laws may represent a substantial weakness. Because of this weakness, one could argue for the passage of "limited licensure" laws that would restrict surgery to those with surgical training in accredited programs,or the use of cancer drugs to oncologists. Obviously, such laws would indeed be complex to administer and might stifle some of the highly beneficial flexibility given to practicing physicians. They presumably would, however, also prevent uncommon but egregious abuse of the medical license. Whether they would produce more good than harm is an open question.

A further weakness of licensure is its static nature, although this situation appears to be changing in many states. Once licensed, individuals need only send in a fee on a regular basis and indicate they had not been convicted of a felony in the past year to be relicensed. Given the rapid changes in medical knowledge and practice, there has been concern that professionals should demonstrate evidence of "keeping up to date" to be licensed. This concern has led to the development of "relicensure" requirements that the individual must show proof of a certain amount of continuing medical education (CME). For instance, in several states, physicians must be able to document 150 hours of CME every three years to be relicensed. These CME credits can be obtained through attendance at special courses, teaching, independent study, and similar activities.

While mandatory continuing education resolves some of the problems inherent in what amounts to lifetime licensure, it does not resolve those related to the general nature of the license itself and, more seriously, does not address the failure of structural mechanisms to guarantee the appropriateness of the process of care.

Licensure has also been applied to hospitals and long term care institutions. In general, such licenses heavily emphasize physical structure with a modicum of required organizatonal structure. To the extent that medical care is provided in organized settings, institutional licensure represents a pervasive mechanism that can contribute to assuring the quality of care; however, given the present form of most licensing mechanisms, this potential might not be realized.

CERTIFICATION AND ACCREDITATION

The second most pervasive structural assurance mechanism has been voluntary professional certification and accreditation. For physicians, this has assumed the form of certification by specialty boards that require completion of at least three years of postgraduate training and the passage of a special examination. Several specialty boards also require one or more years of practice after completion of residency training and/or submission of a series of records of actual cases for review by members of the board.

Specialty certification goes one step beyond licensure in setting minimal standards of quality for the provider's training and knowledge, but has limitations similar to those of licensure. As in the case of relicensure, there has been a trend toward mandatory periodic recertification by many of the specialty boards to assure updating of knowledge. While recertification tends to be structure-oriented and based on tests of knowledge, at least one Board, the Academy of Family Practice, requires that records of selected cases be submitted for review.

At the institutional level, The Joint Commission on Accreditation of Hospitals (JCAH) is the major voluntary accreditation mechanism. In the past the JCAH has relied heavily on assessments of organizational structure and physical environmental standards as a basis of its periodic biannual accreditation program. For example, it has set standards for the organization of the medical staff, mechanisms for peer review, and staffing patterns for nursing care. In recent years, it has also required that hospitals submit actual peer-reviewed "audits" of medical care as a basis for reaccreditation. This latter requirement means that accreditation by the JCAH represents a blend of structural and performance-based assessments. The JCAH is a voluntary review body, but its direct and indirect effects on the organization of most hospitals, and more recently many long term care institutions, should not be underestimated.

PERFORMANCE-BASED ASSURANCE APPROACHES

The structural mechanisms are directed at the providers of care rather than focused on care for selected patients or groups of patients, and generally do not rely on assessments of how the system is actually performing. In view of this deficiency, there is considerable interest in performance-based assurance programs that include utilization review and review of both processes and outcomes of care.

UTILIZATION REVIEW

Utilization review represents one of the earliest forms of process assurance to be instituted on a large scale. In essence, utilization review is directed at assuring that care is actually required and that the care setting is not inappropriately costly for the level of care provided. Not surprisingly, utilization review (UR) developed out of a desire to control the costs of care and was developed through cooperation between insurers and professional groups. UR grew slowly in the private sector in the late 1950s and 1960s and gained considerable attention in the public sector after the passage of Medicare and Medicaid. UR has been embodied into the Professional Standards Review Organization (PSRO) program.

There are three forms of utilization review: review of the necessity of care prior to the provision of a service, review during the care process, and review after the care has beeen provided. These are known as "prospective," "concurrent," and "retrospective" review respectively. In general, utilization review has been directed at costly institutionally-based care, but can also be applied in ambulatory care, dental care, and elsewhere.

How does utilization review relate to the quality of care? While it is true that efforts aimed at controlling inappropriate hospital admissions or lengths-of-stay in hospitals were begun because of interests in cost-containment, they definitely represent a form of quality assurance. Patients spared admission to a hospital for surgical removal of a gallbladder because they do not require surgery as determined by a peer review group are spared the pain, distress, and potential life-threatening hazards of major surgery; this is certainly a quality assurance function. Similarly, patients who might otherwise be kept in a hospital despite the availability of equally appropriate care at home, or in other less intense settings, are spared exposure to a host of nosocomial infections and other risks that can produce injury in the hospital. Because of their orientation toward cost control, utilization review programs are generally designed to avoid unnecessary care and do not specifically promote increased utilization where underprovision of services could occur (i.e., increased access).

The mechanism of review used by utilization review groups and PSROs include establishment of explicit criteria for both appropriate indications for hospitalization and length-of-stay. Cases not meeting these criteria might not be reimbursed by the insurance program. In practice, the review body (e.g., Foundation for Medical Care or PSRO) usually sets explicit criteria that can be applied by review coordinators who most commonly are specially trained nurses or medical records personnel. Cases are reviewed shortly after admission (concurrent review) and periodically during the hospital stay. Cases which do not appear to meet the indications for hospitalization are then formally reviewed by a physician or panel of physicians. Most systems also include an appeal mechanism. Cases that are not found to meet indications for continued stay are then denied payment (after a small grace period) by the insurer for any further duration of stay.

Some utilization review programs have a mechanism for prehospital admission review that is applied to elective hospitalization. "Second-surgical opinion" programs represent such a review mechanism and require approval by an independent physician of the need for the planned surgery (48).

The extent to which utilization review programs have reduced inappropriate utilization or saved money spent for hospital care is unclear at present, and a review of relevant studies suggests mixed results (52). Furthermore, even if hospital costs are reduced, it does not necessarily follow that total costs to individuals or society are reduced.

PEER REVIEW ASSURANCE PROGRAMS

While most utilization review programs represent forms of peer review, they are not designed to monitor patient-specific aspects of care once it has been decided that a certain procedure or level-of-care is appropriate. For example, once a decision has been made that a patient can have a diseased gallbladder removed, utilization review systems are not designed to assess the technical adequacy of the procedure performed or whether there were preventable operative complications. This latter question can only be addressed by peer review systems which focus on specific aspects of quality of care. Examples of peer review programs are provided elsewhere and this discussion will focus primarily on the approach known as "medical audits." (53)

The medical audit concept has been embellished in recent years, but essentially consists of the following six steps: 1) Selection of a topic for study such as care for a specific disease or use of a certain procedure or drug. 2) Selection of explicit criteria for good care using both process and outcome criteria. These might include whether specific diagnostic tests and treatments were performed, whether the status at discharge compared favorably with the expected status, and whether there were avoidable complications or unnecessary lengths-of-stay. 3) Review of medical records to determine if the criteria for good care are met, usually by a medical records analyst. 4) Specific review by professional peers of all cases that do not meet the criteria for good care. 5) Development of specific recommendations for assuring that any deficiencies found will be avoided in the future (e.g., education programs, changes in administrative procedures, requirements for consultations). 6) Re-study of the topic at a future date to ascertain if deficiencies have actually been reduced or eliminated. These elements of quality assurance have been incorporated into two complementary programs—the Professional Standards Review Organization (PSRO) and the Performance Evaluation Program of the JCAH.

PROFESSIONAL STANDARDS REVIEW ORGANIZATION

The PSRO program, also discussed in Chapter 11, represents the most ambitious, publicly mandated performance-based quality assurance program in existence (54, 55). The program incorporates the features of utilization review and medical care evaluation studies carried out at the hospital and nursing home level, as well as an overall analysis of patterns of care by different providers carried on at the agency (i.e., PSRO) level.

The PSRO program was established in 1972 and is administered at the federal level through the U.S. Department of Health, Education, and Welfare as discussed in previous chapters. It is currently under the responsibility of the Health Care Financing Administration, which is also responsible for administering the Medicare and Medicaid programs. The law (P.L. 92-603) establishing PSROs provides that care under the Medicare, Medicaid, and Title V (Maternal and Child Health) programs would be paid for if it met criteria for medical necessity and was provided in the appropriate level of facility. Thus, hospital care would not be covered if the appropriate care could be given on an outpatient basis or in a less costly facility such as a nursing home.

The implementation of the PSRO program was federally mandated, but the actual establishment of the 195 state or area-wide PSROs was left in the hands of practicing physicians. The individual PSRO must assure that the review activities are carried out in its area. It can delegate the review process to hospitals who meet certain requirements or it can elect to perform all of the review activities itself. Under these arrangements, criteria for review of care can vary at the local level so that considerable flexibility exists. The primary activities of utilization review and quality assurance employ the strategies described above. The medical audits tend to be process-oriented but usually include criteria covering avoidance of complications and the expected state of the patient at discharge. Reports of the audit and UR activities are monitored by the PSRO staff who are in turn responsible to the physician board of the PSRO.

In general, PSRO activities are oriented to hospital care, but the legislation provides for review of ambulatory and long term care as well, and a third of the PSROs have begun efforts in the long term care area.

THE PERFORMANCE EVALUATION PROGRAM (PEP) OF THE JCAH

The PEP system of the JCAH, which began in the early 1970s, complements the PSRO program and embodies the features of medical audits (56). It provides for review of care to all patients, not just persons insured by the federal government. Furthermore, it emphasizes more participation by administrators and other hospital personnel, including nurses and social workers, rather than just physicians in the medical audits. It is similar to the PSRO program in that it relies on the local institution to develop the criteria for care and to carry out the actual review. However, just as in the case when PSROs delegate review to individual hospitals, there is a required reporting system so that the JCAH can monitor the quality of the review process itself.

MALPRACTICE AS A QUALITY ASSURANCE MECHANISM

The legal system plays a role in quality assurance because of patients' ability to sue for malpractice, which is to some extent a quality assurance mechanism (57). Despite possible abuses by a minority of patients and lawyers, most malpractice awards do relate to less than optimal care, and all physicians are aware that they are in jeopardy of suit for egregious deficiencies in the quality of care.

ASSESSMENT OF QUALITY OF CARE

This chapter has reviewed salient issues with regard to quality assessment strategies and described basic quality assurance mechanisms. The uncertainty concerning the impact of various medical strategies on the health of individuals places some limitations on our ability to assess and assure the quality of medical care. However, there is sufficient medical knowledge to provide a solid foundation for systems of quality assessment and assurance which, as a minimum, could help us to avoid harmful strategies, promote known helpful strategies, and allow identification of practice patterns which are beyond the realm of reasonable professional practice. While the chapter has dealth primarily with examples of physician and hospital behavior, the concepts are analogous for assessing care by other professionals or institutions.

A final note must be made concerning the importance of personal motivation in improving the quality of health care. No matter how systems are structured, the final, common pathway of assessment will rely on the best professional judgement of a variety of individuals. The development, the quality, and the acceptance of those judgments will be a function of the professional's personal commitment to promoting good care in the context of a supportive organizational framework. Without strong positive commitments by the practicing professionals, all of the structure will prove to be of no avail. Conversely, without the appropriate structural support, the best of professional commitments and energy expenditure will be as efficacious as the sorrowful figure of the lone, would-be knight tilting at windmills.

REFERENCES

1. Knowles JH, editor: *Doing Better and Feeling Worse: Health in the United States.* New York, W.W. Norton and Company, 1977.

2. Donabedian A: *Medical Care Appraisal: A Guide to Medical Care Administration. Volume II.* New York, American Public Health Association, 1969.

3. Williamson JW: *Improving Medical Practice and Health Care: A Bibliographic Guide to Information Management in Quality Assurance and Continuing Education.* Cambridge, Massachusetts, 1977.

4. Barro AR: Survey and evaluation of approaches to physician performance measurement. *JME,* 48: 1047-1093, Supplement 11, 1973.

5. Williams KN, Brook RH: Quality measurement and assurance. *Hlth and Med Care Serv Rev,* 1:3-15, 1978.

6. Shortell SM, Richardson WC: *Health Program Evaluation.* St. Louis, Missouri, C.V. Mosby Company, 1978.

7. Bergman AB, Staemm SJ: The morbidity of cardiac non-disease in school children. *NEJM,* 276:1008–1013, 1967.

8. Sackett DL, Taylor DW, Haynes RB, et al: The short term disadvantage of being labeled hypertensive. *Clinical Research,* 25:266, 1977.

9. Neutra R: Indications for the Surgical Treatment of Suspected Acute Appendicitis: A

Cost-Effectiveness Approach. Chapter 18 in Bunker JP, Barnes BA, Mosteller F, editors: *Costs, Risks and Benefits of Surgery.* New York, Oxford University Press, 1977, pp. 277–307.

10. Watkins RN, Howell L: A population based quality assessment of the treatment of appendicitis. Presentation 105th Annual Meeting American Public Health Association, 1977.

11. Bunker JP, Barnes BA, Mosteller F, editors: *Costs, Risks, and Benefits of Surgery.* New York, Oxford University Press, 1977, pp. 28–76.

12. Bloch D: Evaluation of nursing care in terms of process and outcome: Issues in research and quality assurance. *Nursing Research,* 24:526–563, 1975.

13. Zimmer M, Lang N: Evaluation of patient health/wellness outcomes, Chapter 15, pp 155–172 in Maria Phaneuf: *The Nursing Audit. Self-Regulation in Nursing Practice.* New York: Appleton-Century Crofts, 1976.

14. Payne BC, Lyons TF, Dwarshius L, et al: *The Quality of Medical Care: Evaluation and Improvement.* Chicago, Illinois, Hospital Research and Educational Trust, 1976, pp. 7–19.

15. Kessner DN, Kalk CE: *Contrasts in Health Status, Volume 2: A Strategy for Evaluating Health Services.* Washington, D.C., National Academy of Science, 1973.

16. Koran LM: The reliability of clinical methods, data and judgments (parts 1 and 2). *NEJM,* 293:642–646 and 695–701, 1975.

17. Zuckerman AE, Starfield B, Hochreiter C, et al: Validating the content of pediatric outpatient medical records by means of tape-recording doctor-patient encounters. *Pediatrics,* 56:407–411, 1975.

18. LoGerfo JP, Dynes IN, Frost F, et al: Tonsillectomies, adenoidectomies, audits: have surgical indications been met? *Med Care,* 16:950–955, 1978.

19. Osborne CE, Thompson HC: Criteria for evaluation of ambulatory child health care by chart audit-development and testing of a methodology. *Pediatrics,* S6:625–692, 1975, Supplement Part 2.

20. Demlo LK, Campbell PN, Spaght S: Reliability of information abstracted from patients' medical records. *Med Care,* 16:995–1004, 1978.

21. Shapiro S: End-result measurements of quality of medical care. *Milbank Memorial Fund Quarterly,* 45:7–30, 1967.

22. Brook RH, Davies-Avery A, Greenfield S, et al: *Quality of Medical Care Assessment Using Outcome Measures: An Overview of the Method.* Santa Monica, California, Rand Corporation, 1976.

23. Stewart AL, Ware JE, Brook RH: *Conceptualization and Measurement of Health for Adults in the Health Insurance Study. Volume 2, Physical Health in Terms of Functioning.* Santa Monica, California, Rand Corporation, 1978.

24. Ware JE, Johnston SA, Davies-Avery A, et al: *Conceptualization and Measurement of Health for Adults in the Health Insurance Study. Volume 3, Mental Health.* Santa Monica, California, Rand Corporation, 1978.

25. Donald CA, Ware JE, Brook RH, et al: *Conceptualization and Measurement of Health for Adults in the Health Insurance Study. Volume 4, Social Health.* Santa Monica, California, Rand Corporation, 1978.

26. Ware JE, Davies-Avery A, Donald CA: *Conceptualization and Measurement of Health for Adults in the Health Insurance Study. Volume 5, General Health Perception.* Santa Monica California, Rand Corporation, 1978.

27. Bergner M, Bobbitt RA, Krenel A, et al: The Sickness Impact Profile: conceptual formulation and methodological development of a health status index. *Int J Hlth Serv,* 6:393–415, 1976.

28. Forrest WH, Scott WR, Brown BW: Study of the Institutional Differences in Postoperative Mortality. Project Report, National Center for Health Services Research (PB 250–940). 1974.

29. Gonnella J, Louis DZ, McCord JJ: The staging concept-an approach to the assessment of outcome of ambulatory care. *Med Care,* 14:13–21, 1976.

30. Donabedian A: Promoting quality through evaluating the process of patient care. *Med Care,* 6:181–202, 1968.

31. DeGeyndt W: Five approaches for assessing the quality of care. *Hosp Admin,* 15:21–42, 1970.

32. Brook RH, Williams KN, Davies-Avery A: Quality assurance today and tomorrow: forecast for the future. *Annals Internal Med,* 85:809–817, 1976.

33. Greenfield S, Lewis CE, Kaplan SH, et al: Peer review by criteria mapping: criteria for diabetes mellitus. The use of decision-making in chart audit. *Annals of Internal Med,* 83:761–770, 1975.

34. Tompkins RK, Burnes DC, Cable WE: An analysis of the cost-effectiveness of pharyngitis management and acute rheumatic fever prevention. *Annals of Internal Med,* 86:481–492, 1977.

35. Lee RI, Jones LW: *The Fundamentals of Good Medical Care.* Chicago, Illinois, University of Chicago Press, 1933.

36. Zyzanski SJ, Hulka BS, Cassel JC: Scale for the measurement of "satisfaction" with medical care: modifications in content, format, and scoring. *Med Care,* 12:611–620, 1974.

37. Ware JE, Davies-Avery A, Stewart PE: The measurement and meaning of patient satisfaction. *Health and Medical Care Services Review,* 1:1–15, 1978.

38. Lebow J: Consumer assessments of the quality of medical care. *Med Care,* 12:328–337, 1974.

39. Lyle CB, Applegate WB, Citron DF, et al: Practice habits in a group of eight internists. *Annals of Internal Med,* 84:594–601, 1976.

40. Shapiro S, Jacobziner H, Densen PM, et al: Further observation on prematurity and perinatal mortality in a general population and in the population of a prepaid group practice medical plan. *AJPH,* 50:1304–1317, 1960.

41. Scott WR, Forrest Jr WH, Brown Jr BW: Hospital structure and postoperative mortality and morbidity. *Organizational Research in Hospitals—An Inquiry Book,* 1976.

42. Kessner DM, Snow CK, Singer J: *Contrasts in Health Status. Volume 3, Assessment of Medical Care for Children.* Washington D.C., National Academy of Sciences, 1974.

43. Schroeder SA, Donaldson MS: The feasibility of an outcome approach to quality assurance—a report from one HMO. *Med Care,* 14:49–56, 1976.

44. Peterson OL, Andrews LP, Spain RS, et al: An analytic study of North Carolina general practice 1953–1954, *J Med Ed,* 31:1–165, 1956, number 12, part 2,

45. Lembcke PA: Medical auditing by scientific methods: illustrated by major female pelvic surgery. *JAMA,* 162:646–655, 1956.

46. Doyle JC: Unnecessary hysterectomies—study of 6,248 operations in 75 hospitals during 1948. *JAMA,* 151:360–365, 1953.

47. Dyck FJ, Murphy FA, Murphy JK, et al: Effect of surveillance on the number of hysterectomies in the Province of Saskatchewan. *NEJM,* 296:1326–1328, 1977.

48. McCarthy E, Widmer G: Effects of screening by consultants on recommended elective surgical procedures. *NEJM,* 291:1331–1335, 1974.

49. Payne BC, Lyons TI, Devarshires L, et al: *Quality of Medical Care Evaluation and Improvement.* Chicago, Illinois, Hospital Research and Educational Trust, 1976, pp. 20–28.

50. Ray W, Federspiel CP, Schaffner W: Prescribing of choloramphenicol in ambulatory practice. An epidemiologic study among Tennessee Medicaid recipients *Ann of Internal Med,* 84:266–270, 1976.

51. Brook RH, Williams KN, Rolph JE: Controlling the use and cost of medical services. The New Mexico experimental medical care review organization–a four year case study. *Med Care, 16 (Supplement No. 9):1–76, 1978.*

52. Chassin M: The containment of hospital costs: a strategic assessment. *Med Care,* 16 (Supplement No. 10):1–55, 1978.
53. Ertel PY, Aldredge MG (eds): *Medical Peer Review: Theory and Practice.* C.V. Mosby, St. Louis, 1977.
54. Jessee WF, Munier WB, Fielding JE, et. al.: PSRO: an educational force for improving quality of care. *NEJM,* 292:668–675, 1975.
55. Goran MJ, Roberts JS, Kellogg MA, et. al.: The PSRO hospital review system. *Med Care,* 13 (Supplement No. 4), 1975.
56. Jacobs CM, Christoffel T, Jacobs ND: *Measuring the Quality of Patient Care—The Rationale for Outcome Audit.* Ballinger Publishing Company, Cambridge, 1976.
57. Brook RH, Brutoco RL, Williams KN: The relationship between medical malpractice and quality of care. *Duke Law J,* 1975:1197–1231, 1976.

Index

Access to care, ambulatory services, 120
  quality of care and, 377-378
Accreditation, 160, 383
Almshouses, 126
Ambulatory health services, 25, 93-123
  access to, 120
  emergency medical services, *see* Emergency
      medical services; Emergency rooms
  home health services, 115
  integrated system of, 123
  mental health, 217
  for middle-class, middle-income families, 18
  neighborhood health centers, 113-114
  organization of, 118-123
  outpatient clinics, 111-112
  for the poor, 20-21
  provider satisfaction and, 121-122
  public health services, 116-118
  rural health care, 115-116
  solo practitioners, 96-98
  surgery centers, 112
  types of, 93-95
  utilization of, 56, 76-78
  Veterans Administration system and, 28
  see also Clinics; Community Mental Health
      Centers; Group practice
Ambulatory surgery centers, 112
Ambulatory visits, 56, 76-78
  prepaid group practices and, 109
  see also Physician visits
American Medical Association (AMA), 102, 332,
    346
American Psychiatric Association, 203, 209
American Psychological Association, 210
Anesthesia, 128-129
Antibiotics, 6
Atherosclerosis (arteriosclerosis), 7-8, 40-41, 230,
    232, 248

Behavioral model of health services utilization,
    68-74

Blue Cross/Blue Shield, 13, 16, 154, 159, 161, 310
  development of, 304, 306, 307
  hospital reimbursement by, 297-303, 346-347
  operating expenses of, 307, 308
  utilization of, 77

Cancer, 38, 42-43, 230, 232
Capital expenditures and services (CES) controls,
    344-345
Capitation, 295
Certificate-of-need (CON), 344-345
Certification, 159-160, 383
Chief-of-staff, hospital, 149
Children, utilization of health services by, 82-83
Chronic illnesses, defining, 7
  nursing homes and, 176-177
  prevention of, 7-8
  treatment of, 7, 8
Civilian Health and Medical Program of the
      Uniformed Services (CHAMPUS), 26
Clinics, free, 116, 217
  outpatient, 111-112
  for mental patients, 207
Committee on the Costs of Medical Care, 329-330
Community, ambulatory care system and, 122
  nursing homes and, 191, 192
  see also Ambulatory health services
Community hospitals, *see* Hospitals, community
Community Mental Health Centers, 19, 114, 208,
    212, 219
  ambulatory visits to, 56
  financing of, 215
Community psychiatry, 209
Comprehensive Health Planning (CHP), 160,
    333-335, 337, 338
Computerized axial tomography (CAT scanners),
    238-240, 242
Consumer groups, Veterans Administration
      system and, 27
Continuity of care, 19, 20, 121
Coordination of care, 121

Coronary artery disease, 40
Coronary bypass surgery, 248
Cost-benefit analysis, 364
Cost-effectiveness analysis, 364

Dawson Report, 330
Death, causes of, 5, 6
Degenerative diseases, 39
Dental services, utilization of, 59-61, 69, 72, 82
Dentists, supply of, 266-268
Deviant behavior, definitions of, 199
Diabetes mellitus, 36
Diagnostic technologies, 234-245
    basic research technologies, 234-236
    clinical conversion of basic technologies, 236
    computerized axial tomography (CAT
        scanners), 238-240, 242
    costs of health care and, 242
    diagnostic imperatives and, 243, 245
    electronic industry and, 243
    external energy probes and, 238
    intrinsic energy sources, 236-239
    radioisotopes, 241
    thermography, 241-242
    ultrasound, 240-241
Dialysis machines, 249, 250
Dietary habits, disease patterns and, 43
Disease, changing patterns of, 41-43
    clinical manifestations of, 39
    definition of, 36-37
    epidemics of infectious, 4-6, 9, 126-127
    germ theory of, 129
    pathophysiologic processes of, 37-39
    symptom production and, 39-41
Drugs, psychotropic, 207

Economic Stabilization Program (ESP), 161
Education, see Health education; Training
Elderly, expenditures for, 292
    utilization of health services by, 82
    see also Medicare; Nursing homes
Emergency centers, free-standing, 112
Emergency medical services, 112-113, 245-246
Emergency Medical Service systems, 245-246
Emergency rooms, 21, 112-113
    poor people's use of, 20-22
Emotional problems, of middle-class families,
    18-19. See also Mental health services
Environmental change, disease patterns and,
    42-43
Epidemics of infectious diseases, 4-6, 9, 126-127
Evaluation of health services, 355-364
    cost-benefit and cost-effectiveness analyses,
        364
    population-based rates for program evaluation,
        361-364
    reasons for, 356-357
    relationship between health and medical care,
        359-361
    specification of objectives and, 357-359

    see also Quality of care, evaluation of
Expenditures, health care, 287-292
Experimental Health Services Delivery System
    (EHSDS) program, 355-358

Family planning services, 117
Federal Employees Health Insurance Plan, 216
Federal government, 12-14, 16
    development of hospitals and, 132-133
    ownership of hospitals and, 142
    see also specific agencies and programs
Fee-for-service reimbursement, 294-295
Financing of health services, 4, 22, 31, 287-320
    expenditures, 287-292
    hospital reimbursement mechanisms, 295-303
        allowable costs, 298-299
        equity between classes of patients, 298-299
        insurance, 301-303
        prospective cost reimbursement, 299-301
        prospective rate setting, 346-347
        retrospective per diem reimbursement,
            297-299
        schedule of charges, 296-297
    mental health services, 214-215
    physician-patient relationship and, 293-294
    physician reimbursement, 294-295
    public policy issues in, 316-320
    see also Health insurance; Medicaid; Medicare
Flexner Report, 130, 229, 259
Foreign medical graduates (FMG), 272-275
Free clinics, 116, 217
Frontier Nursing Service, 116

Geriatrics, 182, 190
Germ theory of disease, 129
Governing boards of hospitals, 144-146
Group Health Cooperative of Puget Sound, 101
Group practice, 99-110
    advantages and disadvantages of, 105-108
    history of, 101-102
    neighborhood health centers, 113-114
    organization of, 102-105
    prepaid, see Prepaid group practice

Health behavior, 74, 76
Health Belief Model of health services utilization,
    64-65, 74-76
Health care expenditures, 287-292
Health care financing, see Financing of health
    services
Health Care Financing Administration, 347
Health care personnel, see Personnel, health care
Health care system(s), evaluation of, see
    Evaluation of health services
    free-market approach to, 30
    health planning approach to, 30-31
    historical evolution of, 3-15
        predominant health problems, 4-8
        social organization, 12-14
        summary of historical trends, 14-15

technology, 8-14
incremental tinkering approach to, 31
overview of, 15-32
    economic inefficiency, 29-30
    middle-class, middle-income system, 17-19
    military medical care system, 24-26
    multiplicity of subsystems, 15-17, 29-30
    poor, inner-city minority families, 20-23
    rationalization of health care system, 30-32
    Veterans Administration health care system,
        26-28
planning of, see Planning of health services
public utility approach to, 31
technology available to, 8-14
    social organization for use of, 12-14
utilization of, see Utilization of health services
Health departments, public, 117-118
Health education, 117, 120
Health, Education, and Welfare, Department of,
    160
Health insurance, 16, 131-132, 281, 303-316
    benefit structures, 309-311
    development of, 13, 303-307
    Health Maintenance Organizations, see Health
        Maintenance Organizations (HMO)
    hospital investment and, 344
    hospitals and, 301-303
    for mental health services, 215-216, 222-223
    national, 222
    operating expenses of voluntary plans, 307-309
    see also Medicaid; Medicare
Health Insurance Plan of New York, 101
Health Maintenance Organizations (HMO), 110,
    216
    hospital cost inflation and, 153, 154
    insurance aspects of, 311-313
    utilization of, 78
    see also Prepaid group practice
Health Manpower Act of 1968, 260
Health Professions Education Assistance Act, 260
Health Services and Mental Health
        Administration (HSMHA), 336, 337
Health Systems Agencies (HSA), 338, 345
Heart, totally implantable mechanical, 251-253
Heart disease, 230. See also Atherosclerosis
    (arteriosclerosis)
Hill-Burton program (Hospital Survey and
        Construction Act of 1946), 132-133, 142,
        160, 331-332
Home health services, 115
Hospitals, 125-162
    accreditation of, 160, 383
    administration of, 146-148
    admission rates, 56, 77, 78
    ambulatory surgery centers in, 112
    certification of, 159-160, 383
    city or county, 16, 134
        poor, inner-city families, 20-22
    classification of, 133-134
    community, 138-139

internal organization, 143-150
reimbursement mechanisms, 295-303
cost controls on, 161
cost inflation and, 151-154, 343-347
financing and ownership of, 139, 142
for-profit, investor-owned, or proprietary,
    136-138
governing boards of, 144-146
history of, 9-10, 16, 126-133
    government's role, 132-133
    health insurance, development of hospitals
        and, 131-132
    Hill-Burton program, 132-133, 142, 160,
        331-332
    medical education and, 130-131
    medical science, advances in, 128-129
    nursing, 129-130
    technology, 129
investment and output decisions of, 343-344
lengths of stays in, 56-57, 138
licensure of, 159
medical staff of, 148-150. See also Physicians,
    hospitals and
mental, see Mental hospitals
for middle-class, middle-income families, 18
military, 25
nonprofit (voluntary), 127-128, 138
outpatient clinics of, 111-112
personnel of, 153
    nurses, supply of, 268-272
    unionization of, 157-159
    see also Personnel, health care
primary care group practices in, 112
public, 134-136
Public Health Service, 115
regionalization of, 156-157
regulation of, 159-162, 343-348
    bases of controls, 343-344
    capital expenditures and services (CES)
        controls, 344-345
    certificate-of-need (CON) laws, 344-345
    Professional Standards Review
        Organizations (PSRO), 345-346, 348
    prospective rate setting, 346-347
reimbursement mechanisms, 295-303
    allowable costs, 298-299
    equity between classes of patients, 298-299
    insurance, 301-303
    prospective cost reimbursement, 299-301
    prospective rate setting, 346-347
    retrospective per diem reimbursement,
        297-299
    schedule of charges, 296-297
small and rural, 154-157
teaching, 111
utilization of, 76-78
    control of, 162, 382
    cost inflation, 151-154
    utilization review, 384
see also Inpatient services

Hospital Survey and Construction Act of 1946,
    see Hill-Burton program (Hospital Survey
    and Construction Act of 1946)
Hypertension, 36-37

Illness, chronic, *see* Chronic illnesses
    definition of, 35-36
Illness behavior, 74, 76
Indian Health Service, 115
Individual practice association (IPA), 312, 313
Infectious diseases, 41
    epidemics of, 4-6, 9, 126-127
Inflammation, 38
Inflation, hospitals and, 151-154, 343-347
Inpatient services, for middle-class, middle-
    income families, 18
    for the poor, 21
    prepaid group practices and, 109
    utilization of, 56-57
Insurance, *see* Health insurance

Joint Commission on Accreditation of Hospitals
    (JCAH), 159, 160, 383
    Performance Evaluation Program (PEP) of,
    386

Kaiser Foundation Health Plan, 101, 109
Kidney, artificial, 249, 250
Kidney transplants, 250

Law, mental health, 220-221
Learned helplessness, in nursing homes, 188
Licensure, 381-382
Long-term care, 82
    for middle-class, middle-income families, 18
    military medical system and, 25
    for the poor, 21
    Veterans Administration system and, 27, 28
    see also Nursing homes

Malpractice, 280-281
    hospitals and, 145, 152
    as quality assurance mechanism, 386
Manic depressive syndromes, 198
Mayo Clinic, 101
Medicaid, 78, 85, 133, 134, 304, 313, 315-316
    mental health services and, 216
    nursing homes and, 23, 172, 177, 178, 180, 183
    regulation of hospitals and, 159-162
Medical research, *see* Research, medical
Medical schools 9, 228, 229, 259
Medical staff of hospitals, 148-150
Medicare, 13, 14, 19, 78, 85, 133, 134, 304, 313
    mental health services and, 216
    nursing homes and, 172, 180, 183
    Part A of, 314
    Part B of, 314
    regulation of hospitals and, 159-162
Mental health personnel, 209-214
Mental health services, 197-223

barriers to, 219-220
    comprehensive, 218
    coordinating, 218-219
    development of, 203-208
    for elderly, 191-192
    insurance coverage for, 215-216, 222-223
    for middle-class families, 18-19
    military, 25-26
    organization of, 214-217
    outpatient, 207, 219-220
    planning, 221-222
    for the poor, 21-22
    in private sector, 216-217
    in public sector, 217
    utilization of, 84-85, 202-203, 218-220
    see also Community Mental Health Centers
Mental hospitals, 16, 212
    number and rate of patient care episodes in, 57
    state, 19, 22, 220
Mental illness, definitions of, 197-200
    incidence and prevalence of, 200-202
    see also Mental health services
Mental Retardation Facilities and Community
    Mental Health Centers Construction Act of
    1964, 208
Metabolic diseases, 38-39
Middle-class, middle-income health care system,
    17-19
Military health care system, 13, 16, 24-26, 115.
    See also Veterans Administration (VA)
    health care system
Monitoring methods, 245

National Ambulatory Medical Care Survey
    (NAMCS), 98
National Center for Health Services Research
    and Development (NCHSR&D), 336-337
National health insurance, 222
National Health Planning and Resources
    Development Act of 1974, 14, 160-161,
    338-339
National Health Service Corps, 114
National Institute of Health (NIH), 10, 229, 231,
    232
National Institute of Mental Health, 207
National Mental Health Act of 1946, 207
National Mental Health Study Act of 1955, 207-208
Neighborhood health centers, 113-114
Neoplasms (cancers), 38, 230, 232
    changes in incidence and prevalence of, 42-43
Nurses, changing role of, 279
    geriatric, 182, 190, 191
    history of hospitals and, 129-130
    psychiatric, 211-212
    supply of, 268-272
    training of, 8-10
Nursing homes, 28, 169-193, 220
    admissions to, 57-58, 173, 176
    community and, 191, 192
    convergence of poor and middle-class systems

in, 22
costs of care in 177-180, 291-292
descriptive data on, 172-177
historical development of, 170-172
Medicaid and, 23, 172, 177, 178, 180, 183
medical care in, 182, 190-191
medical versus social models of, 189-192
mental health services in, 191-192
payment for care in, 180-182
quality of care in, 183-187
quality of life in, 187-192
social needs and, 191-192

Occupational medicine, 117
Office-based practice, 96-100
Osteopathy, 278
Outcome measures of quality, 369-371, 378-379
Outpatient clinics, 111-112
for mental patients, 207
see also Ambulatory health services

Pacemakers, 248-249
Partnership for Health Amendments of 1967,
333, 334
Patient compliance, 97, 121
Patient satisfaction, quality of care and, 377
Peer review programs, 385
Penicillin, 6
Performance Evaluation Program (PEP), 386
Personnel, health care, 256-285
certification of, 257, 259
growth in number of, 257
mental health, 209-214
"pool" of, 279-281
productivity of, 281-282
professional versus public control of, 282-285
role conflicts among, 277-278
socialization of, 276
specialization of, 257
supply of, 259-272
dentists, 266-268
determining optimal numbers, 282
distribution, 263-266
nurses, 268-272
pharmacists, 266-268
physicians, 259-266
training of, 275-277
see also Nurses; Physicians
Pesthouses, 126-127
Pharmacists, supply of, 266-268
Physician-patient relationship, 97
efficiency and, 376-377
financial aspects of, 293-295
Physicians, certification and accreditation of,
383
foreign medical graduates (FMG), 272-275
hospitals and, organizational aspects, 145, 146,
148-150
regulation of hospitals, 343-344
licensure of, 381-382

middle-class, middle-income families and,
17-19
nursing homes and, 182, 190
peer review programs and, 385
percentage of population seeing, 53
reimbursement of, 294-295
in solo practice, 96-98
specialization of, 10
supply of, 259-266
training of, 8-10, 45, 152. See also Medical
schools
Physician visits, 54-56, 69, 72, 79. See also
Ambulatory visits
Planning of health services, 30-31, 325-339
assessment of, 347-349
Comprehensive Health Planning, 333-335, 337
definition of, 325-326
Experimental Health Services Delivery
System (EHSDS) program, 335-338
Hill-Burton program, 132-133, 142, 160,
331-332
National Health Planning and Resources
Development Act of 1974, 14, 160-161,
338-339
origins of, 328-330
rationales for, 326-328
Regional Medical Programs, 332-333
Poor, inner-city system of care, 20-23
Prepaid group practice, 108-110, 311, 312
utilization of, 76-78
see also Health Maintenance Organizations
(HMO)
President's Commission on Heart Disease,
Cancer, and Stroke, 332
Prevention, primary, 93, 95
Preventive health services, utilization of, 59
Preventive medicine, 17-18
military medical system and, 24-25
poor families and, 20
Primary care, 95
emergency room, 112-113
by solo practitioners, 97
Primary care network plan, 312-313
Primary prevention, 93, 95
Process measure of quality of care, 371-374,
380-381
Professional Standards Review Organizations
(PSRO), 153-154, 162, 183, 340, 345-346,
348, 384-386
Prognostic adjustment factor (PAF), 182
Psychiatric hospitals, see Mental hospitals
Psychiatric services, see Mental health services
Psychiatrists, 209, 216-217
Psychologists, 209-210
Psychotropic drugs, 207
Public health, 17, 116-118
military medical system and, 24-25
poor families and, 20
Public health departments, 17, 117-118
Public Health Service, United States, 115

Quality assurance, 381-386
Quality of care, in ambulatory care, 121
  evaluation of, 355-356, 365-381
    access to care, 377-378
    choice of what to study, 365
    choice of whom to study, 365
    efficiency of care, 375-377
    illustrative studies, 378-381
    outcome measure, 369-371, 378-379
    patient satisfaction, 377
    process measures, 371-374, 380-381
    quality assurance mechanisms, 381-386
    reliability of secondary data sources,
        367-368
    sources of data, 366
    structural measures of quality, 374-375
    validity and reliability, 366-367
  in for-profit hospitals, 137
  governing boards of hospitals and, 145
  in nursing homes, 183-187
  sensitivity, specificity, and predictive value
      of methods of, 368-369
Quality controls, 159-160, 342

Radioisotopes, 241
Ransdel Act, 229
Rationalization of health care system,
        ambulatory care, 121
  approaches to, 30-32
Regional Advisory Groups (RAG), 332-333
Regionalization, 330
  small and rural hospitals and, 156-157
Regional Medical Programs, 160, 337
Regional Medical Programs Act, 332-333
Regulation of health services, 325
  assessment of, 347-349
  definition of, 326
  hospitals, see Hospitals, regulation of
  rationales for, 326-328
  types of, 340-342
Research, medical, 9, 10, 228, 229
    historical development of, 229-231
    see also Technology (health care)
Rheumatoid arthritis, 37
Role conflicts in health services, 277-278
Rural health care, 115-116
  utilization of, 85
Rural hospitals, 154-157

Schizophrenia, 198, 200
Scientific medicine, 4, 229-230
Secondary care, 95
Self-care, 83-84
Sick role behavior, 74, 76
Socialization of health care personnel, 276
Social organization, of health care, 12-14
  for use of technology, 12-14
Social psychiatry, 209
Social Security Act, nursing homes and, 170, 180
Social Security Amendments of 1972, 160, 162

Social workers, 210-211
Solo practice, 96-98
State Health Coordinating Committee (SHCC),
        338, 339, 345
State Planning and Development Agency
        (SHPDA), 338, 339, 345
State mental hospitals, 19, 22, 220
Structural measures of quality of care, 374-375
Surgery, ambulatory (outpatient), 112
Symptoms, production of, 39-41

Taft-Hartley Act, 158
Technology (health care), 8-14, 227-254
  assessment of, 251-253
  diagnostic technologies, 234-235
    basic research technologies, 234-236
    clinical conversion of basic technologies,
        236
    computerized axial tomography (CAT
        scanners), 238-240, 242
    costs of health care, effect of energy
        probes on, 242
    diagnostic imperative, 243, 245
    electronics industry, 243
    external energy probes, 238
    intrinsic energy sources, 236-239
    radioisotopes, 241
    thermography, 241-242
    ultrasound, 240-241
  emergency medical services, 245-246
  future forecasts, 253-254
  group practice and, 101
  historical development of, 228-234
  history of hospitals and, 129
  hospital cost inflation and, 152-153
  monitoring methods, 245
  patterns of disease and, 42
  pseudo-solutions, 250-254
  social organization for use of, 12-14
  therapeutic technologies, 246-251
Tertiary care, 95
Therapeutic community, 209, 211
Thermography, 241-242
Tomography, 238-240, 242
Toxic diseases, 38
Training, of health personnel, 275-277
  of nurses, 8-10
  of physicians, 8-10, 45, 152. See also Medical
      schools

Ultrasound, diagnostic, 240-241
Unionization of hospital employees, 157-159
Utilization of health services, 43-86
  ambulatory visits to outpatient facilities and
      community mental health centers, 56
  availability of health services and, 45-46
  categories of, 49
  by children, 82-83
  concepts of needs, wants, and demand for
      health services, 50